Introduction to
BASIC CARDIAC DYSRHYTHMIAS

Introduction to
BASIC CARDIAC DYSRHYTHMIAS

Third Edition

Sandra Atwood, RN, BA

Cheryl Stanton, RN, CEN

Jenny Storey-Davenport, RN, BSN, C

Original illustrations by Jenny Storey-Davenport, RN, BSN, C
Modified versions by Mark Wieber

With 672 illustrations

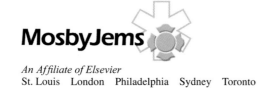

An Affiliate of Elsevier
St. Louis   London   Philadelphia   Sydney   Toronto

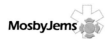

An Affiliate of Elsevier

11830 Westline Industrial Drive
St. Louis, Missouri 63146

INTRODUCTION TO BASIC CARDIAC DYSRHYTHMIAS, THIRD EDITION
Copyright © 2003, Mosby, Inc. All rights reserved.

Notice

CARDIOLOGY is an ever-changing field. Standard safety precautions must be followed, but as new research and clinical experience broaden our knowledge, changes in treatment and drug therapy may become necessary or appropriate. Readers are advised to check the most current product information provided by the manufacturer of each drug to be administered to verify the recommended dose, the method and duration of administration, and contraindications. It is the responsibility of the licensed prescriber, relying on experience and knowledge of the patient, to determine dosages and the best treatment for each individual patient. Neither the publisher nor the editor assumes any liability for any injury and/or damage to persons or property arising from this publication.

The Publisher

Previous editions copyrighted 1990, 1996

ISBN-13: 978-0-323-01864-7
ISBN-10: 0-323-01864-5

Acquisitions Editor: Claire Merrick
Developmental Editor: Laura Bayless
Publishing Services Manager: Deb Vogel
Project Manager: Mary Drone
Design Manager: Bill Drone

TG/CCW

Printed in the United States of America

Last digit is the print number: 9   8   7   6   5   4

We lovingly dedicate this book
to our husbands and children
Phil, Ken, and Tracy
Lee, Alicia, Melynda, Michael, and Jim

PREFACE

Introduction to Basic Cardiac Dysrhythmias was originally written to help the beginning learner unravel the mysteries of those squiggly lines seen on the monitor and rhythm strip. Our intent is to explain what happens inside the heart when a dysrhythmia is seen, as well as how the dysrhythmias appears on a monitor or rhythm strip.

Although the text is designed for students without a medical background, the learner with cardiac knowledge should also find it helpful as a review of dysrhythmias and treatment.

The term **dysrhythmia** is used in the title and throughout the text because we believe it is an accurate description of the information presented. We have used simple medical terminology whenever feasible; numerous illustrations are also included to make learning as easy as possible.

The hearts found in the illustrations are not drawn to scale; the atria, atrioventricular junction, and septum are drawn larger than normal, to show the conduction pathway of the heart clearly. A sequential approach is used, following the normal electrical conduction pathway of the heart.

All rhythm strips appear as from a Lead II placement and reflect examples of cardiac rhythms found in the adult patient.

- **Chapter 1** covers the basic anatomy and physiology of the cardiac, pulmonary, and vascular systems, with corresponding illustrations for additional clarification. Medical terms are introduced with simple explanations and definitions.
- **Chapter 2** explains the equipment and supplies used in telemetry, the components of a cardiac complex, and information for interpreting rhythm strips.
- **Chapter 3 to 7** explain basic cardiac dysrhythmias, following the normal, sequential conduction pathway of the heart (i.e., atrial, junctional, and ventricular dysrhythmias), as well as heart blocks, aberrant and escape beats, followed by pacemaker rhythms.
- **Chapter 8** offers a concise review of all dysrhythmias discussed in the book, providing sample rhythm strips and brief explanations of the criteria involved in identifying each dysrhythmia.
- **Chapter 9** focuses on the treatment of basic dysrhythmias and follows current American Heart Association Standards.
- **Chapter 10** includes at least one example of each dysrhythmia shown in the book, as well as space for the reader to write in the measurements of each component and the name of the dysrhythmia.
- **Chapter 11** provides various case studies for additional review of dysrhythmias and treatment.

Review questions can be found at the end of Chapters 1 to 7, as well as review rhythm strips after Chapters 2 to 7, to assist readers in measuring their progress in learning. Crossword and word puzzles are included throughout the book to assist in learning and "for fun." Two sections of flashcards, abbreviations, glossary, answer section and index can be found at the end of the book.

We gratefully acknowledge the efforts of others who were so instrumental in the completion of this text. Many thanks to all of our nursing friends and colleagues for their encouragement and to all the nurses and monitor technicians who attended our courses and provided such valuable feedback about our original study guide.

Last, but certainly not least, our loving thanks to our families for their patience, understanding, and encouragement.

INTRODUCTION TO THE THIRD EDITION

We have made several changes in the third edition of *Introduction to Basic Cardiac Dysrhythmias*. These changes include the addition of 50 rhythm strips to Chapter 10, and the complete revision of the medication review in Chapter 9, which is based on the year 2000 Cardiovascular Care guidelines.

These changes and additions also include the following new information:
Updated illustrations and materials
Definitions of terminology at the beginning of each chapter
Review questions added to Chapter 1
Wolff-Parkinson-White syndrome added to Chapter 3
Additional crossword puzzles, as requested by many readers
Introduction of word puzzles to aid in terminology recognition
Information about AED units
Over 50 additional practice strips
Seven additional case studies added to Chapter 11
Medication flashcards for review of drug treatments
Expanded glossary, abbreviations, and index

Note to the Reader

While the authors and the publisher have made every attempt to check the accuracy of this text, the possibility of error can never be eliminated. The information presented here represents accepted practices in the United States, but is not offered as a standard of care. It is the reader's responsibility to learn and follow the protocols of their locality, and to follow the direction of a licensed physician. It is also the reader's responsibility to stay informed of procedural changes and new drugs used in emergency care.

CONTENTS

Introduction to
BASIC CARDIAC DYSRHYTHMIAS

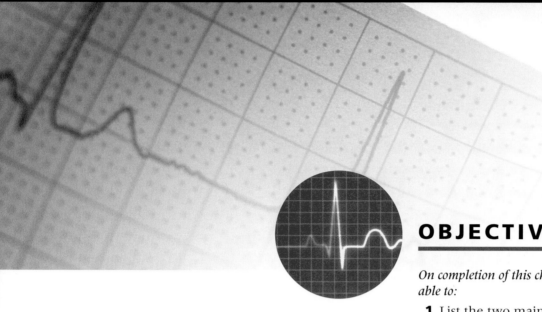

OBJECTIVES

On completion of this chapter, the reader should be able to:

1 List the two main organs of the cardiopulmonary system.

2 Identify the four heart chambers, three cardiac muscle layers, and four main heart valves.

3 Explain the basic function of the lungs.

4 Describe the three main types of blood vessels.

5 Describe the flow of a drop of blood from the vena cava through the heart and lungs to the aorta.

6 Explain how to measure cardiac output.

7 Explain the four common characteristics of all cardiac cells.

8 Define the following terms: polarization, depolarization, and repolarization.

9 Describe the movement of an electrical impulse, following the normal cardiac conduction pathways.

10 Explain the actions of the sympathetic and parasympathetic nervous systems on the heart rate.

ANATOMY AND PHYSIOLOGY

OUTLINE

DEFINITIONS

Automaticity The ability of cardiac cells to initiate or generate an electrical impulse

Autonomic Nervous System Part of the nervous system that regulates many organs, such as the heart and blood vessels

Cardiac Pertaining to the heart

Cardiac Output The amount of blood pumped by the left ventricle in 1 minute

Conductivity The ability of cardiac cells to transmit an electrical impulse

Contractility The ability of cardiac cells to respond to an electrical impulse by contracting

Cyanosis Bluish-gray color of the lips, skin, and nail beds, caused by a lack of oxygen

Depolarization Conduction of an electrical impulse through the heart muscle; normally causes a cardiac contraction

Dyspnea Difficult or painful breathing

Excitability The ability of cardiac cells to respond to an electrical impulse

Heart Muscular organ that pumps blood to the body cells

Heart/Lung Circulation The transportation of blood from the body cells, through the heart and lungs, and back to the body cells

Hypotension Decreased blood pressure; below patient's normal blood pressure

Lungs Two organs that remove carbon dioxide from the blood, replacing it with oxygen

Polarization Cardiac ready state; the cells are ready to receive an electrical impulse

Pulmonary Pertaining to the lungs

Repolarization Cardiac recovery phase; the cells are returning to the ready state

ANATOMY

The main organs of the cardiopulmonary system are the heart and lungs. These organs work together to circulate oxygenated blood through blood vessels to all body cells.

HEART

The adult heart is a hollow, muscular organ that is located in the chest cavity, between the sternum (breastbone) and the spinal column. The normal adult heart weighs about 1 lb (0.45 kg) and is approximately the size of an adult fist (Fig. 1-1).

The heart functions as a double-sided pump. The pumping action of the right and left sides occurs when the muscular walls of each heart chamber contract (squeeze), causing blood to be forced out of the chambers.

> NOTE: The following hearts are drawn for simplicity and ease of illustration. They are **not** drawn to scale.

Heart Chambers

The heart has four chambers: right atrium, left atrium, right ventricle, and left ventricle (Fig. 1-2). The *atria* (plural for atrium) are thin-walled, upper chambers that function as reservoirs, or holding areas, for blood. *Ventricles* are the lower chambers of the heart. The right ventricle has a thin muscular wall. The muscle of the left ventricular wall is much thicker, because it has to pump blood throughout the body, to all body cells.

The heart is further divided by a muscular wall called the *septum.* The septum separates the atria (interatrial septum) and ventricles (interventricular septum) into right and left sides (Fig. 1-3). The right ventricle pumps blood to the lungs, while the left ventricle pumps blood throughout the body.

The atria contract at the same time, followed by the ventricles contracting at the same time. These contractions usually occur in a rhythmic beat. The pumping action of the left ventricle produces a pulse, or wave of pressure, which can be

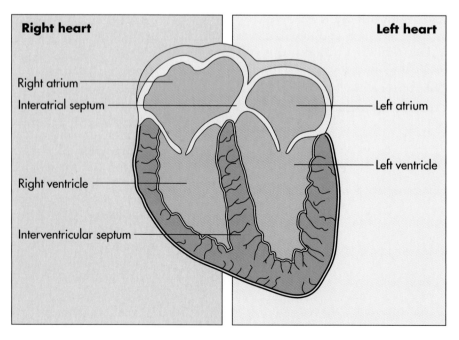

FIG. 1-1 Adult heart.

counted. This pulse is called the heart rate (HR) and usually is measured as heart beats per minute.

Heart Muscle

The heart is made of specialized muscle tissue that is not found anywhere else in the body. This specialized tissue forms the cardiac wall and has three main layers. The inner layer of the cardiac wall is called the *endocardium* and lines the chambers of the heart and covers the valves.

The middle layer of the cardiac wall is the *myocardium*. This layer is the heart muscle and provides the pumping action needed to circulate blood. The *epicardium* is the outer layer of the cardiac muscle and is a thin, protective membrane that covers the outside of the heart.

The heart is contained in a loose-fitting sac called the *pericardium* or *pericardial* sac (Fig. 1-4). A small amount of fluid (10 to 30 ml) can be found in the space be-

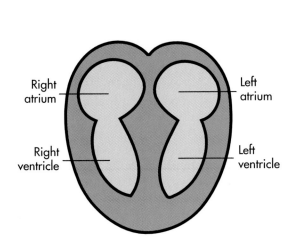

FIG. 1-2 The four chambers of the heart.

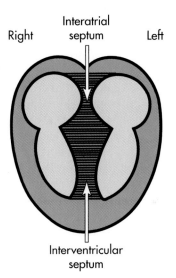

FIG. 1-3 Septum divides the right and left sides of the heart.

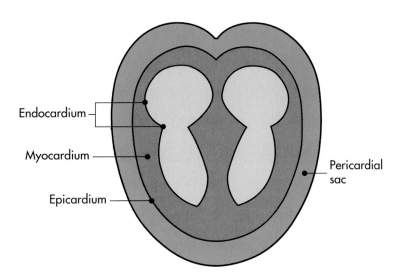

FIG. 1-4 Three layers of cardiac tissue and pericardial sac.

tween the epicardium and pericardium. This fluid *(pericardial fluid)* acts as a lubricant, allowing the heart to move within the sac as it beats.

The myocardium and pericardium are further divided into sublayers, which are discussed in 12-Lead electrocardiogram courses.

Heart Valves

The heart has four valves that are covered with endocardial tissue. These four valves are located in the following areas of the heart:

> *Tricuspid valve*—Between the right atrium and the right ventricle
> *Pulmonic valve*—Between the right ventricle and the pulmonary artery
> *Mitral valve*—Between the left atrium and the left ventricle
> *Aortic valve*—Between the left ventricle and the aorta (Fig. 1-5)

These valves are flaplike structures that open and close in response to the pumping action of the heart. The opening and closing of the heart valves permit the flow of blood in a forward direction and prevent blood from flowing backward.

For example, in the left side of the heart, as the blood enters the empty left atrium, the blood causes increased pressure against the atrial walls. When the atrial pressure becomes greater than the ventricular pressure, the mitral valve opens, allowing most of the blood to flow into the left ventricle. The atrium then gives a mild contraction (atrial kick), emptying the remaining blood into the left ventricle.

As the left ventricle contracts, the mitral valve closes and the aortic valve opens. The closed mitral valve prevents the flow of blood back into the left atrium. The open aortic valve allows the blood to be pumped from the heart and then carried throughout the body, to all body cells.

The "lub dub, lub dub" noises caused by the normal closing of the valves are known as *heart sounds.* In an adult, a *murmur* is an abnormal sound made by blood flowing through a valve that is not functioning correctly. This sound can be heard when listening to the heart with a stethoscope. Heart murmurs are usually caused by an improperly functioning mitral valve.

Lungs

The main organs of the pulmonary system are the right and left lungs. They are large, spongy organs that are located in the chest cavity, slightly behind and on

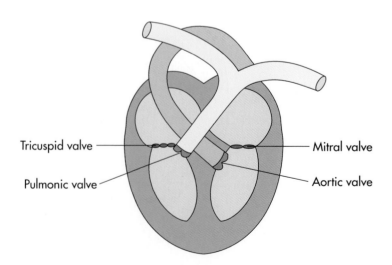

FIG. 1-5 Heart valves.

either side of the heart. Each lung is encased in a protective sac called the *pleural sac.* The main function of the lungs is to remove carbon dioxide from the blood and to replace it with oxygen (Fig. 1-6).

This exchange begins when air, containing oxygen, is inhaled through the nose or mouth into the trachea. The trachea is a hollow tube that extends downward for approximately 4½ inches, when it divides into two slightly smaller tubes, called *bronchi,* one for each lung. After the bronchi enter the lungs, each bronchus further divides into smaller tubes, called the *bronchioles.* The air continues traveling through the bronchioles, as they further divide into smaller and smaller tubes, and finally end in the alveoli (see Fig. 1-6).

The *alveoli* are tiny sacs of tissue that are arranged in grapelike clusters. The alveoli are surrounded by very small blood vessels called *capillaries.* The actual exchange of carbon dioxide from the capillary blood for oxygen from the inhaled air takes place in these tiny sacs. Because the walls of both the alveoli and the capillaries are only one cell thick, the exchange of carbon dioxide for oxygen takes place easily.

BLOOD VESSELS

Blood vessels are located throughout the body, and their primary purpose is transportation. They carry oxygenated blood to all body cells and then transport blood with carbon dioxide from the body cells to the lungs.

The three main types of blood vessels are *arteries, veins,* and *capillaries* (Fig. 1-7). Arteries carry blood away from the heart, and veins carry blood to the heart. The

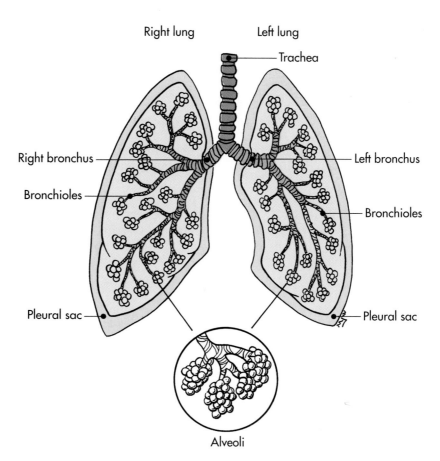

FIG. 1-6 Lungs and air pathways from trachea to alveoli.

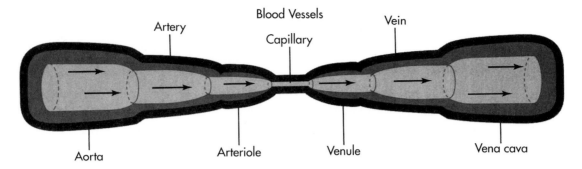

FIG. 1-7 Gradual change in the size of blood vessels and vessel walls.

exchange of nutrients and waste products for the body cells takes place in the capillaries.

Arteries

Arteries are blood vessels that carry oxygenated blood away from the heart to all parts of the body. Arteries have the thickest walls of all blood vessels because they must withstand the pumping pressure of the heart. The *aorta* is the largest artery in the body.

The arteries divide into *arterioles,* which are smaller blood vessels with thinner walls. The arterioles connect arteries to capillaries.

Veins

Veins are vessels that carry blood with carbon dioxide from the body cells back to the heart. The venous walls are thinner than the arterial walls and contain tiny valves (similar to cardiac valves) that prevent the backward flow of blood. The *vena cava* is the largest vein in the body. The smallest veins are called *venules,* which connect veins to capillaries.

> NOTE: **The one exception to the definition of arteries and veins is found in the heart/lung circulation. The pulmonary arteries carry blood with carbon dioxide to the lungs, and the pulmonary veins carry blood with oxygen to the heart.**

Capillaries

Capillaries, the smallest blood vessels in the body, also have the thinnest walls of any blood vessel. The exchange of oxygen and waste products between the blood and the body cells takes place through the capillary walls, which are only one cell thick.

Coronary Arteries

The heart muscle receives its blood supply from *coronary arteries.* These special arteries branch off the aorta and supply oxygenated blood to each portion of the heart muscle.

For example, the right coronary artery divides into the marginal artery and the right anterior and right posterior descending arteries, which again divide into smaller arteries (Fig. 1-8). Therefore the right coronary artery and its branches are able to provide oxygenated blood to the muscle tissue of the right atrium, the left ventricle, and the right ventricle. The left coronary artery branches (divides) into the left anterior descending artery and the circumflex artery, which both divide into smaller arteries. The left coronary artery and its branches provide oxygenated blood to the muscle tissue of the left atrium, left ventricle, and right ventricle.

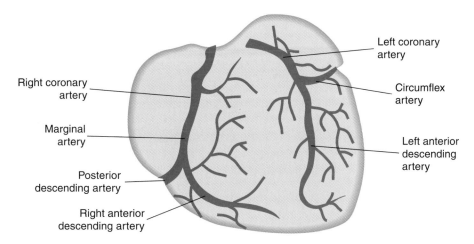

FIG. 1-8 Coronary vessels: arteries that supply oxygen and nutrients to cardiac muscle cells.

Most of this oxygenated blood flows to the cardiac muscle between heart beats (contractions) while the myocardium is resting.

MYOCARDIAL INFARCTION

A coronary artery may become partially or completely blocked by blood clots or a build-up of cholesterol on the inside of the artery wall. When a blockage occurs, the cardiac muscle usually nourished by that artery does not receive enough oxygen.

The decreased supply of oxygen to tissue is called *ischemia*. Ischemia that occurs in the cardiac muscle and is not diagnosed and treated usually leads to *myocardial infarction* (MI; death of cardiac tissue). The death of cardiac tissue usually lessens the ability of the cardiac muscle to contract and pump blood efficiently.

A myocardial infarction (MI, heart attack, or coronary) can affect any area of the heart muscle or myocardium.

The location of the MI may cause an interruption in the cardiac electrical conduction pathways. This interruption may cause dysrhythmias (abnormal cardiac rhythms), which are discussed in Chapters 3 through 7.

Symptoms of an MI may include chest pain or pressure that is described as a heavy feeling, a dull ache, a feeling of being squeezed, or a discomfort similar to indigestion. The pain or pressure may radiate (move) down the left arm or up into the neck, jaw, back, or shoulders. Other signs include nausea; vomiting; difficulty breathing; and pale, cool, sweating skin. Confusion or loss of consciousness may also be present.

Some patients, who may include those with heart transplants, severe diabetes, or different types of paralysis, may have symptoms that vary from very mild to no symptoms at all.

MECHANICAL PHYSIOLOGY

HEART/LUNG CIRCULATION

The right side of the heart receives blood from the vena cava and sends this blood to the lungs. The lungs filter carbon dioxide from the blood and exchange it for oxygen. The oxygenated blood then flows to the left side of the heart, which

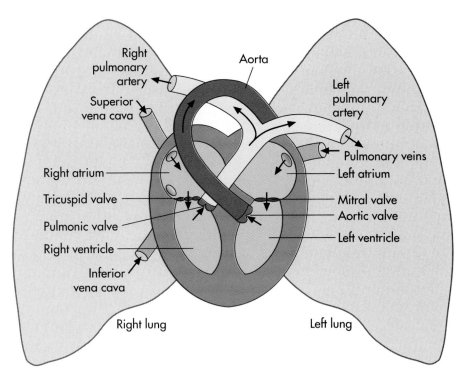

FIG. 1-9 Heart/lung circulation.

pumps the blood into the aorta. Blood is circulated through the heart and lungs in the following order:

vena cava → right atrium → tricuspid valve → right ventricle → pulmonic valve → pulmonary arteries → lungs → pulmonary veins → left atrium → mitral valve → left ventricle → aortic valve → aorta → rest of the body, including the heart (Fig. 1-9).

CARDIAC OUTPUT

One method of measuring how efficiently the heart is pumping and circulating blood to the body cells is by determining the *cardiac output (CO)*. Cardiac output is the amount of blood pumped by the left ventricle in 1 minute.

Cardiac output is measured by multiplying the heart rate (HR) by the stroke volume (SV), which is the amount of blood pumped by the left ventricle with each beat. The formula is: CO = SV × HR.

CO—Cardiac output is the amount of blood pumped by the left ventricle in 1 minute. The normal amount is usually 5000 to 6000 ml.
SV—Stroke volume is the amount of blood pumped by the left ventricle with each contraction or beat, approximately 70 ml.
HR—Heart rate is the number of times the left ventricle contracts in 1 minute; the normal rate is 60 to 100.
Example: CO = SV × HR; the stroke volume is 70 ml and the heart rate is 80: CO = 70 × 80 = 5600 ml = normal cardiac output.

When the cardiac output is abnormal, the heart will try to balance it by changing either the stroke volume or the heart rate. For example, if a person exercises and becomes physically fit, the stroke volume usually increases because the heart muscle is stronger and pumps more blood with each beat. The heart rate then decreases to keep the cardiac output within the normal range.

Example: CO = SV × HR; with an increased SV of 90 ml and a decreased HR of 60: CO = 90 × 60 = 5400 ml = normal cardiac output.

The opposite is also true. When the heart cannot pump the usual amount of blood because of injury or disease, the stroke volume decreases. The heart rate then increases to maintain a normal cardiac output.

Example: CO = SV × HR; with a decreased SV of 50 ml and an increased HR of 110: CO = 50 × 110 = 5500 ml = normal cardiac output.

If the heart is unable to increase the stroke volume or the heart rate, the cardiac output will decrease.

Example: CO = SV × HR; with a decreased SV of 50 ml and a HR of 60: CO = 50 × 60 = 3000 ml = decreased cardiac output.

A decreased (poor) cardiac output may cause damage to major organs such as the heart and brain. This damage occurs because there is not enough blood being circulated to carry oxygen to the body cells.

Poor cardiac output may be indicated by any combination of the following signs and symptoms:

- Pale, cool, clammy skin
- Nausea and vomiting (N/V)
- Dizziness, weakness, faintness
- Shortness of breath (SOB)
- Sudden change in blood pressure
- Dyspnea (difficulty breathing)
- Severe chest pain
- Confusion or disorientation
- Cyanosis (bluish-gray color to skin)
- Decreased urinary output
- Unresponsiveness

ELECTROPHYSIOLOGY

All muscle tissue contracts in response to an electrical stimulus or impulse. For example, skeletal muscle will contract after receiving stimulation from a nerve. However, *cardiac muscle* is unique; not only can it respond to an electrical impulse, cardiac muscle also has pacemaker cells that can generate electrical impulses.

The following definitions explain four common characteristics of cardiac cells:

Automaticity—the ability of cardiac pacemaker cells to generate or initiate their own electrical impulses

Excitability—irritability; the ability of cardiac cells to respond to an electrical stimulus; when a cardiac cell is highly irritable, less stimulus is required to cause a contraction

Conductivity—the ability of cardiac cells to transmit an electrical stimulus to other cardiac cells

Contractility—the ability of cardiac cells to shorten, causing cardiac muscle contraction in response to an electrical stimulus

Contractility is a mechanical function of the heart. Automaticity, excitability, and conductivity are electrical functions.

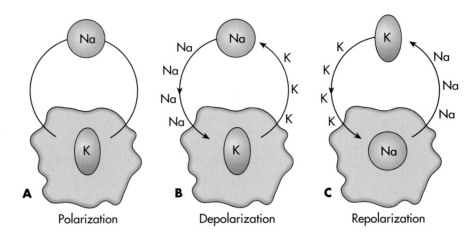

FIG. 1-10 A to **C,** Electrical conduction within cardiac cells showing exchange of sodium and potassium.

DEPOLARIZATION AND REPOLARIZATION

The following terms explain the phases of the normal electrical activity of the heart:

Polarization—the phase of readiness; the muscle is relaxed and the cardiac cells are ready to receive an electrical impulse

Depolarization—the phase of contraction; the cardiac cells have transmitted an electrical impulse, causing the cardiac muscle to contract

Repolarization—the recovery phase; the muscle has contracted and the cells are returning to a ready state

All tissue, including cardiac muscle, is made of many single cells that contain chemicals such as potassium and sodium. The cells normally have *potassium* (K) on the inside of the cell and *sodium* (Na) on the outside, making the cells negatively charged. These cells are *polarized,* or in the ready state (Fig. 1-10, *A*).

When a pacemaker cell generates an electrical impulse to a polarized cardiac cell, most of the potassium moves to the outside of the cell and most of the sodium moves to the inside of the cell, making the cells positively charged. This movement of the potassium and sodium through the cell wall causes a "spark" of electricity. The electrical spark is then conducted to the remaining cells in that part of the heart, causing *depolarization* (Fig. 1-10, *B*). While in this state, the cardiac cells contract. They cannot respond to any further electrical impulses until they have repolarized and become negatively charged again.

After the electrical impulse has passed through the cells, the potassium reenters the cells and the sodium leaves, causing *repolarization* (Fig. 1-10, *C*). However, all cells do not repolarize at the same time. Therefore some cardiac cells are able to conduct an additional electrical impulse sooner than others.

ELECTRICAL CONDUCTION PATHWAY

Although any cardiac pacemaker cell is capable of initiating an electrical impulse, the normal pacemaker is the *sinoatrial (SA) node.* The normal electrical conduction pathway of the heart occurs in the following order:

sinoatrial node → internodal and intraatrial pathways → atrioventricular node → bundle of His → bundle branches → Purkinje's fibers → ventricular muscle (Fig. 1-11).

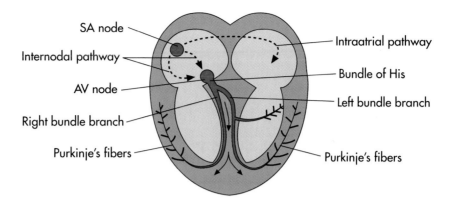

FIG. 1-11 Normal electrical conduction pathway of the heart.

Sinoatrial node (SA node)	The SA node is located in the upper portion of the right atrium and is called the *pacemaker of the heart*. The SA node initiates an electrical impulse that travels downward, throughout the muscle of both atria. This impulse travels through the atrial muscles by way of the *intraatrial conduction pathways,* causing depolarization of the atrium. The same impulse is also transmitted from the SA node to the atrioventricular (AV) node through the *internodal conduction pathways.* The SA node usually generates 60 to 100 electrical impulses per minute.
Atrioventricular node (AV node)	The AV node is located in the general area of the lower right atrium near the septum. The AV node continues transmitting the impulse from the atria to the bundle of His. If the SA node fails to function, pacemaker cells between the atria and the AV node *(AV junction)* are capable of functioning as a *secondary pacemaker.* This area of the electrical conduction system usually generates 40 to 60 electrical impulses per minute.
Bundle of His	The bundle of His, located below the AV node, continues transmitting the electrical impulse to the bundle branches.
Bundle branches (BB)	The lower portion of the bundle of His divides into a *right bundle branch* (leading into the right ventricle) and a *left bundle branch* (leading into the left ventricle). The bundle branches continue transmitting the electrical impulse to the Purkinje's fibers.
Purkinje's fibers	Extending from the bundle branches into the muscular walls of the ventricles, the Purkinje's fibers conduct the electrical impulse from the bundle branches to cells of the ventricular muscle.
Ventricular muscle	The cells of the ventricular muscle receive an electrical stimulus from the Purkinje's fibers and contract. If the SA node **and** the AV junction do not initiate an electrical impulse, an impulse can be generated from any pacemaker cell in the ventricles, including the Purkinje's fibers or the bundle branches. Impulses initiated below the AV node are usually generated at a rate of 20 to 40 impulses per minute.

AUTONOMIC NERVOUS SYSTEM

The electrical conduction system of the heart is affected by the *autonomic nervous system*. The function of the autonomic nervous system is to maintain the body in a normal state by controlling several organs, including the heart, as well as the blood vessels. This control is done automatically, without a person being aware it is happening.

The autonomic nervous system is divided into two parts: the *sympathetic* and the *parasympathetic* systems.

The sympathetic nervous system prepares the body to react in times of stress or emergencies, increasing cardiac output by increasing the heart rate, blood pressure, and force of cardiac contractions. This is known as the "fight or flight response." The sympathetic nerves can be stimulated by anger, pain, fright, caffeine, and some drugs.

The parasympathetic nervous system affects the heart in the opposite way by decreasing the rate of cardiac contractions. This reaction usually occurs after the stress or emergency is over, allowing the body to restore energy. The parasympathetic nerves can be stimulated by straining to have bowel movement, a urinary bladder that is too full, vomiting, and some drugs.

Medications are available to reverse the effects of the sympathetic and parasympathetic nervous systems on the heart, when necessary. For example, when the parasympathetic nerves have been stimulated and decrease the heart rate too much, drugs such as atropine block the parasympathetic nerves and allow the heart rate to increase.

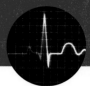

REVIEW QUESTIONS

TRUE ~~FALSE~~ (circled)   1. The main organs of the cardiopulmonary system are the heart and blood vessels.

~~TRUE~~ (circled) FALSE   2. The heart is a double-sided pump.

~~TRUE~~ (circled) FALSE   3. The ventricles function as reservoirs for blood.

TRUE FALSE   4. Contractility is an electrical function of the heart.

5. The upper chambers of the heart are known as the _Atria_, and the lower chambers of the heart are known as the _Venr_.

6. List the three main layers of cardiac muscle:
   a. _____
   b. _____
   c. _____

7. Identify the four valves of the heart:
   a. _Tricuspid_
   b. _Pulmonary_
   c. _Mitral (Bicuspid)_
   d. _Aortic_

8. a. What type of blood vessels carry blood away from the heart?
      Artery
   b. What type of blood vessels carry blood back to the heart?
      Vein
   c. What type of blood vessels allow the exchange of oxygen and nutrients for waste products at the cell level? _Capillaries_

9. The layer of the heart that contracts to pump blood to the lungs and throughout the body to all body cells is the:
   a. endocardial.
   b. myocardial. (circled)
   c. epithelial.
   d. epicardial.

10. Cardiac muscle tissue receives its blood supply from the:
    a. pulmonary arteries.
    b. coronary arteries. (circled)
    c. myocardial arteries.
    d. coronary veins.

11. In the lungs, the exchange of oxygen from inhaled air and carbon dioxide from capillary blood takes place inside tiny sacs called _alveoli_.

12. Cardiac output is determined by:
    a. stroke volume multiplied by the respiratory rate.
    b. stroke volume divided by the heart rate.
    c. heart rate divided by the stroke volume.
    d. heart rate multiplied by the stroke volume. (circled)

13. Automaticity is the ability of cardiac cells to:
    a. contract.
    b. respond to an electrical impulse.
    c. regenerate themselves.
    d. initiate their own electrical impulse. (circled)

14. The sympathetic nervous system:
    a. increases cardiac output and blood pressure.
    b. decreases heart rate and blood pressure.
    c. controls the autonomic nervous system.
    d. increases heart rate, blood pressure, and the force of cardiac contractions.

15. The ability of cardiac cells to transmit an electrical impulse is:
    a. excitability.
    b. conductivity.
    c. contractility.
    d. automaticity.

16. Explain the terms:
    a. depolarization:

    _____
    _____
    _____
    _____

    b. repolarization:

    _____
    _____
    _____
    _____

17. Trace a drop of blood from the vena cava throughout the rest of the body including the heart.
    Vena cava → _____
    _____
    _____
    _____
    _____

18. Trace the normal electrical conduction pathway system of the heart:
    _____
    _____
    _____
    _____
    _____

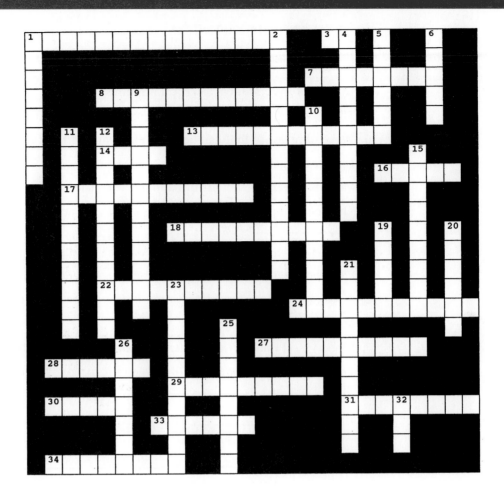

CROSSWORD PUZZLE CLUES

Across

1. Part of autonomic nervous system that decreases heart rate.

3. The _____ node transmits electrical impulses between the SA node and the bundle of His.

7. Atrioventricular area known as the secondary pacemaker of the heart.

8. Ability of cardiac cells to respond to electrical impulses.

13. Ability of cardiac cells to generate electrical impulses.

14. The SA _____ is the primary pacemaker of the heart.

16. Largest artery in the body.

17. Tissue forming the sac that surrounds the heart.

18. The SA node initiates _____ impulses.

22. Conduction pathway between the SA node and the AV junction is the _____ pathway.

24. First or inner layer of heart wall.

27. Cardiac cells _____ after they have transmitted an electrical impulse.

28. Bundle of His conducts electrical impulses to the _____ branches.

29. The _____ nervous system maintains the body in a normal state.

30. Wave of pressure that can be counted; heartbeats per minute.

31. Lack of oxygen to tissue.

33. Valve between the left atrium and left ventricle.

34. The ventricular muscle cells receive electrical impulses from the _____'s fibers.

Down

1. Valve between the right ventricle and artery leading to lungs.

2. Ability of cardiac muscle to shorten in response to an electrical impulse.

4. Lower chambers of the heart.

5. Blood vessel that carries oxygenated blood away from the heart.

6. Two organs where exchange of oxygen for carbon dioxide takes place.

9. Ability of cardiac cells to transmit electrical impulses.

10. Heart/lung _____ describes the way blood travels between the heart and lungs.

11. Part of the autonomic nervous system that increases heart rate.

12. Conduction pathway between the right and the left atrium is the _____ pathway.

15. Valve between the right atria and the right ventricle.

19. Upper chambers of the heart.

20. Abnormal sound made by blood passing through damaged valves.

21. Layer of cardiac muscle that contracts.

23. When cardiac cells _____, they are able to conduct an electrical impulse again.

25. Arteries that supply the heart muscle with oxygen; also another name for a myocardial infarction.

26. Small, grapelike clusters in the lungs where the exchange of oxygen for carbon dioxide takes place.

32. The AV node transmits electrical impulses to the bundle of _____.

The solution to this crossword puzzle is in the answer section.

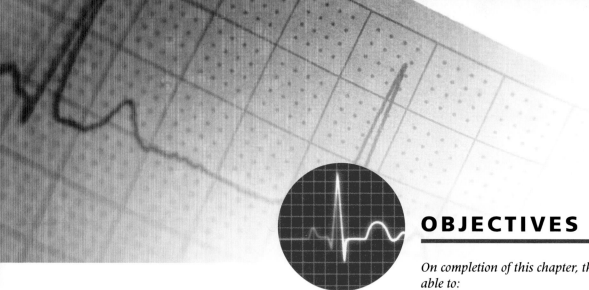

OBJECTIVES

On completion of this chapter, the reader should be able to:

1 Define the terms monitor, electrodes, leads, Lead II, baseline, rate, rhythm, and artifact.

2 Describe the electrode placement for Lead II.

3 Identify the components of a cardiac cycle.

4 Define the terms refractory period, absolute refractory period, and relative refractory period.

5 State five questions to ask when evaluating P waves and QRS complexes.

6 State three questions to ask when evaluating PR intervals.

7 Describe the use of calipers when measuring the rhythm (regularity) of a cardiac rhythm.

8 Explain how to calculate the heart rate using the 3-second rhythm strip method, 6-second rhythm strip method, and two division methods.

9 List four causes of artifact.

MONITORING AND TELEMETRY

OUTLINE

DEFINITIONS

Absolute Refractory Period The period of time when the cardiac cells have not completed repolarization and cannot contract again

Artifact Interference or static seen on the monitor

Complex Components A set of waves seen on a monitor, which represent an electrical impulse traveling through the electrical conduction pathway of the heart; it includes P, Q, R, S, and T waves

Electrode Adhesive pads that are attached to the patient's skin

leads Wires that connect the electrodes to the monitor or telemetry unit

Leads The specific placement of electrodes on the patient's skin

Monitor A TV-like screen that shows the conduction of electrical impulses as they travel through the electrical conduction pathway of the heart

P to P Interval Length of time between one P wave and the next P wave

Rate The number of electrical impulses conducted in 1 minute

Refractory Period The time between depolarization and repolarization

Relative Refractory Period The period of time when cardiac cells have repolarized enough that some cells can be stimulated to depolarize

Rhythm The regularity of the appearance of the complex components

R to R Interval Length of time between one R wave and the next R wave

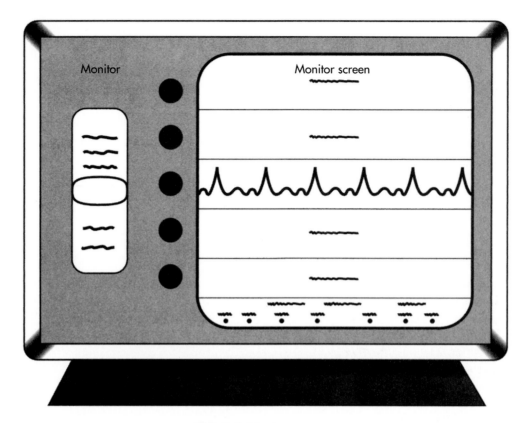

FIG. 2-1 Monitor screen.

Telemetry refers to the process of monitoring cardiac electrical activity by transmitting the information to a monitor or telemetry unit. This process includes a machine, graph paper, the identification of complex components, and the interpretation of rhythm strips.

MONITORS AND TELEMETRY UNITS

The movement of electrical impulses through the heart can be seen by using a machine that is called an *electrocardiograph* or *monitor*. The monitor shows the electrical impulses as a pattern of waves on the monitor screen (Fig. 2-1).

These wave patterns can also be transferred to graph paper for a printed record of the electrical impulses as they travel through the heart. This printed record is called a *rhythm strip* (Fig. 2-2).

Many monitors feature a *freeze mode* to stop the action on the screen. A *delay mode* may also be available to print a specific part of the wave pattern that has already been seen. These special features allow the observer to study the wave pattern more closely.

> NOTE: Remember that the monitor does **not** show the actual **contraction** of the cardiac muscle, only the conduction of the electrical impulses through the heart. Cardiac contractions can only be confirmed by the presence of a pulse.

ELECTRODES AND LEADS

The monitor receives electrical impulses from the patient's heart through a system of electrodes placed on the body. *Electrodes* are adhesive pads that contain a conductive gel and are attached to the patient's skin.

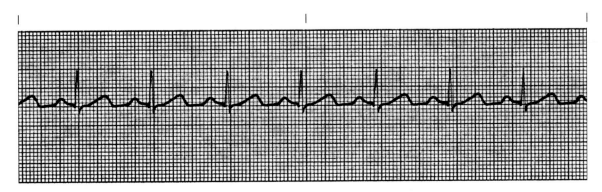

FIG. 2-2 Rhythm strip.

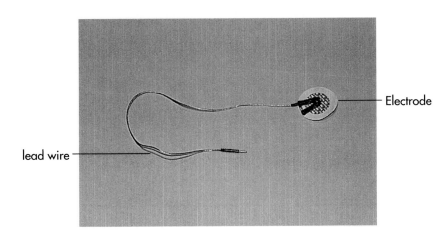

FIG. 2-3 Monitor lead wire and electrode.

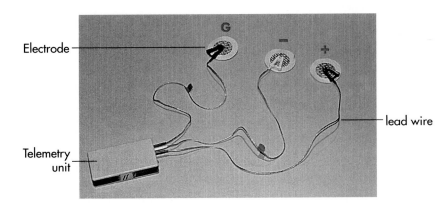

FIG. 2-4 Telemetry unit with lead wires and electrodes.

Electrodes are connected to the monitor by clearly marked wires called *leads* (Fig. 2-3). A positive, a negative, and a ground lead must be used for the monitor to receive a clear picture of the cardiac electrical impulses.

The leads from the electrodes may be connected either directly to a monitor or to a telemetry unit. The *telemetry unit* is a small, battery-operated box that resembles a transistor radio. It transmits the electrical impulses to a monitor at a nursing station or other central location (Fig. 2-4).

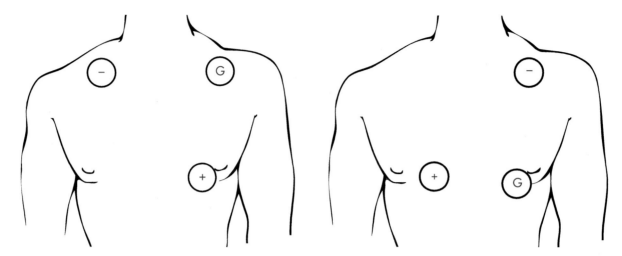

FIG. 2-5 Placement of electrodes for Lead II monitoring.

FIG. 2-6 Placement of electrodes for modified chest Lead I (MCL I) monitoring.

LEAD PLACEMENT

The placement of the electrodes on the patient's body determines the angle at which the electrical impulses are received and therefore the part of the heart being observed. The 12-Lead *electrocardiogram (ECG, EKG)* "looks" at the heart from 12 different viewing angles. However, most patients are monitored using only one or two "viewing angles." The patterns of the electrodes on the patient are called *Leads.*

> **NOTE:** The term *leads* is used in two different ways:
> 1. **The wires leading from electrodes to the monitor. The word "leads" is not capitalized in this definition.**
> 2. **The different types of electrode placements. In this definition, the word "Leads" is capitalized.**

The standard ECG Leads are I, II, III, aVR, aVL, aVF, V_1, V_2, V_3, V_4, V_5, and V_6. Leads I, II, III, aVR, aVL, and aVF are known as *limb* or *peripheral* Leads. Leads V_1, V_2, V_3, V_4, V_5, and V_6 are known as *chest* or *precordial* Leads. In limb Leads, electrodes are placed on the arms and legs or outer areas of the chest. In chest Leads, electrodes are attached to very specific areas of the chest.

The placement of electrodes for the chest Leads is sometimes changed slightly to "see" a specific area of the heart more clearly. The chest Leads (V_1 through V_6) are then referred to as *modified chest Leads (MCL)* and become MCL I through MCL VI. These leads are discussed in more detail in the study of 12-Lead ECG.

Patients are usually monitored in Lead II or MCL I. Lead II shows the movement of the electrical impulse (depolarization) through the ventricles most clearly, and MCL I shows the depolarization of the atria.

In Lead II, the negative electrode is placed on the patient's right upper chest and the positive electrode on the left lower chest. The ground electrode is usually positioned on the left upper chest; however, the ground lead may be placed anywhere on the body because its purpose is to reduce static (Fig. 2-5).

In the MCL I Lead, the positive electrode is placed on the patient's midchest to the right of the sternum and the negative electrode on the left upper chest. The ground electrode may be applied anywhere on the body, but is usually positioned on the left lower chest (Fig. 2-6).

> **NOTE:** Rhythms included in this book are described as they appear in Lead II on an adult patient.

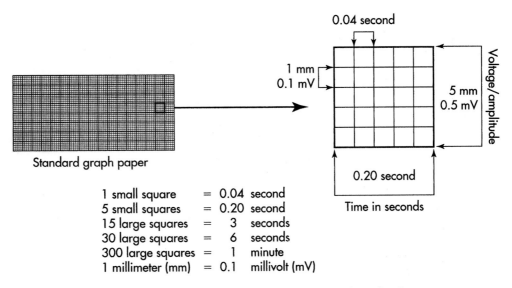

1 small square   = 0.04 second
5 small squares   = 0.20 second
15 large squares   = 3   seconds
30 large squares   = 6   seconds
300 large squares   = 1   minute
1 millimeter (mm)   = 0.1   millivolt (mV)

FIG. 2-7 Standard monitoring graph paper illustrating time and amplitude measurements.

GRAPH PAPER

The rhythm strip provides a printed record of cardiac electrical activity and is printed on ruled *graph paper.* Graph paper is divided into small squares that are 1 mm in height and width. The paper is further divided by darker lines every fifth square, both vertically (top to bottom) and horizontally (side to side). Each large square is 5 mm high and 5 mm wide.

Graph paper measures both time and amplitude. *Time* is measured on the horizontal line. Each small square is equal to **0.04 second** and each large square (5 small squares) is **0.20 second.** These squares measure the length of time it takes an electrical impulse to pass through a specific part of the heart (Fig. 2-7).

The force of the electrical impulse is measured by *amplitude.* Amplitude is measured on the vertical line. Each small square on the graph paper is equal to **0.1 millivolt** (mV), and each large square (5 small squares) is **0.5 mV.**

COMPLEX COMPONENTS

Each *wave* seen on the graph paper or monitor screen represents an electrical impulse in a specific part of the heart. (Wave components used in this book are described as they appear in Lead II.)

BASELINE

The *baseline, or isoelectric line,* is the straight line, without any waves, that can be seen on either the monitor or the graph paper. It represents the absence of electrical activity in the cardiac tissue. All waves begin and end at the baseline. A *deflection* (wave) above the baseline is positive (+) and indicates electrical flow **toward** a positive electrode. A deflection below the baseline is negative (–) and indicates an electrical flow **away from** a positive electrode (Fig. 2-8).

The conduction of an electrical impulse for a single heart beat normally contains five major waves: P, Q, R, S, and T. The combination of these five waves, including the baseline, represents a single heartbeat, or one *cardiac cycle.* A cardiac cycle is measured from the beginning of one P wave to the beginning of the next P wave (Fig. 2-9).

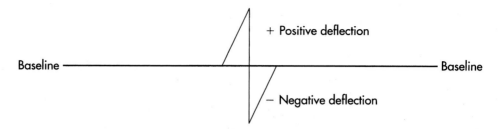

FIG. 2-8 Baseline (isoelectric line) with positive and negative deflections.

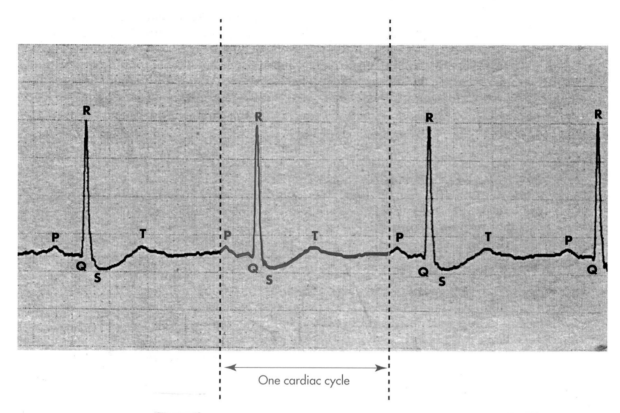

FIG. 2-9 Cardiac cycle with P, Q, R, S, T waves, and baseline.

P WAVE

The *P wave* is the first positive (upward) deflection before the QRS complex. The P wave represents the depolarization of both the right and the left atria (Fig. 2-10). The repolarization of the atria is not usually seen on the rhythm strip because the wave that shows the recovery of the atrial cells is buried in the QRS complex.

PR INTERVAL

The *PR interval (PRI)* represents the time it takes an electrical impulse to be conducted through the atria and the atrioventricular node until the impulse begins to cause ventricular depolarization. The PR interval is measured from the beginning of the P wave to the beginning of the next deflection of the baseline. The normal PR interval is **0.12 to 0.20 second,** or three to five small squares on the graph paper (Fig. 2-11). An abnormal PR interval indicates a disturbance in the electrical conduction pathway.

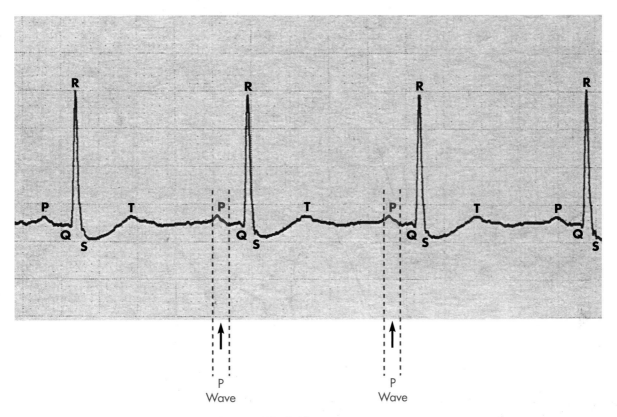

FIG. 2-10 P waves.

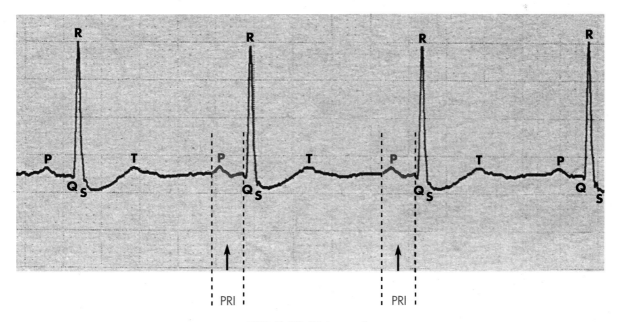

FIG. 2-11 PR intervals.

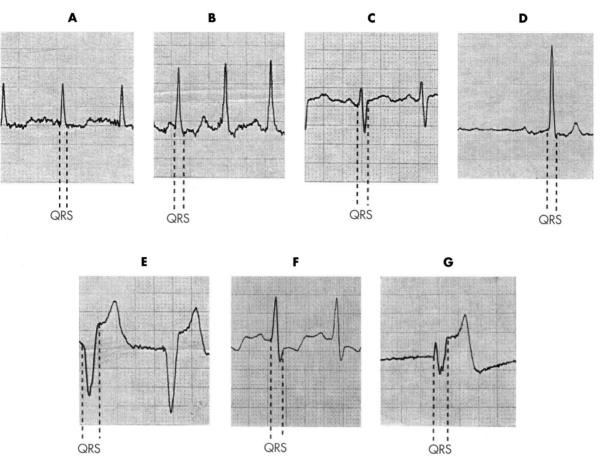

FIG. 2-12 **A** to **G,** QRS complexes.

QRS COMPLEX

The *QRS complex* usually contains three waves: the Q, R, and S. The *Q wave* is the first negative (downward) deflection following the PR interval. The *R wave* is the first positive deflection after the P wave. The *S wave* is the first negative deflection that follows the R wave (Fig. 2-12). Although the Q wave may not be present in all Leads, this combination of waves is still called a **QRS complex.**

The QRS complex represents ventricular depolarization, or the conduction of an electrical impulse from the bundle of His through the ventricular muscle.

The measurement of the QRS complex starts at the beginning of the Q wave (or the R wave if the Q wave is not present). The QRS measurement ends where the S wave meets the baseline, or where the S wave would meet the baseline if it did not curve into the ST segment.

The QRS complex normally measures less than **0.12 second,** or less than three small squares on the graph paper. A QRS complex that measures greater than 0.12 second indicates a disturbance in the electrical conduction pathway.

ST SEGMENT

The portion of the line that leads from the end of the S wave to the beginning of the T wave is the *ST segment* (Fig. 2-13, *A*). The ST segment may be normal (flat), elevated (above the baseline), or depressed (below the baseline) (Fig. 2-13, *B* and *C*). The beginning of the T wave may be difficult to determine in elevated ST segments.

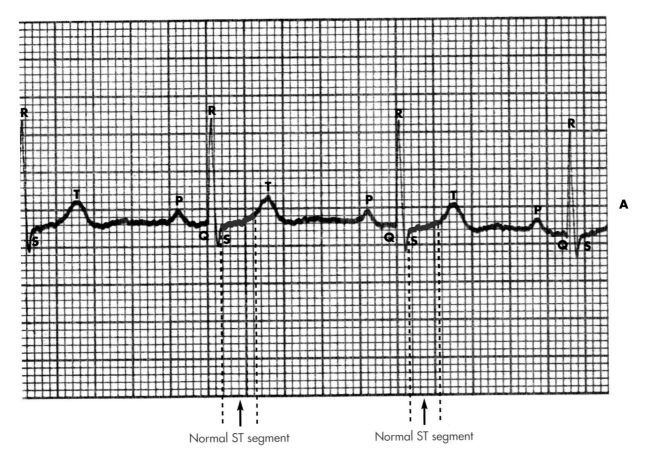

Normal ST segment   Normal ST segment

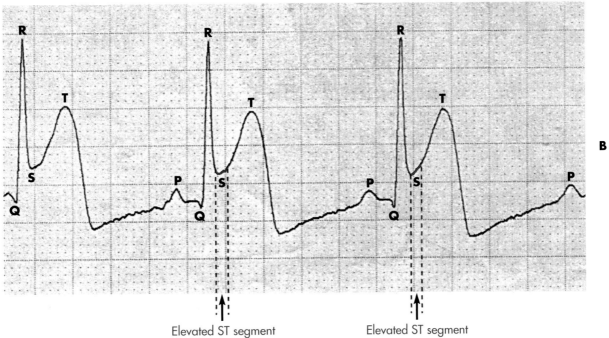

Elevated ST segment   Elevated ST segment

FIG. 2-13 A, Normal ST segments. **B,** Elevated (peaked) ST segments.

Continued

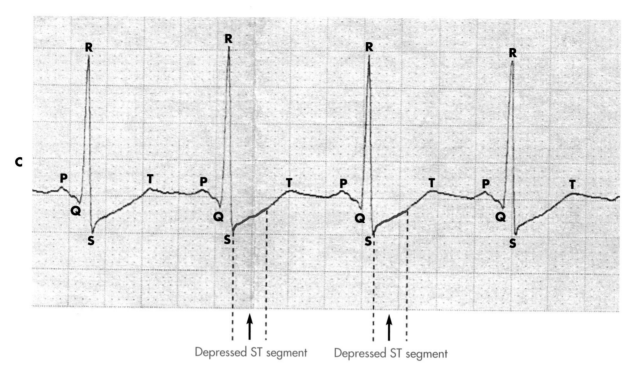

C

Depressed ST segment   Depressed ST segment

FIG. 2-13, cont'd C, Depressed ST segments.

Changes in the ST segment can be used to diagnose a cardiac problem only when seen in a 12-Lead ECG.

T WAVE

The *T wave* follows the ST segment and indicates the repolarization of the ventricular myocardial cells (Fig. 2-14, *A*). The T wave may be either above or below the isoelectric line.

A T wave greater than half the height of the QRS complex is *elevated* (peaked) and may indicate new ischemia (lack of oxygen) of the cardiac muscle (Fig. 2-14, *B*). A *depressed* (inverted) T wave follows an upright QRS complex, is below the isoelectric line, and looks upside down (Fig. 2-14, *C*). An inverted T wave is frequently an indication of previous cardiac ischemia.

P TO P INTERVALS AND R TO R INTERVALS

The P to P interval is the length of time from one P wave to the next P wave. It is usually measured from the beginning of the P wave to the beginning of the next P wave. However, any part of the P wave can be used for measurement, as long as the identical part of each P wave is used.

The R to R interval is the length of time from one R wave to the next R wave. It is usually measured from the peak of one R wave to the peak of the next R wave. However, as when measuring P waves, any point on the R wave may be used, as long as the identical point is used on each R wave. These intervals can be measured by using either calipers or paper and pencil (see "Rhythm," p 33).

The measurements of these intervals are used to determine if the rhythm of a strip is regular or irregular.

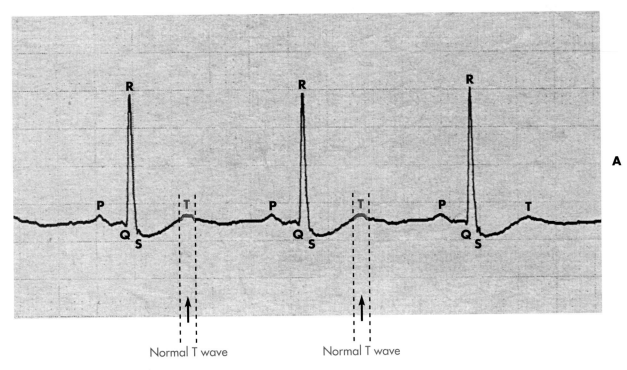

Normal T wave   Normal T wave

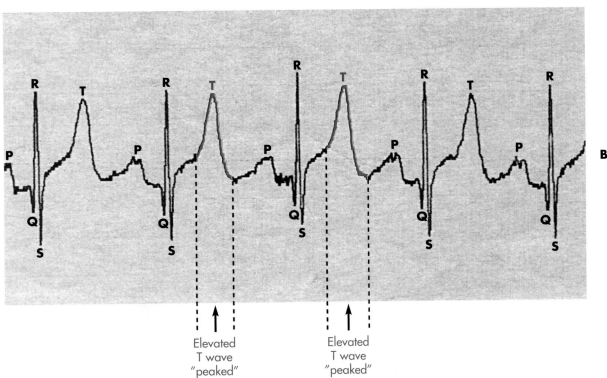

Elevated
T wave
"peaked"

Elevated
T wave
"peaked"

FIG. 2-14 A, Normal T waves. **B,** Elevated T waves.

Continued

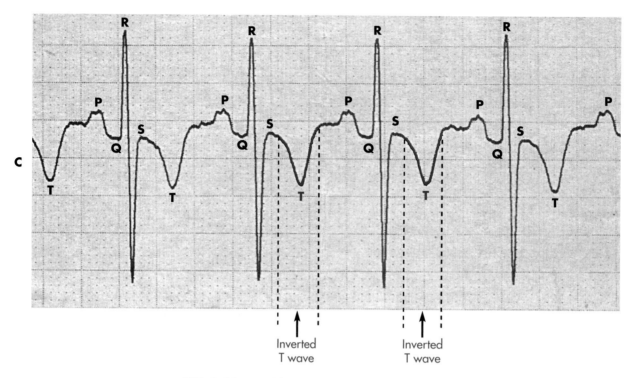

Inverted
T wave

Inverted
T wave

FIG. 2-14, cont'd C, Depressed (inverted) T waves.

QT INTERVAL

The depolarization and repolarization of the ventricles are shown by the *QT interval.* The QT interval is measured from the beginning of the QRS complex to the end of the T wave.

QT intervals are either normal or prolonged. A normal QT interval is less than one half the R to R interval of that complex and the R wave of the following complex (Fig. 2-15, *A*). A QT interval that is greater than one half the R to R interval of that complex and the R wave of the following complex is *prolonged* (Fig. 2-15, *B*). A prolonged QT interval usually indicates a problem within the electrical conduction pathway of the heart.

> **NOTE:** The rhythm strip represents **only** the conduction of electrical impulses through the myocardial cells. Normally, it also represents the contraction of the heart muscle. However, this is not always true, so **you must treat the patient** and any symptoms that are present, **not the monitor.**

REFRACTORY PERIODS

In addition to identifying wave and complex formations, it will be helpful to understand refractory periods.

The *refractory period* is the time between depolarization and the return of the cardiac cells to the ready or polarized state. While the cells are recovering, the atria and ventricles are refilling with blood, preparing to contract again. The refractory period is divided into two phases:

1. *Absolute refractory period*—the cardiac cells have not completed repolarization and **cannot** be stimulated to conduct an electrical impulse and contract again (depolarize). This period is measured from the beginning of the QRS complex through approximately the first half of the T wave.

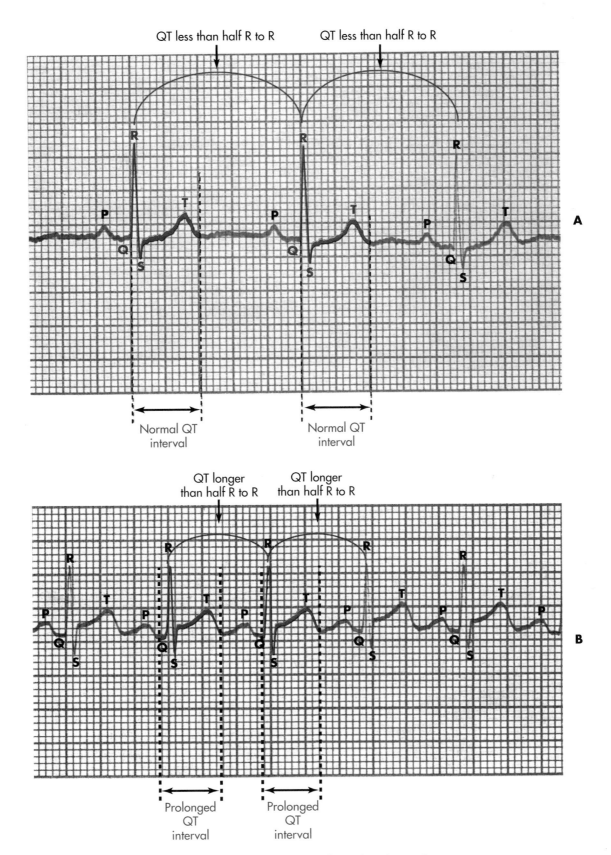

FIG. 2-15 A, Normal QT intervals. **B,** Prolonged QT intervals.

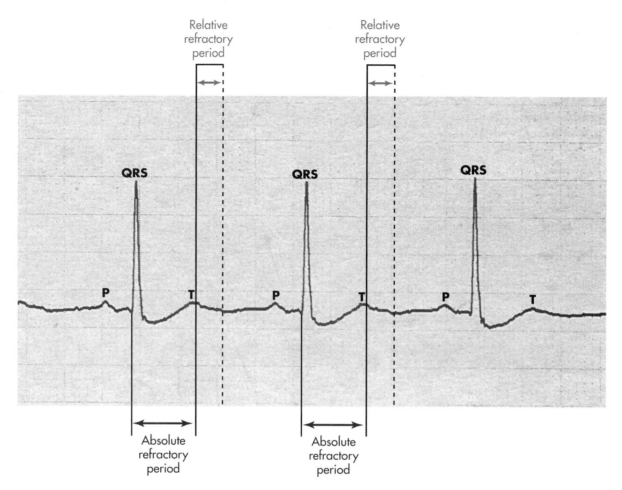

FIG. 2-16 Absolute and relative refractory periods.

2. *Relative refractory period*—the cardiac cells have repolarized to the point that **some** cells can again be stimulated to depolarize, if the stimulus is strong enough. However, if these cells are stimulated during this period, they will probably conduct the electrical impulse in a slow, abnormal pattern. This period is measured from the end of the absolute refractory period to the end of the T wave. The relative refractory period is also known as the *vulnerable period of repolarization* (Fig. 2-16).

This information allows more accurate interpretation of dysrhythmias, particularly those involving premature ventricular contractions (see Chapter 6).

INTERPRETING A RHYTHM STRIP

A *rhythm strip* is a tool that assists the observer in the interpretation of a patient's cardiac rhythm. It also is useful to monitor changes in the cardiac cycle. However, a 12-Lead ECG is necessary to diagnose a cardiac problem.

To interpret a cardiac rhythm accurately, you must evaluate P waves (including the ratio of P waves to QRS complexes), PR intervals, QRS complexes, rhythm (regularity), and rate.

These components may be evaluated in any order; however, they must all be evaluated on every rhythm strip. Rhythm interpretation is easier if each component is examined in the same order with each strip.

First, look at the general appearance of the entire rhythm strip, then examine each individual component.

COMPLEX FORMATION

The **appearance** of the P, Q, R, S, and T waves, and the **ratio** of P waves to QRS complexes should be evaluated. Examine each cardiac cycle from the beginning to its end.

1. *P waves*—examine each P wave.
   a. Are P waves present?
   b. Are they all upright?
   c. Do all P waves look alike?
   d. Is there a P wave before every QRS complex?
   e. Are the P to P intervals equal?
2. *PR intervals*—measure each PRI.
   a. Are PRIs present?
   b. Are all PRIs equal?
   c. Are all PRIs within the normal range of 0.12 to 0.20 second?
3. *QRS complexes*—examine and measure each QRS complex.
   a. Are QRS complexes present?
   b. Do all QRS complexes look alike?
   c. Is there a QRS complex after every P wave?
   d. Are the R to R intervals equal?
   e. Are all QRS complexes within the normal range of less than 0.12 second?

ST segments, T waves, and QT intervals are not required for the interpretation of cardiac rhythms. However, they can be important as indicators of changes in a patient's cardiac condition, such as new ischemia. Therefore any change in the ST segment, T wave, or QT interval should be included in the interpretation of a cardiac rhythm strip.

RHYTHM

The term *rhythm* is used to describe how regularly the complexes occur. To determine if the complexes occur regularly, measure the R to R intervals and the P to P intervals (if P waves are present). If the R to R intervals are equal, the rhythm is regular (Fig. 2-17). If the P to P, R to R, or both intervals vary by less than 0.06 second (1.5 small squares), the rhythm can be considered regular. If the intervals vary by more than 0.06 second, the rhythm is irregular. The P to P intervals are also measured to determine if the atrial rhythm is regular.

Calipers provide the most accurate method of measuring rhythm. Place the point of one caliper leg on the top of an R wave (Fig. 2-18, *A*). Adjust the caliper so the point of the second caliper leg is on the top of the next R wave. Then twist the caliper so that the point of the first leg is going toward the third R wave. If the rhythm is regular, the second caliper point will be on the top of the third R wave (Fig. 2-18, *B*). Continue moving the calipers across the rhythm strip, measuring the distance between each two R waves, to check the regularity of the R waves (Fig. 2-18, *C*). The rhythm is irregular if the measurement differs by more than 0.06 second. The P to P rhythm can be checked in the same way using P waves instead of R waves.

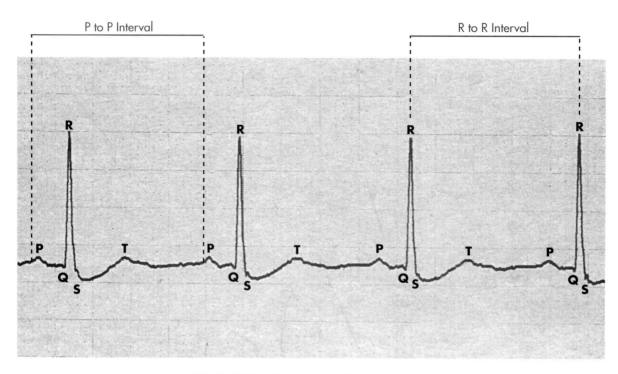

FIG. 2-17 P to P interval and R to R interval.

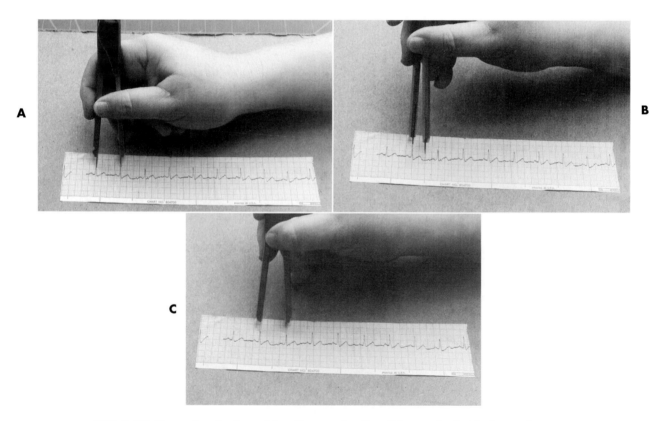

FIG. 2-18 Measuring rhythm with calipers, using R to R intervals: **A,** Mark two R waves. **B,** Twist caliper to next R wave. **C,** Continue checking remaining R waves for regularity.

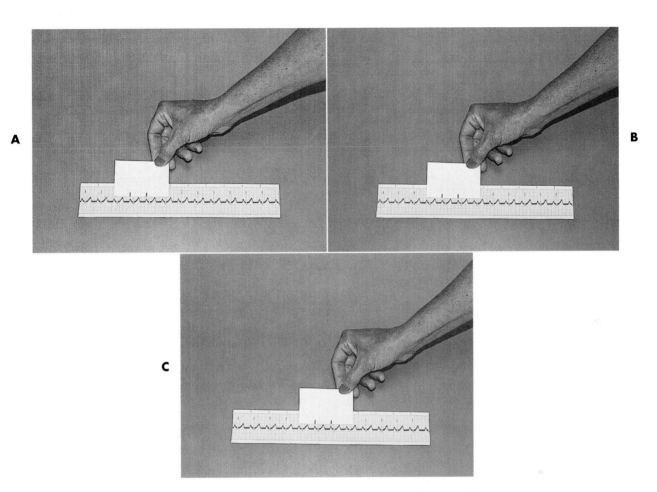

FIG. 2-19 Measuring rhythm with paper, using P to P intervals. **A,** Mark two P waves. **B,** Move paper to next P wave. **C,** Continue checking remaining P waves for regularity.

When calipers are not available, an acceptable alternative involves the use of a blank piece of paper and a pencil. Place the paper over the rhythm strip so only the tips of the R waves are showing. Mark small dots on the paper where the first two R waves occur. Then move the paper so the first dot is now on the second R wave. If the rhythm is regular, the second dot will fall on the next R wave. Continue moving the paper across the rhythm strip in this manner to check the regularity of each R wave. The P to P rhythm can be checked in the same way (Fig. 2-19, *A, B,* and *C*).

RATE

Rate is the number of electrical impulses conducted through the myocardium in 1 minute. **Atrial rate** is determined by the number of P waves seen, while the **ventricular rate** is determined by the number of R waves. The ventricular rate should be the same as the patient's pulse, if the myocardium is contracting with each QRS complex and if the cardiac output is within normal limits.

Many methods of calculating rate exist, but the following are the methods used most frequently:

1. *Calculation by a 6-second rhythm strip.* The graph paper may have small indicator lines (vertical lines) in the top margin of the paper, which measure 1-second intervals. Every 3 seconds, the indicator line is longer or darker. The space

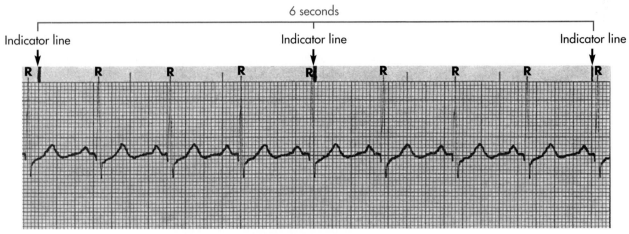

7 R waves × 10 = 70 heart rate
30 large squares (30 × 0.20 sec) = 6 seconds = 6 inches
10 × 6 = 60 seconds or 1 minute
1 second = 1 inch

FIG. 2-20 Six-second rhythm strip method of calculating heart rate.

between three long lines equals 6 seconds. To calculate the heart rate, count the number of R waves in a 6-second rhythm strip and multiply that number by 10. If a QRS complex falls directly under the beginning or ending indicator line, it is included in the total number of R waves counted. This calculation gives an *approximate* heart rate per minute (Fig. 2-20). If the graph paper does not have 1- or 3-second interval lines, you can:

a. Measure 6 inches of the paper to get a 6-second strip, since 1 inch of graph paper equals 1 second. Then count the number of R waves in the strip and multiply that number by 10.

b. Count the number of R waves in 30 large squares and multiply that number by 10, since 30 large squares equal 6 seconds.

2. *Calculation by a 3-second rhythm strip.* The space between two long indicator lines equals 3 seconds (3 inches). Count the number of R waves between the two long lines and multiply by 20, or count the number of R waves in 15 large squares and multiply by 20. This calculation gives an *approximate* heart rate per minute (Fig. 2-21).

3. *Calculation by division.* This method is more precise than the first two methods; however, **it should only be used when the rhythm is regular.** To use this method, count the number of large squares between two R waves and divide 300 by this number to determine the heart rate. For example, 300 divided by 3 (number of large squares between two R waves) equals 100. The heart rate is 100.

    When counting the number of large squares between two R waves, if part of a large square is included, count each small square as 0.2. Add the number of large and small squares and then divide 300 by that number. For example, 4 large and 4 small squares equal 4.8 squares; 300 divided by 4.8 equals 62.5. The heart rate is approximately 63 (Fig. 2-22).

    An additional method using calculation by division involves counting the number of small squares between two R waves. Then divide 1500 by that number to determine the rate. For example, in Figure 2-22, 24 small squares are between the two R waves. 1500 divided by 24 equals 62.5, or a heart rate of approximately 63.

4. *Calculation by a 1-minute rhythm strip.* This method is the most accurate for calculating rate. Count the number of R waves in a 1-minute rhythm strip.

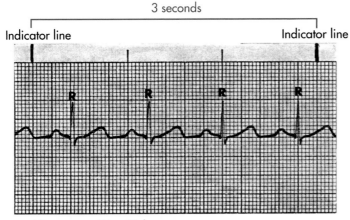

4 R waves × 20 = 80 heart rate
15 large squares (15 × 0.20 sec) = 3 seconds = 3 inches
20 × 3 = 60 seconds or 1 minute

FIG. 2-21 Three-second rhythm strip method of calculating heart rate.

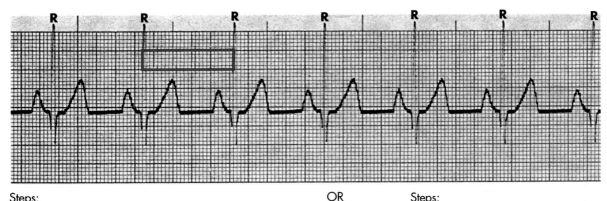

Steps: OR   Steps:
1. 4 large and 4 small squares between R waves   1. 24 small squares between R waves
2. 4 small squares × 0.2 = 0.8   2. 1500 ÷ 24 = 62.5
3. 300 ÷ 4.8 = 63   3. Approximate heart rate = 63
   Approximate heart rate = 63

FIG. 2-22 Two division methods of calculating heart rate.

This method is rarely used because it requires a relatively long period of time to perform.

All heart rates in this book have been calculated by the 6-second rhythm strip method unless stated otherwise and are only approximate rates.

Take time to practice identifying the various components of many rhythm strips. These components are the *basic building blocks* needed for future identification of rhythms and dysrhythmias. The more you practice, the easier it will become to identify each component.

ARTIFACT

Artifact is interference or static seen on the monitor screen or rhythm strip. This interference may be caused by the electrode losing contact with the patient's skin, patient movement or shivering, a broken cable or lead wire, or improper grounding.

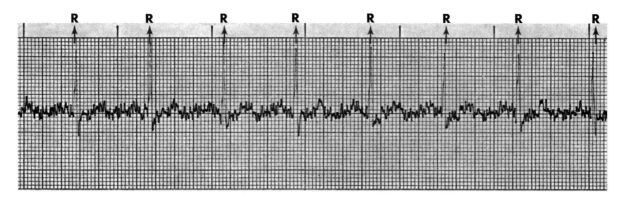

FIG. 2-23 60 cycle interference.

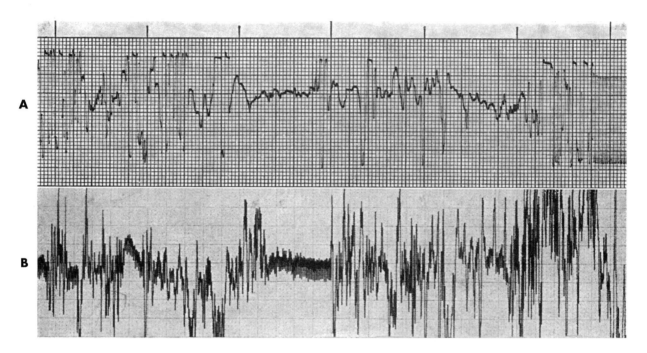

FIG. 2-24 A, Artifact: rhythm not measurable. **B,** Artifact: rhythm not visible.

One type of artifact is *60-cycle interference,* which appears as a fuzziness of the baseline. The P wave may not be seen because of this interference, but the QRS is usually visible (Fig. 2-23).

The 60-cycle interference is usually seen when the electrodes have lost contact with the patient's skin. This situation may result from excessive chest hair, sweaty skin, or the loss of conductive gel.

NOTE: The conductive gel of the electrodes may dry out with prolonged use or improper storage. Be sure that the conductive gel is still moist and the electrodes are firmly attached to the patient's skin.

The 60-cycle interference also may be caused by either the patient or the lead cable touching a metal object, such as a bed rail. A blanket between the metal object and the patient or lead wire should correct the interference.

Artifact that completely hides both the P wave and the QRS complex may be caused by either a loose lead or patient movement (Fig. 2-24, *A* and *B*). Patient as-

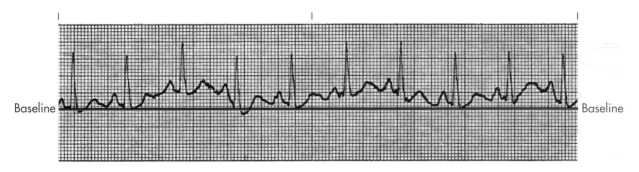

FIG. 2-25 Wandering baseline.

sessment is very important because this artifact can mimic a lethal dysrhythmia on the monitor or rhythm strip.

Patient movement or deep, rapid breathing also may cause an artifact in which the baseline moves up and down rapidly on the monitor screen or rhythm strip. This type of artifact is called a *wandering baseline* and is usually corrected when the patient lies still or when the electrode placement is changed (Fig. 2-25).

REVIEW QUESTIONS

TRUE FALSE   1. The monitor shows the conduction of the electrical impulses through the heart, not the actual contraction of the heart muscle.

TRUE **FALSE**   2. Leads are color-coded wires that connect the telemetry unit to the patient's cardiac muscle.

TRUE **FALSE**   3. Lead II and MCL I are the two Leads most often used to monitor patients.

TRUE FALSE   4. It is important to check complex formation, rhythm, and rate when interpreting a rhythm strip.

5. The P wave represents the depolarization of both the right and left:
a. ventricles
b. atria and ventricles
c. valves
d. atria

6. The normal PR interval measures _____ to _____ second.
a. 0.04 to 0.12
b. 0.4 to 0.12
c. 0.12 to 0.20
d. 0.04 to 0.20

7. The measurement of a normal QRS complex is:
a. 0.4 to 0.12 second
b. 0.12 to 0.20 second
c. 0.4 to 0.20 second
d. 0.04 to 0.12 second

8. Identify the components and intervals included in one complete cardiac cycle:
a. _P wave_
b. _PR interval_
c. _QRS complex_
d. _ST segment_
e. _T wave_
f. _Q-T interval_
g. _U wave_

9. A T wave represents:
a. depolarization of the ventricles
b. repolarization of the atria
c. polarization of all cardiac cells
d. repolarization of the ventricles

10. A normal QT interval measures: _Total Time for Vent de + re polarization_

11. Explain how to calculate heart rate using the 6-second rhythm strip method: _# of cycles in 6 seconds (30 large boxes) X 10_

12. Calculate the heart rate using both division methods when the distance between two R waves is:
    a. Three large squares:

    _____

    _____

    _____

    _____

    b. Four large and two small squares:

    _____

    _____

    _____

    _____

13. List two facts about PR intervals that are important to measure when interpreting a rhythm strip:
    a. _____

    _____

    b. _____

    _____

14. List five facts about QRS complexes that are important to evaluate when interpreting a rhythm strip:
    a. _____

    _____

    b. _____

    _____

    c. _____

    _____

    d. _____

    _____

    e. _____

    _____

15. Three common causes of artifact are:
    a. patient movement; low amplitude; 60-cycle interference
    b. patient movement; slow respirations; loose leads
    c. patient movement; chest Leads; 60-cycle interference
    d. patient movement; loose leads; 60-cycle interference

16. Explain the difference between relative and absolute refractory periods.

    _____

    _____

    _____

    _____

    _____

RHYTHM STRIP REVIEW

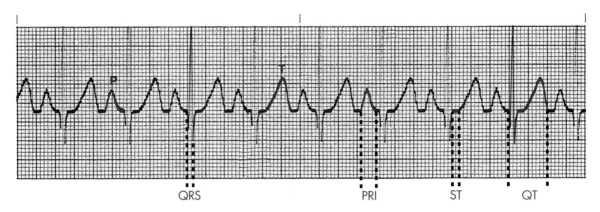

IDENTIFY: P wave, PR interval, QRS complex, ST segment, T wave, and QT interval

MEASURE: PR interval _____0.20_____   Rhythm _____regular_____
QRS complex _____0.06-0.08_____   Heart rate _____90_____
QT interval _____prolonged_____

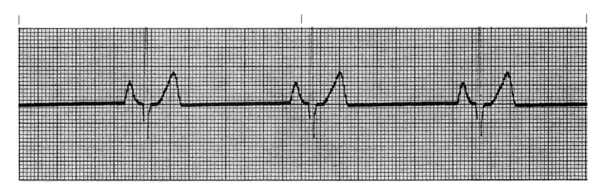

1. IDENTIFY: P wave, PR interval, QRS complex, ST segment, T wave, and QT interval
   MEASURE: PR interval _____   Rhythm _____
   QRS complex _____   Heart rate _____
   QT interval _____

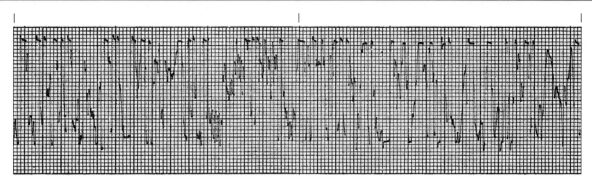

2. IDENTIFY: P wave, PR interval, QRS complex, ST segment, T wave, and QT interval
   MEASURE: PR interval _____ Rhythm _____
   QRS complex _____ Heart rate _____
   QT interval _____

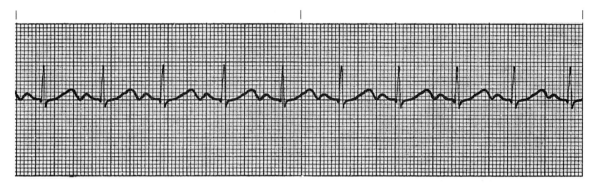

3. IDENTIFY: P wave, PR interval, QRS complex, ST segment, T wave, and QT interval
   MEASURE: PR interval _____ Rhythm _____
   QRS complex _____ Heart rate _____
   QT interval _____

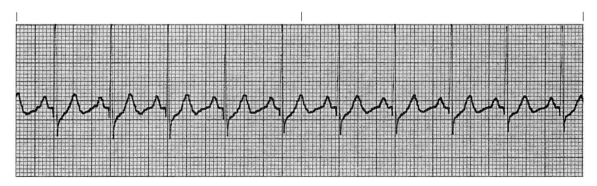

4. IDENTIFY: P wave, PR interval, QRS complex, ST segment, T wave, and QT interval
   MEASURE: PR interval _____ Rhythm _____
   QRS complex _____ Heart rate _____
   QT interval _____

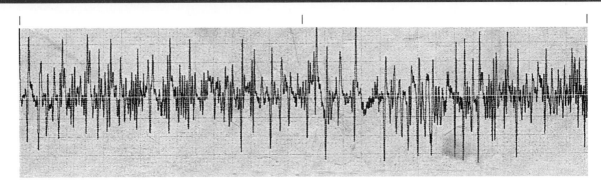

5. IDENTIFY: P wave, PR interval, QRS complex, ST segment, T wave, and QT interval
    MEASURE: PR interval _____ Rhythm _____
    QRS complex _____ Heart rate _____
    QT interval _____

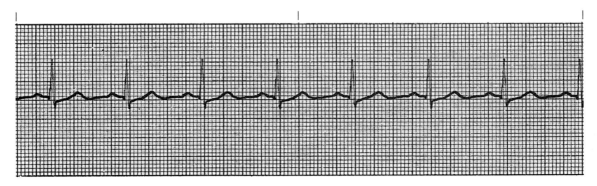

6. IDENTIFY: P wave, PR interval, QRS complex, ST segment, T wave, and QT interval
    MEASURE: PR interval _____ Rhythm _____
    QRS complex _____ Heart rate _____
    QT interval _____

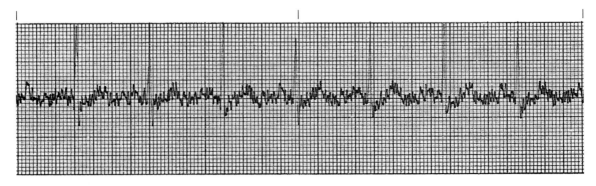

7. IDENTIFY: P wave, PR interval, QRS complex, ST segment, T wave, and QT interval
    MEASURE: PR interval _____ Rhythm _____
    QRS complex _____ Heart rate _____
    QT interval _____

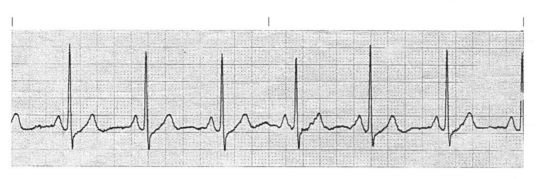

8. IDENTIFY: P wave, PR interval, QRS complex, ST segment, T wave, and QT interval
    MEASURE: PR interval _____ Rhythm _____
    QRS complex _____ Heart rate _____
    QT interval _____

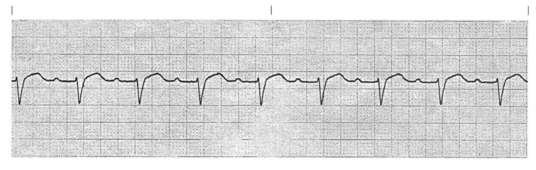

9. IDENTIFY: P wave, PR interval, QRS complex, ST segment, T wave, and QT interval
    MEASURE: PR interval _____ Rhythm _____
    QRS complex _____ Heart rate _____
    QT interval _____

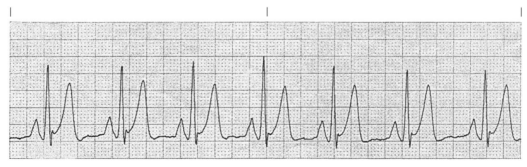

10. IDENTIFY: P wave, PR interval, QRS complex, ST segment, T wave, and QT interval
    MEASURE: PR interval _____ Rhythm _____
    QRS complex _____ Heart rate _____
    QT interval _____

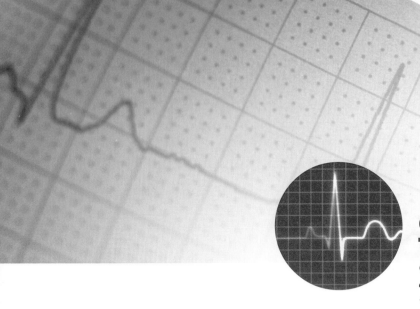

OBJECTIVES

On completion of this chapter, the reader should be able to:

1 Describe the conduction of a normal electrical impulse from the sinoatrial node to the ventricular muscle.

2 Describe a normal sinus rhythm, including measurements of the components.

3 Identify sinus bradycardia, sinus tachycardia, and sinus arrhythmia.

4 Explain the differences between a sinus exit block and a sinus arrest, including measurements of the components.

5 Describe the appearance of a premature atrial contraction, including measurements of the components.

6 Explain the primary difference between paroxysmal atrial tachycardia and supraventricular tachycardia.

7 Describe the appearance of atrial flutter, including measurements of the components and types of blocks (ratios).

8 Describe atrial fibrillation, including measurements of the components.

9 Describe Wolff-Parkinson-White syndrome, including measurements of the components.

SINUS AND ATRIAL DYSRHYTHMIAS

OUTLINE

DEFINITIONS

Accessory Pathway An additional or abnormal electrical conduction pathway; the bundle of Kent (Kent bundle) is one accessory pathway

Antegrade Downward movement of an electrical impulse from atria to ventricles

Atrial Dysrhythmia A rhythm that is initiated from any pacemaker site in the atria, when the sinoatrial (SA) node fails to initiate an electrical impulse

Bradycardia Heart rate slower than 60 electrical impulses per minute

Compensatory Pause A pause in the rhythm that measures two times the R to R interval of the underlying rhythm

Delta Wave An extra "bump" seen in the slurred section at the beginning of a QRS complex; seen in Wolff-Parkinson-White syndrome

Dysrhythmia Abnormal cardiac rhythm

Inherent Heart Rate Normal rate at which electrical impulses are generated; the inherent heart rate for the sinoatrial node is 60 to 100 heartbeats per minute

Noncompensatory Pause A pause in the rhythm that measures less than two times the R to R interval of the underlying rhythm

Normal Electrical Conduction Pathway Sinoatrial (SA) node to atrioventricular (AV) node, through the bundle of His and bundle branches, to the Purkinje's fibers, ending in the ventricular muscle

Paroxysmal Sudden, intermittent start and stop of symptoms or dysrhythmias; usually used to describe a type of atrial tachycardia

Premature Contraction A complex that occurs earlier than expected in the underlying rhythm

Sinoatrial (SA) Node The pacemaker of the heart; it usually initiates the electrical impulses that travel through the electrical conduction pathway of the heart.

Sinus Rhythm Cardiac rhythm that shows the movement of an electrical impulse traveling from the sinoatrial node to the ventricles, following the normal electrical conduction pathway.

Tachycardia Heart rate faster than 100 electrical impulses per minute.

SINUS RHYTHMS

The sinoatrial (SA) node is located in the upper portion of the right atrium and is referred to as the *pacemaker of the heart* (see Chapter 1). The SA node normally initiates the electrical impulse that travels throughout the heart, leading to depolarization of the atria and ventricles (Fig. 3-1). If the SA node fails to generate an electrical impulse, any other pacemaker cell within the atria is capable of initiating an impulse.

The SA node, as well as other pacemaker cells in the atria, normally generates 60 to 100 electrical impulses per minute. This is known as the *inherent* heart rate of the atria. In sinus rhythms, the electrical impulse travels from the SA node, through the atria to the atrioventricular (AV) node, continuing through the bundle of His and bundle branches, to the Purkinje's fibers, and ending in the ventricular muscle.

Because the electrical impulse follows this normal pathway throughout the heart, an upright P wave is present, representing atrial depolarization. The PR interval is within the normal limits of 0.12 to 0.20 second. The QRS complex, representing ventricular depolarization, measures less than 0.12 second (Fig. 3-2). However, in some sinus rhythms, the length of PR intervals may vary within the normal limits.

Rhythms originating from the SA node are *sinus rhythms* or *sinus dysrhythmias* (abnormal rhythms), and rhythms originating from other atrial sites are *atrial dysrhythmias.* The term *dysrhythmia* is used with all cardiac rhythms except normal sinus rhythm.

Sinus dysrhythmias are usually not serious. However, as with any rhythm, **patient assessment** is essential to determine the patient's tolerance of the dysrhythmia.

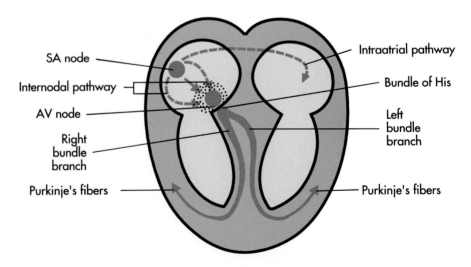

FIG. 3-1 Normal cardiac electrical conduction pathway.

NOTE: The patient is considered medically unstable if any combination of the following occur: weakness, faintness, sudden change in blood pressure, chest pain, confusion, unresponsiveness, or other signs or symptoms of poor cardiac output.

NORMAL SINUS RHYTHM

Normal sinus rhythm (NSR) is the ONLY rhythm considered "normal." In this rhythm, the SA node initiates all the electrical impulses that are transmitted throughout the heart. The SA node generates an impulse that travels downward, throughout both the right and the left atria, causing atrial depolarization. The impulse is then transmitted through the AV node, the bundle of His, and both bundle branches to the Purkinje's fibers and ends in the ventricular muscle, where it causes ventricular depolarization (Fig. 3-3).

Because the electrical impulse follows the normal conduction pathway, an upright P wave precedes every QRS complex. All PR intervals range from 0.12 to 0.20 second, and the QRS complex is less than 0.12 second. All P waves look alike, and all QRS complexes are the same size and shape.

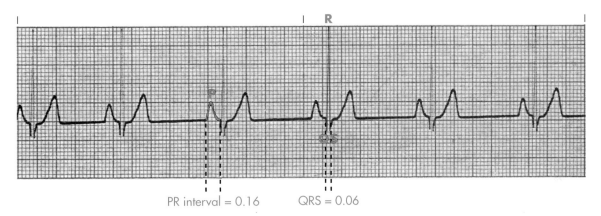

PR interval = 0.16   QRS = 0.06

FIG. 3-2 Atrial rhythm strip with PR interval and QRS complex.

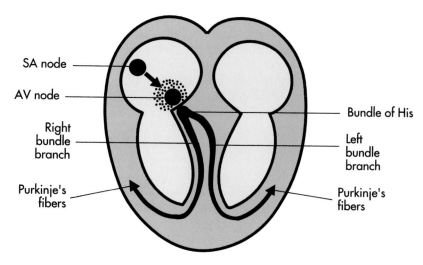

FIG. 3-3 Normal electrical conduction pathway.

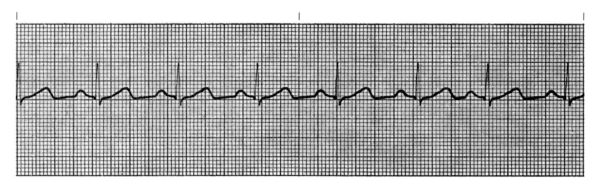

FIG. 3-4 Normal sinus rhythm; heart rate, 80.

In normal sinus rhythm, both the atria and the ventricles depolarize at regular intervals. Therefore the P to P intervals and R to R intervals are regular. In addition, the P to P intervals are the same length as the R to R intervals. Normal sinus rhythm is very regular, and the rate is 60 to 100 electrical impulses per minute (Fig. 3-4).

NOTE: Rhythms included in this book are described as they appear in Lead II on an adult patient.

SINUS BRADYCARDIA

Sinus bradycardia (sinus brady) is a dysrhythmia that occurs when all electrical impulses originate from the SA node and follow the normal conduction pathway. However, the rate is slower than 60 impulses per minute (see Fig. 3-3).

An upright P wave occurs before every QRS complex. The PR intervals remain within the normal range of 0.12 to 0.20 second, and the QRS complexes are less than 0.12 second. All P waves look alike, and QRS complexes are the same size and shape. Because the P to P intervals and the R to R intervals are regular and equal in length, the rhythm is regular. The rate can vary, but it must be slower than 60 electrical impulses per minute in sinus bradycardia (Fig. 3-5).

Sinus bradycardia may be normal for sleeping individuals and athletes. However, it may become a dangerous dysrhythmia if the rate falls significantly **or** if the patient begins to show signs of poor cardiac output. These signs and symptoms include any combination of the following: pale, cool, clammy skin; cyanosis; dyspnea; confusion or disorientation; dizziness, weakness, or faintness; sudden change in blood pressure; shortness of breath; nausea or vomiting; decreased urinary output; severe chest pain; and/or unresponsiveness.

Some common causes of sinus bradycardia are vomiting and/or drugs such as digitalis, morphine, and sedatives.

SINUS TACHYCARDIA

Sinus tachycardia (sinus tach) occurs when all electrical impulses originate from the SA node at a rate between 101 and 150 beats per minute (see Fig. 3-3).

Because the impulse follows the normal electrical conduction pathway, an upright P wave occurs before every QRS complex. PR intervals remain within the normal range of 0.12 to 0.20 second, and QRS complexes are less than 0.12 second (Fig. 3-6, *A*). All P waves look alike, and all QRS complexes are the same size and shape.

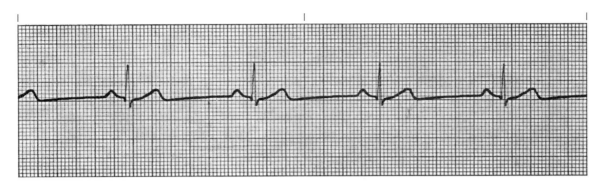

FIG. 3-5 Sinus bradycardia; heart rate, 40.

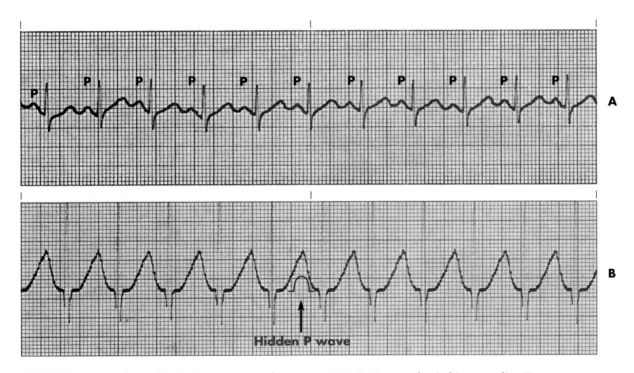

FIG. 3-6 Sinus tachycardia. **A,** P waves seen; heart rate, 110. **B,** P waves buried in preceding T waves; heart rate, 110.

As the rate of the tachycardia increases, the P waves are frequently hidden in the T wave of the preceding QRS complex, causing a slight change in the appearance of the T wave (Fig. 3-6, *B*).

Because the P to P intervals and R to R intervals are usually regular and equal in length, the rhythm usually is regular. The rate can vary, but it usually falls between 101 and 150 electrical impulses per minute.

Sinus tachycardia may become a serious dysrhythmia if the patient becomes *medically unstable* (poor cardiac output).

The most common causes of sinus tachycardia are pain, fever, acute anemia, hemorrhage, exercise, fear, sudden excitement, anxiety, or the effects of drugs such as atropine, nicotine, caffeine, or amphetamines.

SINUS ARRHYTHMIA

Sinus arrhythmia occurs when the SA node initiates all the electrical impulses but at irregular intervals. The P to P intervals and the R to R intervals change with respirations, producing an irregular rhythm (see Fig. 3-3).

Because the impulses are all generated by the SA node and follow the normal conduction pathway, an upright P wave still occurs before every QRS complex. The PR intervals remain within 0.12 to 0.20 second, and the QRS complexes are less than 0.12 second. All P waves look alike, and the QRS complexes are the same in size and shape.

Because the heart rate increases as the patient inhales and decreases as the patient exhales, the 6-second rhythm strip is a more reliable method of determining heart rate. However, the overall heart rate will usually be 60 to 100 electrical impulses per minute. P to P and R to R intervals are irregular, causing the rhythm to be irregular. The longest R to R interval will be **less** than twice the length of any of the remaining R to R intervals (Fig. 3-7).

Although sinus arrhythmia is normal for infants and young children, it may be a warning of a diseased SA node or coronary artery disease in the adult patient. Sinus arrhythmia is usually not serious unless the patient's cardiac output decreases and the patient becomes medically unstable.

As with any rhythm, **patient assessment** is essential to determine the patient's tolerance of the dysrhythmia.

> NOTE: Normal sinus rhythm, sinus bradycardia, sinus tachycardia, and sinus arrhythmia all follow the normal electrical conduction pathway of the heart; only the rate or rhythm varies.

SINUS EXIT BLOCK AND SINUS ARREST

Sinus exit block (sinus block) occurs when the SA node initiates an electrical impulse that is blocked and **not** conducted to the atria. The atria and ventricles do not depolarize, and a P wave will not be seen until the next conducted complex.

Sinus arrest occurs when the SA node does **not** initiate an electrical impulse. Because an impulse is not generated, depolarization will not occur and the next expected complex will not be seen.

Both dysrhythmias appear similar on the monitor screen or rhythm strip. P waves are absent, and QRS complexes are not seen because an impulse is not conducted to

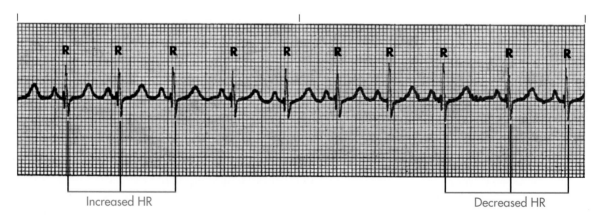

FIG. 3-7 Sinus arrhythmia. Heart rate increases with inspiration and decreases with expiration; overall heart rate, 100.

the ventricles to cause depolarization. The lack of a P wave and QRS complex forms a *pause* on the monitor and rhythm strip.

The length of the pause may help determine whether the dysrhythmia is a sinus exit block or a sinus arrest. The pause of a sinus exit block is equal to **exactly** two or more previous cardiac cycles of the underlying rhythm. For example, the P to P interval of the underlying rhythm will fit into the pause of a sinus exit block exactly two times, or exactly three times, and so forth (Fig. 3-8). The SA node continues to fire at its normal rate, so the rhythm will usually be regular except where the pause occurs.

The pause of a sinus arrest is not equal to exactly two or more cardiac cycles of the underlying rhythm. It will be **more** than two times the cardiac cycle of the underlying rhythm. For example, the P to P interval of the underlying rhythm will not fit into the pause of a sinus arrest exactly two times, or exactly three times, and so forth. Because the SA node is not firing, any pacemaker cell in the heart can begin to initiate electrical impulses. Therefore the complex that ends the sinus arrest may be either atrial, junctional, or ventricular (Fig. 3-9). The rhythm after the sinus arrest may be different than the rhythm before the pause.

Both dysrhythmias may be caused by myocardial infarction (MI), ischemia (lack of oxygen), or drugs such as digitalis or quinidine.

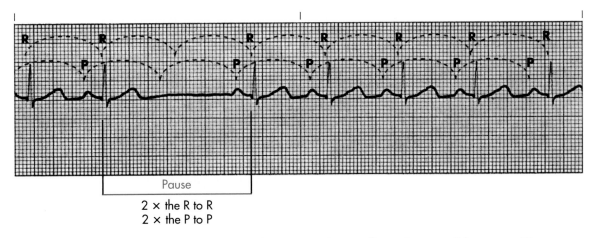

FIG. 3-8 Sinus exit block; pause equal to two previous cardiac cycles; overall heart rate, 70.

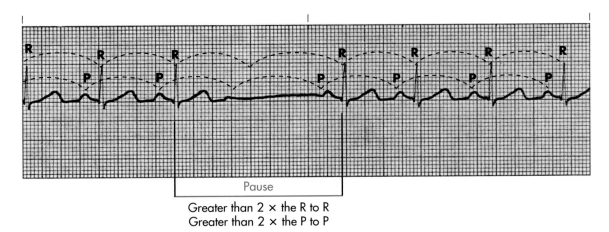

FIG. 3-9 Sinus arrest. Pause will be more than two times the previous cardiac cycle of the underlying rhythm; overall heart rate, 70.

As with any rhythm, **patient assessment** is essential to determine the patient's tolerance of the dysrhythmia. Treatment should be started if the patient is medically unstable (i.e., if the patient has any combination of the following signs and symptoms: pale, sweaty skin; weakness; sudden change in blood pressure; chest pain, or any other symptoms of poor cardiac output).

NOTE: *Sick sinus syndrome (SSS)* has been used in the past to describe a sinus rhythm with a pause. However, sick sinus syndrome is currently used to refer to any dysrhythmia caused by a disruption in the electrical conduction pathway of the atria.

ATRIAL DYSRHYTHMIAS

When the SA node fails to generate an electrical impulse, any other pacemaker site within the atria is capable of initiating the impulse. Cardiac rhythms originating from atrial sites are *atrial dysrhythmias*.

In atrial dysrhythmias, the electrical impulse travels through the atria to the AV node, continues through the bundle of His and bundle branches to the Purkinje's fibers, and ends in the ventricular muscle. Although the depolarization of the atria will vary, depending on the atrial dysrhythmia, the ventricles usually depolarize in a normal manner.

Most atrial dysrhythmias are usually not *lethal* (death producing). However, as with any rhythm, **patient assessment** is essential to determine the patient's tolerance of the dysrhythmia.

PREMATURE ATRIAL CONTRACTION

A *premature atrial contraction (PAC)* is an individual complex that occurs earlier than the next expected complex of the underlying rhythm. It originates from any atrial site outside the SA node (Fig. 3-10). PACs usually occur in an underlying sinus rhythm, which may be regular except for the PAC.

NOTE: Although the term **contraction** is used with a PAC, remember this complex represents electrical activity of cardiac muscle and may **not** reflect an actual contraction.

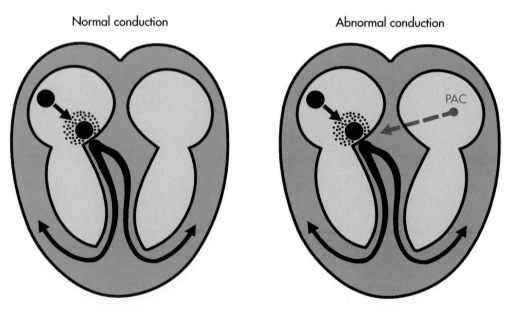

Normal conduction

Abnormal conduction

FIG. 3-10 *Left heart* shows normal electrical conduction pathway. *Right heart* shows conduction pathway of a premature atrial contraction (PAC).

A PAC usually has the same characteristics as other atrial complexes. However, the P wave may appear different in size or shape than the P waves of the underlying rhythm, or it may be hidden in the T wave of the preceding complex.

The PAC is followed by a pause before the underlying rhythm returns. Two different types of pauses follow a premature complex: noncompensatory or compensatory. To determine the type of pause on the rhythm strip, measure the R to R intervals before and after the PAC in the following manner:

1. *Noncompensatory pause:* Measure from the R wave of the complex before the PAC to the R wave of the complex after the PAC. This measurement will be **less** than two times the R to R interval of the underlying rhythm. A noncompensatory pause could indicate the development of increased irritability in the SA node, causing it to generate an impulse sooner than expected in response to the premature beat. This increase in irritability could lead to sinus tachycardia. (This type of pause may also be called an *incomplete compensatory pause.*)

2. *Compensatory pause:* Measure from the R wave of the complex before the PAC to the R wave of the complex after the PAC. This measurement will **equal** two times the R to R interval of the underlying rhythm. In a compensatory pause, the SA node does not respond to the premature beat. Therefore there is no change in the rate or regularity of the underlying rhythm. (This type of pause may also be called a *complete compensatory pause.*)

A PAC is usually followed by a noncompensatory pause.

The underlying rhythm **must** also be identified when interpreting rhythm strips containing a PAC. Although a premature atrial contraction may occur in any rhythm, it is easier to identify in a sinus rhythm or any rhythm with a bradycardia rate (Fig. 3-11, *A* and *B*). When determining the rate of a rhythm containing a PAC, the R wave of the PAC is included in the total count of R waves.

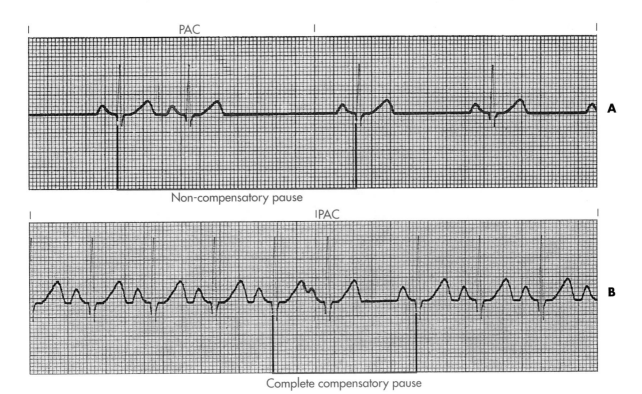

FIG. 3-11 A, Premature atrial contraction (PAC) with a noncompensatory pause in a sinus bradycardic rhythm; heart rate, 40. **B,** PAC with a complete compensatory pause in a sinus rhythm; heart rate, 80 to 90.

A PAC represents increased irritability of the atria. Increased irritability indicates that the cardiac cells are able to respond to even a mild electrical stimulus and may depolarize in an unpredictable rate or manner. PACs may be caused by pain, fever, fear, anxiety, sudden excitement, exercise, or the effects of drugs such as digitalis, atropine, nicotine, caffeine, and amphetamines.

A PAC by itself is not a serious dysrhythmia. However, PACs are frequently monitored, since they may lead to a more serious dysrhythmia, such as paroxysmal atrial tachycardia.

Although a PAC is **not** a true atrial dysrhythmia but an individual complex, it is included in this chapter because it originates from the atria.

PAROXYSMAL ATRIAL TACHYCARDIA/ PAROXYSMAL SUPRAVENTRICULAR TACHYCARDIA

Paroxysmal atrial tachycardia (PAT) is the sudden onset of a tachycardia with a rate greater than 150 electrical impulses per minute. The most recent term for this dysrhythmia is *paroxysmal supraventricular tachycardia (PSVT)*. PAT/PSVT frequently is triggered by a PAC.

Because PAT/PSVT is usually initiated by an irritable site in the atria, a P wave occurs before every QRS complex (Fig. 3-12). However, because of the rapid rate of PAT/PSVT, the P wave may be hidden in the T wave of the preceding complex. If P waves are seen, the PR intervals range from 0.12 to 0.20 second and the QRS complexes are usually less than 0.12 second.

The rhythm is regular because the P to P intervals and R to R intervals are regular and equal in length. The rate may vary from 151 to 250, or more, electrical impulses per minute. Because the rate is so rapid, the ventricles do not have time to fill completely before each contraction, causing a decrease in cardiac output.

Because most of the blood flow through the coronary arteries occurs between heartbeats, the rapid heart rate of a PAT/PSVT may also decrease the amount of oxygenated blood circulated to the heart muscle (myocardium).

The patient may complain of symptoms such as weakness, dizziness, palpitations, or a feeling that the heart is doing "flip-flops." PAT/PSVT may stop as suddenly as it starts, or it may require medical treatment if the patient becomes medically unstable.

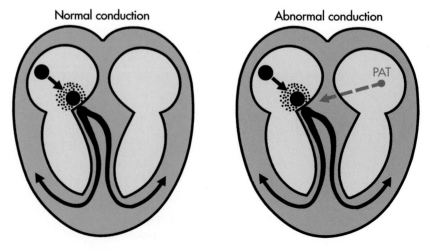

FIG. 3-12 *Left heart* shows normal electrical conduction pathway. *Right heart* shows conduction pathway of paroxysmal atrial tachycardia/paroxysmal supraventricular tachycardia.

A paroxysmal atrial tachycardia is not a lethal dysrhythmia but should be monitored closely, since this rapid rate cannot be tolerated for long periods of time.

To interpret a PAT/PSVT, the **beginning** of the PAT/PSVT **must** be seen, and the underlying rhythm that precedes the PAT must be identified (Fig. 3-13). If the onset of the PAT/PSVT is not seen, the dysrhythmia is called *supraventricular tachycardia,* providing it fits the other characteristics of PAT/PSVT.

A PAT/PSVT may be caused by stimulants such as caffeine, nicotine, or amphetamines.

SUPRAVENTRICULAR TACHYCARDIA

Supraventricular tachycardia (SVT) is the term used when a dysrhythmia fits all the characteristics of a PAT/PSVT, but the beginning of the dysrhythmia is not seen. SVT is a general term that refers to **any** dysrhythmia that cannot be identified by other means, originates from an irritable site **above the bundle of His,** and has a rate **greater** than 150 (Fig. 3-14).

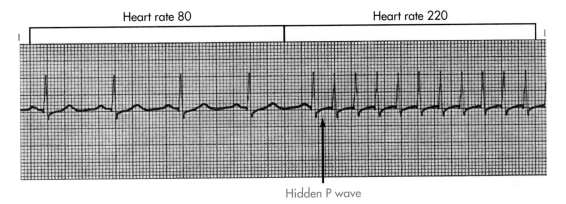

FIG. 3-13 Normal sinus rhythm (NSR) progressing to paroxysmal atrial tachycardia/paroxysmal supraventricular tachycardia; NSR: heart rate, 80; PAT/PSVT: heart rate, 220.

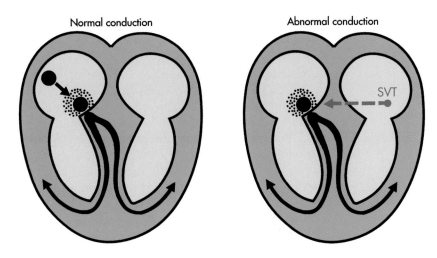

FIG. 3-14 *Left heart* shows normal electrical conduction pathway. *Right heart* shows conduction pathway of supraventricular tachycardia (SVT).

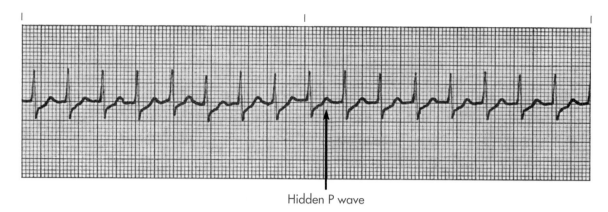

Hidden P wave

FIG. 3-15 Supraventricular tachycardia (SVT): P waves hidden in preceding T waves; onset not seen; heart rate, 160.

A P wave usually occurs before every QRS complex. However, the P wave may be hidden in the T wave of the preceding complex because of the rapid rate of the SVT. If P waves are seen, the PR intervals usually range from 0.12 to 0.20 second, and the QRS complexes usually measure less than 0.12 second. Any P waves that can be seen usually look alike, and the QRS complexes are usually the same size and shape. The P to P intervals and R to R intervals are regular and equal in length, and the rhythm is regular (Fig. 3-15).

The rate of the SVT varies from 151 to 250, or more, electrical impulses per minute. A rhythm resembling SVT but with a heart rate less than 151 is called *sinus tachycardia.*

SVT usually is triggered by an irritable site within the atria. This irritability can be caused by stimulants such as caffeine, nicotine, or amphetamines.

SVT is treated if the patient becomes medically unstable. This dysrhythmia is usually not lethal, but the patient should be assessed frequently because the rapid rate cannot be tolerated for long periods of time.

ATRIAL FLUTTER

Atrial flutter occurs when a single irritable site in the atria initiates many electrical impulses at a rapid rate (Fig. 3-16). The electrical impulses are conducted throughout the atria so rapidly that normal P waves are not produced. Instead of P waves, *flutter waves* (F waves) are formed.

Flutter waves have a typical "saw-toothed" or jagged appearance on the rhythm strip. They may not all look exactly the same, since some F waves may be buried in the QRS complex, ST segment, or T wave.

The negative (downward) stroke of the F wave represents atrial depolarization conducted through an abnormal electrical pathway. The positive (upward) stroke of the F wave indicates atrial repolarization.

During atrial flutter, the atria depolarize more rapidly than normal, but the AV node delays some of the electrical impulses, allowing the ventricles to depolarize at a normal rate. Therefore every atrial impulse cannot be conducted to the ventricles, and a QRS complex is not present for every F wave.

The ventricles usually depolarize and repolarize at regular intervals, allowing them to respond to the atrial impulse at a regular rate, which may result in a regular ventricular rhythm.

The QRS complexes typically measure less than 0.12 second and usually occur at regular intervals. The ventricular rate, as measured by the number of QRS com-

Normal conduction   Abnormal conduction

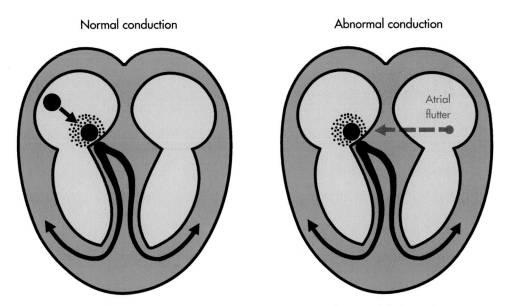

FIG. 3-16 *Left heart* shows normal electrical conduction pathway. *Right heart* shows conduction pathway of atrial flutter.

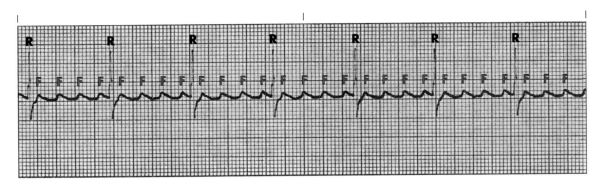

FIG. 3-17 Atrial flutter: atrial heart rate, 280; ventricular heart rate, 70.

plexes, is usually 60 to 100 electrical impulses per minute. However, the atrial rate (F waves) usually ranges from 250 to 350 impulses per minute (Fig. 3-17).

When an atrial flutter has a ventricular rate of less than 60 impulses per minute, it is called *atrial flutter with a slow ventricular response*. When the ventricular rate is 100 to 150 impulses per minute, it is called *atrial flutter with a rapid ventricular response*.

Because the ratio of flutter waves to each QRS complex further describes the dysrhythmia, it is important to determine the number of flutter waves for every QRS complex (Fig. 3-18).

Example: Two F waves with one QRS complex = 2:1 block (ratio)
Three F waves with one QRS complex = 3:1 block (ratio)
Four F waves with one QRS complex = 4:1 block (ratio)
Five F waves with one QRS complex = 5:1 block (ratio)

If the number of flutter waves is the same before every QRS complex, the R to R intervals are equal throughout, and the rhythm is regular. When the number of

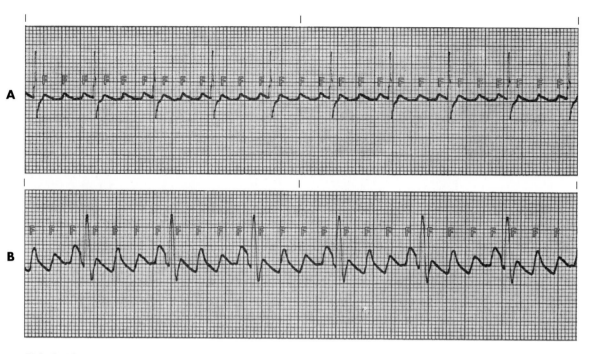

FIG. 3-18 Atrial flutter. **A,** Atrial flutter with a ventricular heart rate of 100, 3:1 block; atrial heart rate of 270, if counting F waves (or 300 if calculated by 3 × 100). **B,** Atrial flutter with a ventricular heart rate of 60, 4:1 block; Atrial heart rate of 260, if counting F waves (or 240 if calculated by 4 × 60).

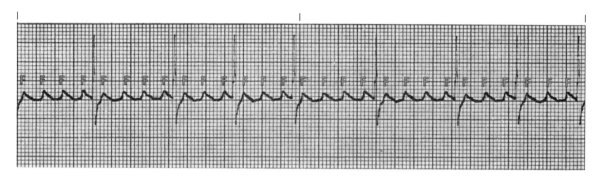

FIG. 3-19 Atrial flutter with variable block; atrial heart rate, 280; ventricular heart rate, 80.

F waves before each QRS complex varies, the R to R interval is irregular, and the rhythm is called *atrial flutter with a variable ventricular response* (Fig. 3-19).

It is not always necessary to determine the actual atrial rate in atrial flutter. However, when an atrial rate does need to be calculated, there are two common methods that can be used:

1. Count the number of F waves in a 6-second strip and multiply that number by 10.
2. Multiply the number of F waves in the ratio by the ventricular heart rate, for example:
   a. In a 3:1 block, with a ventricular rate of 100, use the following shortcut:
      3 F waves (3:1 block) × 100 (ventricular heart rate) = 300 F waves or an atrial heart rate of 300
   b. In a 4:1 block, with a ventricular rate of 60:
      4 F waves (4:1 block) × 60 (ventricular heart rate) = 240 F waves or an atrial heart rate of 240

Normal conduction   Abnormal conduction

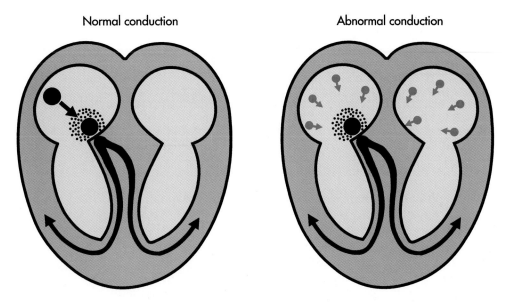

FIG. 3-20 *Left heart* shows normal electrical conduction pathway. *Right heart* shows conduction pathway of atrial fibrillation.

The second method of calculating atrial heart rate in atrial flutter can be used **only** if the ratio does not vary.

Atrial flutter may be caused by heart disease, myocardial infarction, or drug toxicity. This dysrhythmia is usually not lethal. However, it is frequently treated because it indicates increased irritability within the atria. This increased irritability may cause the dysrhythmia to progress to a more serious dysrhythmia.

The patient's symptoms vary depending on the cause of the atrial flutter, the ventricular response, and the patient's tolerance of the dysrhythmia.

ATRIAL FIBRILLATION

In *atrial fibrillation* (A Fib), an increased irritability of all the cardiac cells in the atria exists. Because of this increased atrial irritability, many sites within the atria attempt to initiate electrical impulses at the same time (Fig. 3-20).

Because so many electrical impulses are initiated, most of the impulses are not conducted; therefore the atria is not completely depolarized with each impulse. The atria do not contract forcefully; only a quivering movement *(fibrillatory waves)* occurs. These fibrillatory waves (fib waves) appear on the rhythm strip or monitor screen as a wavy baseline between each QRS complex. No true P waves or PR intervals exist.

At irregular intervals, one electrical impulse **is** conducted through the AV junction and ventricles, resulting in ventricular depolarization and a QRS complex. QRS complexes usually remain within the normal range of less than 0.12 second, and the R to R intervals are irregular throughout the rhythm strip. Frequently, one of the first clues that a dysrhythmia might be atrial fibrillation is seeing R to R intervals that are irregularly irregular (with no pattern to the irregularity).

The atrial heart rate is usually 350 to 500, or more, electrical impulses per minute. However, the AV node delays some of these electrical impulses, allowing the ventricular heart rate to usually remain within the normal limits of 60 to 100 impulses per minute. This dysrhythmia is known as *controlled atrial fibrillation* (Fig. 3-21).

Atrial fibrillation with a ventricular rate of less than 60 impulses per minute is called *atrial fibrillation with a slow ventricular response.* When this dysrhythmia has a

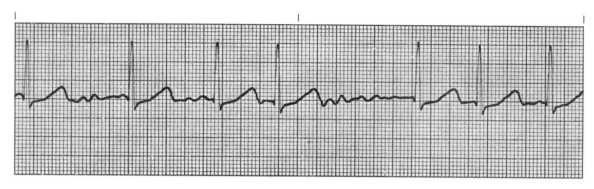

FIG. 3-21 Controlled atrial fibrillation; atrial heart rate, 350 to 500; ventricular heart rate, 70.

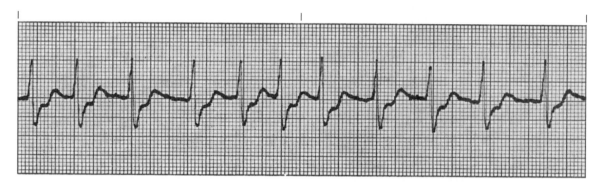

FIG. 3-22 Atrial fibrillation with a rapid ventricular response: no distinguishable P waves; atrial heart rate, 350 to 500; ventricular heart rate, 110.

ventricular rate of 101 to 150 impulses per minute, it is called *atrial fibrillation with rapid ventricular response* (Fig. 3-22). Atrial fibrillation with a ventricular rate greater than 150 impulses per minute is called *uncontrolled atrial fibrillation.*

Atrial fibrillation is not usually considered lethal and may be normal in elderly patients. However, a new occurrence of atrial fibrillation is frequently treated because it indicates an increased irritability within the atria and may progress to a more serious dysrhythmia.

Treatment depends on the patient's tolerance of the dysrhythmia and the patient's symptoms. For example, a patient with atrial fibrillation and a ventricular response of 50 impulses per minute, with stable vital signs, may not require treatment. However, a patient with atrial fibrillation with a ventricular response of 50, who is medically unstable, requires treatment immediately.

Signs and symptoms of a patient who is medically unstable include any combination of the following:

- Pale, cool, clammy skin
- Nausea and vomiting (N/V)
- Dizziness, weakness, faintness
- Shortness of breath (SOB)
- Sudden change in blood pressure
- Dyspnea (shortness of breath)
- Severe chest pain

- Confusion or disorientation
- Cyanosis (bluish gray color to skin)
- Decreased urinary output
- Unresponsiveness

Atrial fibrillation may be caused by severe heart disease or myocardial infarction. It may also occur with excessive use of alcohol or caffeine.

1. Atrial fibrillation and atrial flutter may occasionally be combined in the same dysrhythmia on a rhythm strip. It is then called *atrial fib/flutter.*
2. Atrial fibrillation is usually not a lethal dysrhythmia. However, it **must not** be confused with *ventricular fibrillation,* which **is** a lethal dysrhythmia (see Chapter 6).

WOLFF-PARKINSON-WHITE SYNDROME

Wolff-Parkinson-White (WPW) syndrome is a dysrhythmia that occurs when an electrical impulse follows an additional or abnormal electrical conduction pathway, called the *bundle of Kent* (Kent bundle). Although the normal conduction pathway is working, the impulse from the different pathway, known as an "accessory pathway," also reaches the ventricles after bypassing the AV node. Electrical impulses can travel through the accessory pathway (bundle of Kent) in any one of the following ways:

1. Downward from the atria to the ventricles (antegrade)
2. Upward from the ventricles to the atria (retrograde)
3. Both downward and upward, in a continuous cycle (Fig. 3-23)

Wolff-Parkinson-White (WPW) syndrome is seen on the rhythm strip or monitor screen with the following characteristics:

1. PR interval shorter than 0.12 second if a P wave is present
2. Usually a widened QRS complex, greater than 0.12 second
3. Delta wave

The PR interval is shorter than normal because the electrical impulse does not travel through the AV node, but goes directly from the atria to the ventricles.

The QRS is usually widened if the electrical impulse travels in a retrograde manner, or in a continuous cycle. The QRS complex is usually within the normal limits of 0.04 to 0.12 second when the electrical impulse travels from the atria to the ventricles. The R wave of the QRS complex usually is "slurred," or curved, at the beginning of the R wave.

The *delta wave* is an extra "bump" seen in the slurred section of the QRS complex. The delta wave is formed by depolarization of the ventricles through the accessory pathway, before the normally conducted electrical impulse can reach the ventricles.

The P to P intervals and R to R intervals of WPW syndrome vary, depending on the underlying rhythm.

The rate of WPW syndrome may also vary, depending on the underlying rhythm. However, because the ventricles are receiving impulses from both the normal and accessory pathways, the ventricles usually depolarize quickly, causing tachycardia (Fig. 3-24).

This is usually not a dangerous dysrhythmia, and WPW syndrome is often undiagnosed in many patients until it is found on a routine electrocardiogram (ECG). However, it can become lethal if the ventricular rate increases to 200 to 300 beats

Normal conduction

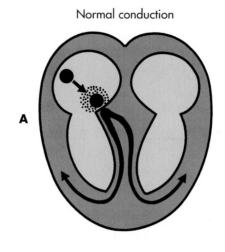

Abnormal conduction

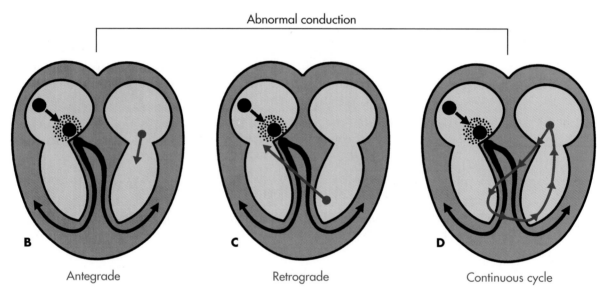

| Antegrade | Retrograde | Continuous cycle |

FIG. 3-23 Wolff-Parkinson-White (WPW) syndrome. **A,** Normal conduction pathway. **B,** Antegrade conduction pathway. **C,** Retrograde conduction pathway. **D,** Continuous cycle pathway. These show only three of many possible abnormal conduction pathways in WPW syndrome.

per minute or greater. WPW syndrome is associated with supraventricular tachycardia and atrial flutter, as well as atrial fibrillation, with uncontrolled ventricular response. It can sometimes mimic *ventricular tachycardia* (see Chapter 6), if the QRS complex is wide and the rate is rapid.

The patient may have no symptoms or may complain of palpitations; racing heart; dizziness, weakness, or faintness; SOB; and/or chest pain.

NOTE: One of the concerns with Wolff-Parkinson-White syndrome, atrial flutter, and especially atrial fibrillation is that clots may form in the atria because the rapid rate may not allow the atria to empty completely. This could lead to stroke, pulmonary emboli, and/or MI.

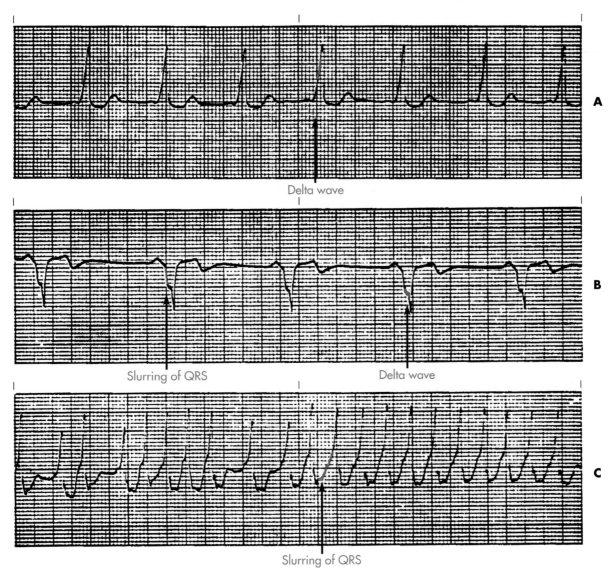

FIG. 3-24 Wolff-Parkinson-White (WPW) syndrome. **A,** Sinus rhythm with WPW syndrome showing delta waves; heart rate, 70. **B,** Sinus bradycardia with WPW syndrome showing slurring of QRS and delta waves; heart rate, 50. **C,** Uncontrolled atrial fibrillation with WPW syndrome mimicking ventricular tachycardia and showing slurring of QRS; atrial heart rate 350 to 500; ventricular heart rate, 210.

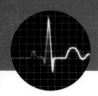

REVIEW QUESTIONS

TRUE   FALSE   1. The SA node normally generates 60 to 100 electrical impulses per minute.

TRUE   FALSE   2. Sinus bradycardia may become dangerous if the heart rate decreases significantly or the patient becomes medically unstable.

TRUE   FALSE   3. The complex that ends a sinus arrest can only be initiated from the SA node.

TRUE   FALSE   4. A PAC is an atrial complex that occurs later than the next expected complex of the underlying rhythm.

TRUE   FALSE   5. In a sinus arrhythmia, the heart rate increases with inspirations and decreases with expirations.

6. The number of electrical impulses in sinus tachycardia is between _____ and _____ per minute.

7. In atrial fibrillation, the QRS complexes usually measure less than _____ second.

8. Sinus exit block occurs when the SA node fails to initiate an electrical impulse for a length of time equal to _____ previous cardiac cycles.

9. If the onset of PAT is not seen, the dysrhythmia is called:
   a. sinus tachycardia
   b. supraventricular tachycardia
   c. premature atrial tachycardia
   d. atrial tachycardia

10. SVT is a dysrhythmia that originates from an irritable site located:
   a. above the bundle of His
   b. within the ventricles
   c. within the bundle branches
   d. below the bundle of His

11. Wolff-Parkinson-White syndrome can be identified by a shortened PR interval and the presence of a(n):
   a. alpha wave
   b. P wave
   c. delta wave
   d. beta wave

12. Atrial flutter has:
   a. P waves
   b. Q waves
   c. F waves
   d. T waves

13. Atrial fibrillation has fib waves that are:
   a. distinct and regular
   b. notched and regular
   c. wavy and irregular
   d. absent

14. Define "variable ventricular response" in atrial flutter:

   _____

   _____

   _____

15. Trace the path of an electrical impulse from the SA node to the ventricular muscle:

_____

_____

_____

16. Describe the components and intervals of a complex in normal sinus rhythm, including measurements as seen on a rhythm strip:

_____

_____

_____

_____

_____

17. What are the heart rates usually found in:
    a. sinus bradycardia? _____
    b. SVT? _____
    c. sinus arrhythmia? _____

18. What is the atrial heart rate in:
    a. atrial flutter? _____
    b. atrial fibrillation? _____

19. What is the difference between the pause of a sinus exit block and a sinus arrest, including the length of the pause?

_____

_____

_____

_____

_____

RHYTHM STRIP REVIEW

1. MEASURE: PR interval _____ Rhythm _____
             QRS complex _____ Heart rate _____
   INTERPRETATION: _____

2. MEASURE: PR interval _____ Rhythm _____
             QRS complex _____ Heart rate _____
   INTERPRETATION: _____

3. MEASURE: PR interval _____ Rhythm _____
             QRS complex _____ Heart rate _____
   INTERPRETATION: _____

4. MEASURE: PR interval _____ Rhythm _____
             QRS complex _____ Heart rate _____
   INTERPRETATION: _____

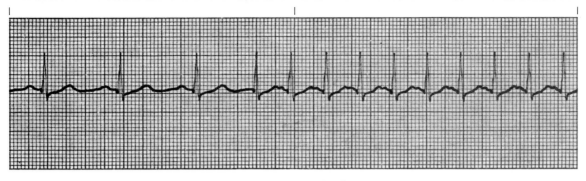

5. MEASURE: PR interval _____ Rhythm _____
                  QRS complex _____ Heart rate _____
INTERPRETATION: _____

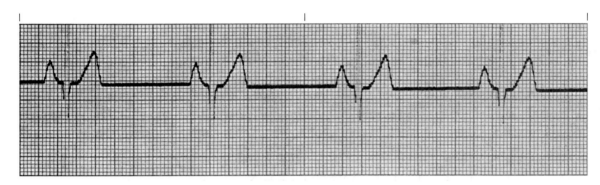

6. MEASURE: PR interval _____ Rhythm _____
                  QRS complex _____ Heart rate _____
INTERPRETATION: _____

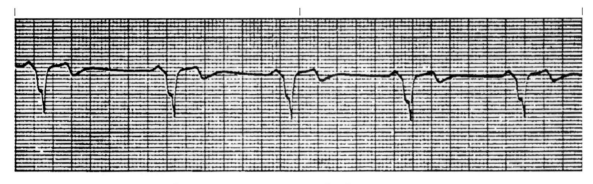

7. MEASURE: PR interval _____ Rhythm _____
                  QRS complex _____ Heart rate _____
INTERPRETATION: _____

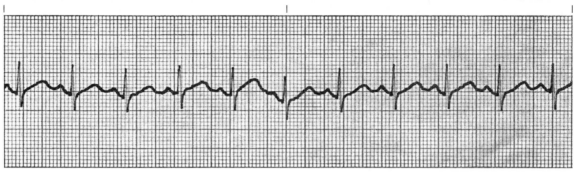

8. MEASURE: PR interval _____ Rhythm _____
   QRS complex _____ Heart rate _____
   INTERPRETATION: _____

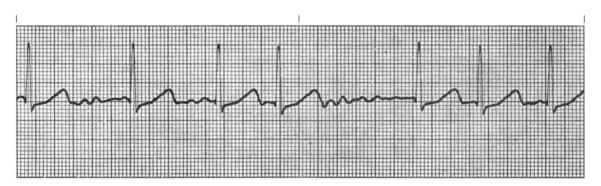

9. MEASURE: PR interval _____ Rhythm _____
   QRS complex _____ Heart rate _____
   INTERPRETATION: _____

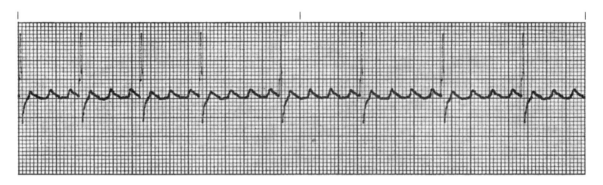

10. MEASURE: PR interval _____ Rhythm _____
    QRS complex _____ Heart rate _____
    INTERPRETATION: _____

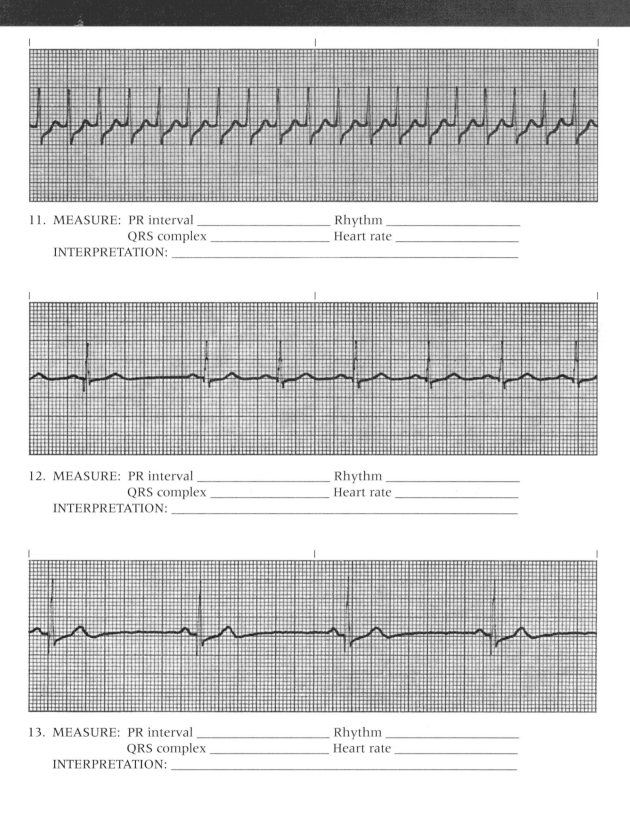

11. MEASURE: PR interval _____ Rhythm _____
    QRS complex _____ Heart rate _____
    INTERPRETATION: _____

12. MEASURE: PR interval _____ Rhythm _____
    QRS complex _____ Heart rate _____
    INTERPRETATION: _____

13. MEASURE: PR interval _____ Rhythm _____
    QRS complex _____ Heart rate _____
    INTERPRETATION: _____

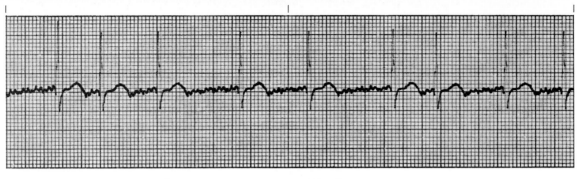

14. MEASURE: PR interval _____ Rhythm _____

   QRS complex _____ Heart rate _____

   INTERPRETATION: _____

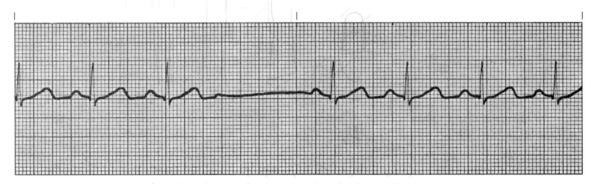

15. MEASURE: PR interval _____ Rhythm _____

   QRS complex _____ Heart rate _____

   INTERPRETATION: _____

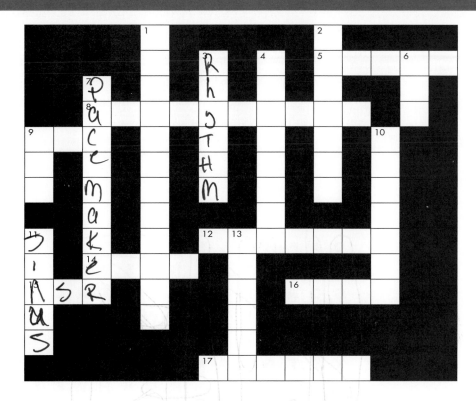

CROSSWORD PUZZLE CLUES

Across

5. Both sinus arrest and sinus exit block are followed by a _____ on the rhythm strip.

8. Sinus _____ changes rate with respirations.

9. A _____ complex occurs earlier than expected.

12. Assessment of the _____ is always important.

14. Sinus _____ block looks like sinus arrest.

15. Only "normal" rhythm.

16. Unstable symptoms indicate _____ cardiac output.

17. _____ dysrhythmias originate outside the SA node above the AV junction.

Down

1. Causes quivering atrium.

2. Sinus rhythms have _____ P waves.

3. NRS has a regular rate and _____.

4. The _____ rate of the atrium is 60 to 100 electrical impulses per minute.

6. Heart rate greater than 150; onset not seen.

7. SA node is normally the _____ of the heart.

9. Sudden onset; heart rate greater than 150.

10. Atrial _____ contains F waves instead of P waves.

11. _____ bradycardia has a heart rate of less than 60 impulses per minute.

13. Sinus _____ forms a pause on the monitor and rhythm strip.

The solution to this crossword puzzle is in the answer section.

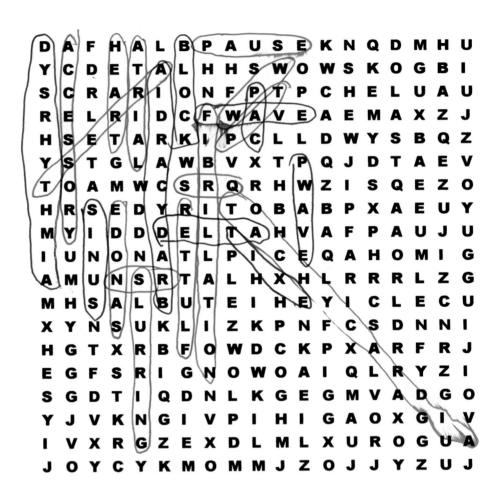

WORD PUZZLE

This word puzzle is designed to help familiarize you with some of the new terminology found in this chapter. Have fun finding all the words on this list. The words will always be in upper case and found in a straight line. The words may be spelled forward (normal), backward, up, down, or diagonally in any direction. Some phrases will not have any spaces between the words; for example, SA node will appear as SANODE. Good luck and enjoy.

ACCESSORY
ARREST
ATRIAL
BLOCK
BRADYCARDIA
DELTA
DYSRHYTHMIA
EXIT
FIBRILLATION
FLUTTER
FWAVE
HEART

NSR
PAC
PAT
PAUSE
PWAVE
QRS
SANODE
SINUS
SLURRING
TACHYCARDIA
WPW

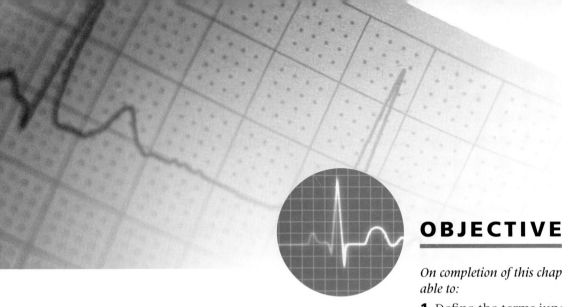

OBJECTIVES

JUNCTIONAL DYSRHYTHMIAS

OUTLINE

DEFINITIONS

AV Node Atrioventricular node; part of the normal electrical conduction pathway of the heart; may function as a secondary pacemaker of the heart

Buried P Wave The P wave is hidden, or buried, within the QRS complex and therefore not seen

Inherent Heart Rate Normal rate at which electrical impulses are generated; the inherent heart rate for the AV junction is 40 to 60 impulses per minute

Inverted P Wave An inverted, or upside-down, P wave before the QRS complex

Junctional Dysrhythmia A cardiac dysrhythmia that is initiated in the AV node (AV junctional area), when the SA node and atrial sites fail to initiate an electrical impulse

Retrograde P Wave A P wave that is seen after the QRS complex; it is also inverted

JUNCTIONAL DYSRHYTHMIAS

As discussed in Chapter 3, the sinoatrial (SA) node and the atria may fail to generate the electrical impulses needed to begin depolarization for many reasons, such as drug toxicity, myocardial infarction, or heart disease. When this failure occurs, the atrioventricular (AV) node may assume its role of the secondary cardiac pacemaker of the heart (see Chapter 1).

The AV node is located in the general area of the lower right atrium, near the septum. It is an indistinct area and difficult to pinpoint exactly. The cardiac tissue immediately surrounding the AV node is usually called the *AV junction* and is also capable of initiating electrical impulses (Fig. 4-1).

Rhythms that start in either the AV node or the AV junctional area are called *junctional dysrhythmias,* or nodal dysrhythmias. The term *nodal* is rarely used today, since junctional is more accurate.

Because the AV junction is not the primary pacemaker of the heart, it is not as efficient as the SA node and has a slower rate. The AV junctional rate is 40 to 60 electrical impulses per minute. This rate is also known as *the inherent heart rate* of the AV junctional area.

A junctional dysrhythmia is not usually lethal. However, as with any rhythm, **patient assessment** is essential to determine the patient's tolerance of the dysrhythmia.

In a junctional dysrhythmia, the electrical impulse travels through the normal conduction pathway from the AV junction, through the bundle of His and bundle branches, to the Purkinje's fibers, ending in the ventricular muscle.

Because the electrical impulse follows the normal conduction pathway through the ventricles, the QRS complex usually measures less than 0.12 second (Fig. 4-2).

However, the electrical impulse that depolarizes the atria must travel in a backward, or *retrograde,* motion from the AV junction up through the atria (Fig. 4-3). This retrograde motion accounts for all three characteristic changes in the P wave, which identify an AV junctional dysrhythmia: *inverted, buried (hidden),* or *retrograde* (Fig. 4-4).

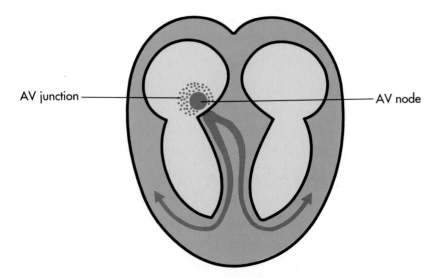

FIG. 4-1 Atrioventricular (AV) node and AV junctional area.

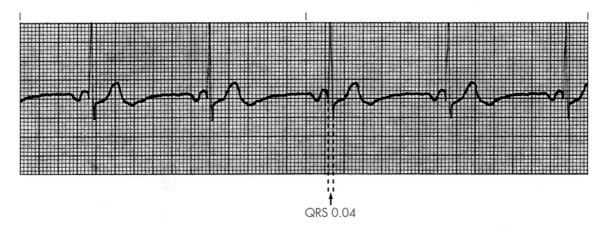

FIG. 4-2 Junctional dysrhythmia showing normal ventricular depolarization.

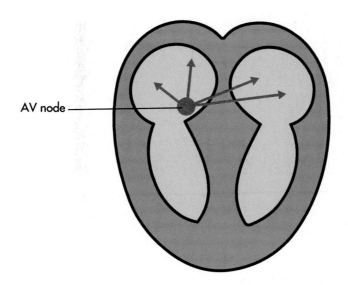

FIG. 4-3 Retrograde electrical conduction pathway from AV node to atria.

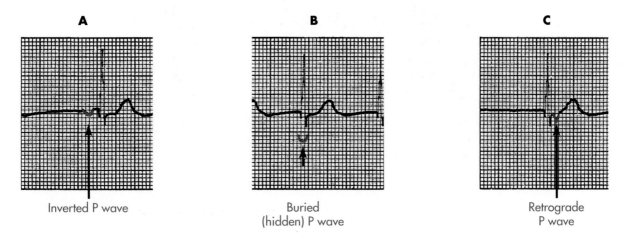

FIG. 4-4 P waves. **A,** Inverted. **B,** Buried. **C,** Retrograde.

INVERTED P WAVE

If the electrical impulse originates high in the AV junctional area, the atria are depolarized quickly, although in a retrograde manner (Fig. 4-5). This retrograde depolarization causes the P wave to be inverted, or upside down (Fig. 4-6). It will be seen on the monitor or rhythm strip as an inverted P wave before the QRS complex.

Because the electrical impulse originates in the AV junction, the distance the impulse must travel to depolarize the ventricles is shorter than normal. The depolarization of the ventricles, reflected by the QRS complex, occurs quickly and may cause a shortened PR interval of less than 0.12 second.

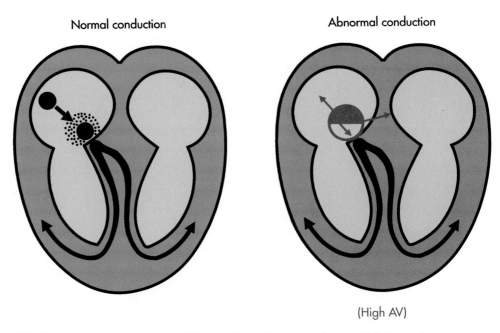

Normal conduction

Abnormal conduction

(High AV)

FIG. 4-5 *Left heart* shows normal electrical conduction pathway. *Right heart* shows conduction pathway of high AV junctional area.

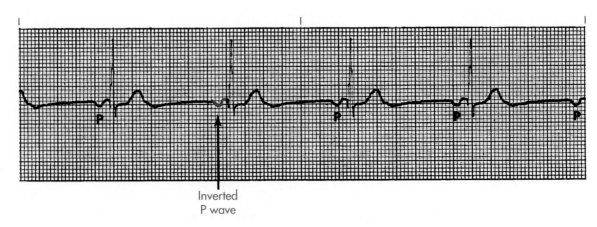

Inverted
P wave

FIG. 4-6 Junctional dysrhythmia with inverted P waves.

BURIED P WAVE

When the electrical impulse originates in the mid-AV junctional area, the distance the impulse must travel up through the atria (retrograde) and down through the ventricles is almost the same. This similar distance causes the atria and the ventricles to depolarize at almost the same time (Fig. 4-7).

Because the force of the atrial depolarization is less than the force of the ventricular depolarization, the P wave is hidden by the QRS complex. This P wave is described as buried, or hidden, and consequently a P wave and a PR interval are not seen (Fig. 4-8).

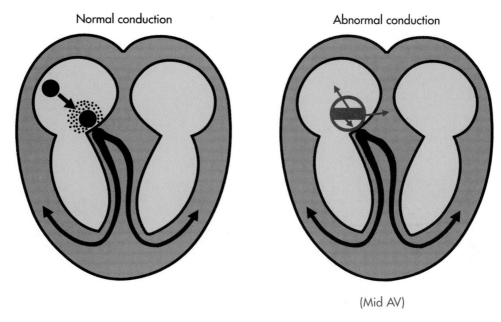

Normal conduction   Abnormal conduction

(Mid AV)

FIG. 4-7 *Left heart* shows normal electrical conduction pathway. *Right heart* shows conduction pathway of mid-AV junctional area.

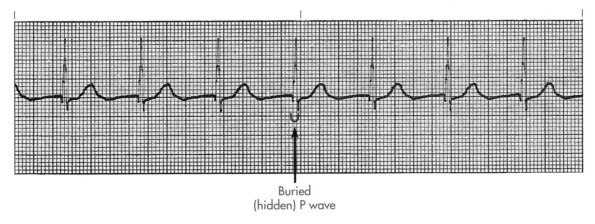

Buried
(hidden) P wave

FIG. 4-8 Junctional dysrhythmia with buried (hidden) P waves.

RETROGRADE P WAVE

When the electrical impulse originates in the lower part of the AV junctional area, the distance the impulse must travel to the atria is greater than the distance to the ventricles (Fig. 4-9). Therefore the atria depolarize slightly later than the ventricles, producing a retrograde P wave after the QRS complex.

The P wave is said to be retrograde because it appears after the QRS complex; no measurable PR interval is present. The P wave is inverted because the atria are depolarized in a retrograde manner (Fig. 4-10).

> NOTE: The term *retrograde* is used in two different ways:
> 1. To appear behind or after
> 2. To occur in a backward or reverse motion

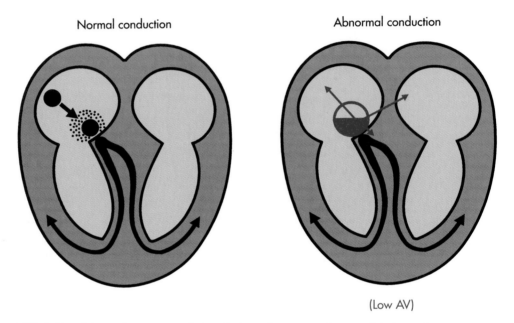

Normal conduction   Abnormal conduction

(Low AV)

FIG. 4-9 *Left heart* shows normal electrical conduction pathway. *Right heart* shows conduction pathway of lower AV junctional area.

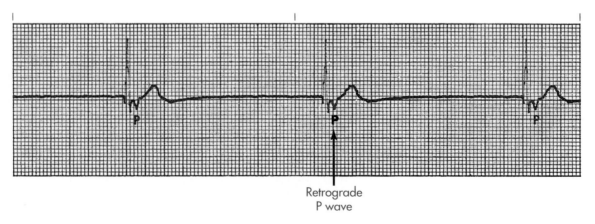

Retrograde
P wave

FIG. 4-10 Junctional dysrhythmia with retrograde P waves.

JUNCTIONAL BRADYCARDIA

Junctional bradycardia occurs when all the electrical impulses originate from a single site within the AV junctional area, at a rate less than 40 impulses per minute.

The P wave is either inverted, buried, or retrograde. The PR interval, if present, is usually less than 0.12 second. However, the QRS complex usually remains less than 0.12 second. Because the P to P intervals, if seen, and the R to R intervals are regular and equal in length, the rhythm is regular. The rate can vary, but it must be less than 40 electrical impulses per minute (Fig. 4-11).

Junctional bradycardia may be caused by heart disease or drugs such as digitalis, quinidine, or sedatives.

A junctional bradycardia may become a serious dysrhythmia if the rate falls significantly or the patient becomes medically unstable.

Remember: any patient with a heart rate of less than 60 electrical impulses per minute has a bradycardic rate. This is known as an *absolute bradycardia*. However, because the inherent rate of the AV junction is 40 to 60 electrical impulses per minute, only a junctional rhythm with a rate below 40 impulses per minute can be called a junctional bradycardia.

ACCELERATED JUNCTIONAL DYSRHYTHMIA/ JUNCTIONAL TACHYCARDIA

Accelerated junctional dysrhythmia occurs when all the electrical impulses originate from a single site within the AV junctional area, at a rate between 61 and 100 impulses per minute.

The P wave is either inverted, buried, or retrograde. The PR interval, if present, is usually less than 0.12 second. Because the electrical impulse follows the normal conduction pathway through the ventricles, the QRS complex usually remains normal, measuring less than 0.12 second.

Because the P to P intervals, if seen, and the R to R intervals are regular and equal in length, the rhythm is regular. The rate can vary, but it must be between 61 and 100 electrical impulses per minute (Fig. 4-12).

Any patient with a heart rate greater than 100 electrical impulses per minute has a tachycardic rate. However, only those rhythms that are junctional and have a rate between 61 and 100 impulses per minute can be called accelerated junctional dysrhythmias. A junctional dysrhythmia with a rate between 101 and 150 impulses per minute is called *junctional tachycardia.*

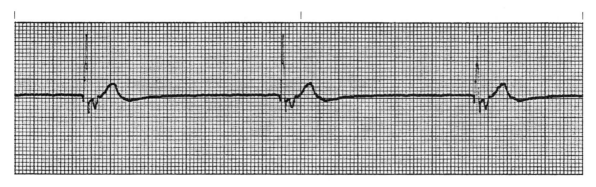

FIG. 4-11 Junctional bradycardia with retrograde P waves; heart rate, 30.

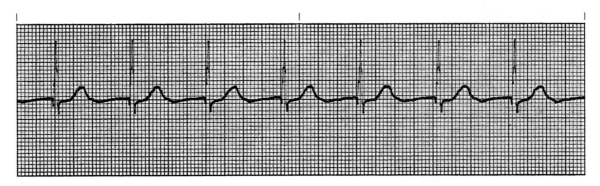

FIG. 4-12 Accelerated junctional dysrhythmia with hidden P waves; heart rate, 70.

Both accelerated junctional dysrhythmia and junctional tachycardia may be caused by heart disease or drugs such as atropine, caffeine, or amphetamines. They also may result from pain, fever, or acute anemia. Exercise or street drugs can also cause these dysrhythmias if heart disease is present.

Either accelerated junctional dysrhythmia or junctional tachycardia may become a serious dysrhythmia if the rate increases significantly or the patient becomes medically unstable. Assessment is required to determine the patient's tolerance of the dysrhythmia and the appropriate treatment.

PREMATURE JUNCTIONAL CONTRACTION

A *premature junctional contraction (PJC)* is an individual complex that originates from a single site in the AV junctional area and occurs earlier than the next expected complex of the underlying rhythm (Fig. 4-13). PJCs are common and can occur in any rhythm.

Although PJCs are **individual** complexes and **not** true rhythms, they are included in this chapter because they originate from the AV junctional area.

A premature junctional contraction has the same characteristics as other junctional complexes. The P wave is either inverted, buried, or retrograde. The PR interval, if seen, may be less than 0.12 second, but the QRS complex is usually normal; less than 0.12 second.

The P to P and the R to R intervals of the underlying rhythm vary, depending on that rhythm. The occurrence of a PJC, in even the most regular rhythm, causes the P to P and the R to R intervals to be irregular.

The premature junctional contraction may be followed by a complete compensatory pause, which allows the underlying rhythm to depolarize at its normal rate, as though the PJC had never occurred. The R to R interval from the complex before the PJC to the complex after the PJC is at least two times the R to R interval of the underlying rhythm.

Although a PJC may occur in any rhythm, it is easier to identify in a sinus or bradycardic rhythm. When determining the rate of any rhythm containing a PJC, the R wave of the PJC is included in the total count of the R waves.

The underlying rhythm must be identified when interpreting a rhythm strip containing a PJC. For example, the underlying rhythm might be a sinus rhythm or a junctional dysrhythmia with a PJCs (Fig. 4-14).

Premature junctional contraction may be caused by pain, fever, fear, anxiety, sudden excitement, exercise, or the effects of drugs such as digitalis, atropine, nicotine, caffeine, and amphetamines. PJCs also may be caused by an increased irri-

Normal conduction   Abnormal conduction

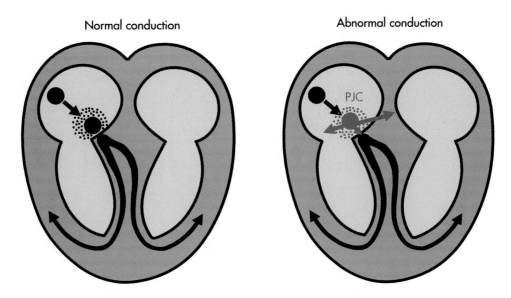

FIG. 4-13 *Left heart* shows normal electrical conduction pathway. *Right heart* shows conduction pathway of a premature junctional contraction (PJC).

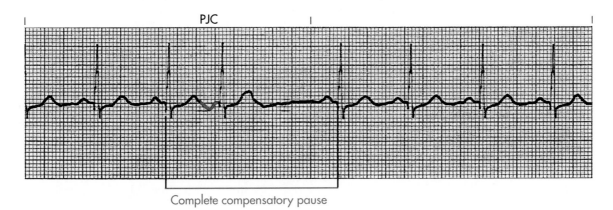

FIG. 4-14 Sinus rhythm with a PJC and a complete compensatory pause; heart rate, 70.

tability of the myocardium. This increased irritability indicates that the cardiac cells are able to respond to even a mild electrical stimulus and may depolarize in an unpredictable rate or manner.

A PJC by itself is not a lethal dysrhythmia. However, it should be monitored closely, since it may trigger a more serious dysrhythmia.

WANDERING JUNCTIONAL PACEMAKER

A *wandering junctional pacemaker dysrhythmia* originates from at least **three** sites within the junctional area (Fig. 4-15). The size and shape of each complex is determined by the site of origin for each complex.

The individual complexes are characterized by P waves that are inverted, buried, or retrograde. Any PR intervals that are seen are usually less than 0.12 second, but the QRS complexes are usually normal; less than 0.12 second.

The rhythm is irregular with varying P to P intervals and R to R intervals. The rate may also vary but is usually 40 to 60 impulses per minute (Fig. 4-16).

Normal conduction   Abnormal conduction

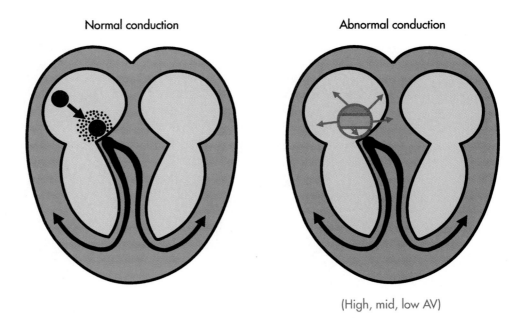

(High, mid, low AV)

FIG. 4-15 *Left heart* shows normal electrical conduction pathway. *Right heart* shows conduction pathway of a wandering junctional pacemaker dysrhythmia.

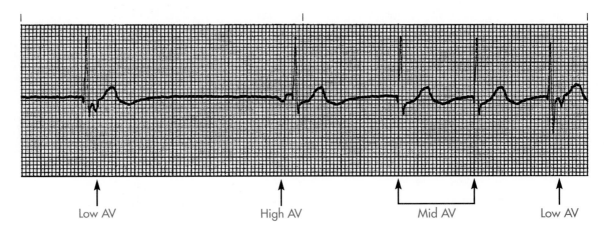

Low AV   High AV   Mid AV   Low AV

FIG. 4-16 Wandering junctional pacemaker dysrhythmia originating in the high, middle, and low AV junctional areas; heart rate, 50.

This dysrhythmia is not usually lethal. However, it is frequently treated, because it indicates increased irritability within the junctional area that may progress to a more serious dysrhythmia.

A wandering junctional pacemaker dysrhythmia may be caused by heart disease, myocardial infarction, or drug toxicity.

A wandering junctional pacemaker dysrhythmia has three or more **junctional** sites. However, a rhythm that has both atrial and junctional sites is identified as a wandering atrial pacemaker dysrhythmia.

WANDERING ATRIAL PACEMAKER

A *wandering atrial pacemaker dysrhythmia* originates from at least **three** different sites above the bundle of His. These sites may include the SA node, any pacemaker site in the atria, the AV junction, or a combination of these areas (Fig. 4-17). Although

Normal conduction   Abnormal conduction

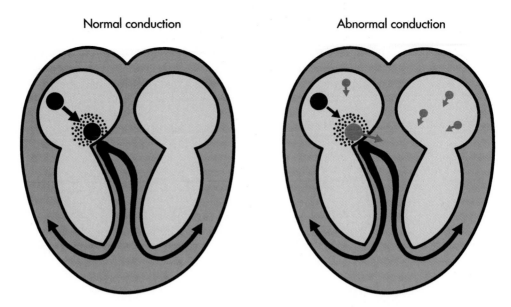

FIG. 4-17 *Left heart* shows normal electrical conduction pathway. *Right heart* shows conduction pathway of wandering atrial pacemaker dysrhythmia.

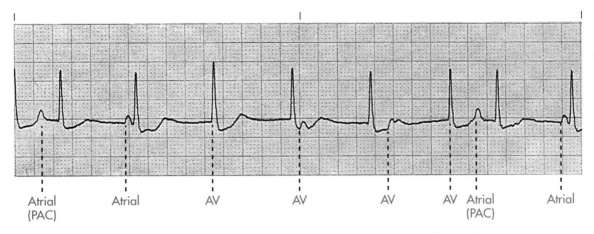

| Atrial (PAC) | Atrial | AV | AV | AV | AV | Atrial (PAC) | Atrial |

FIG. 4-18 Wandering atrial pacemaker dysrhythmia showing different sites of origin; heart rate, 80 to 90.

this is an atrial dysrhythmia, it is included in this chapter because it usually includes some junctional complexes.

The size and shape of each individual complex is determined by the site of origin for that complex. If the site is from the atria, a P wave occurs, followed by a QRS complex that measures less than 0.12 second. The PR interval is usually 0.12 to 0.20 second but may vary because the atrial point of origin varies.

If the complex is from the AV junctional area, the P waves may be inverted, may be buried, or may follow the QRS complex (retrograde). Therefore P waves may not be seen before every QRS complex, and the PR intervals may vary or be absent.

The P to P intervals (if present) and R to R intervals vary, producing an irregular rhythm. The rate may also vary but usually remains between 60 and 100 electrical impulses per minute (Fig. 4-18).

A wandering atrial pacemaker dysrhythmia may be caused by heart disease, myocardial infarction, or drug toxicity.

This dysrhythmia is usually not lethal. However, it is frequently treated because it indicates increased irritability within the cardiac muscle. This increased irritability may cause the dysrhythmia to progress to a more serious dysrhythmia.

The patient's symptoms vary, depending on the rate of the wandering atrial pacemaker and the patient's tolerance of the dysrhythmia.

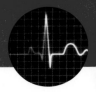

REVIEW QUESTIONS

TRUE FALSE   1. The AV node is located in the lower left atrium, near the septum.

TRUE FALSE   2. A junctional bradycardia has a heart rate of less than 40 electrical impulses per minute.

TRUE FALSE   3. A wandering junctional pacemaker dysrhythmia originates from both the atria and the AV junctional area.

TRUE FALSE   4. In a junctional rhythm, the P wave will be buried if the electrical impulse is initiated high in the AV junctional area.

5. The inherent heart rate of the AV junctional area is _____ to _____ electrical impulses per minute.

6. The QRS complex in a junctional dysrhythmia usually measures _____ second.
   a. 0.12 to 0.20
   b. 0.4 to 0.12
   c. 0.04 to 0.20
   d. 0.04 to 0.12

7. Junctional tachycardia has a heart rate of _____ to _____ electrical impulses per minute.

8. What are the two definitions of the term *retrograde*, as used when describing junctional dysrhythmias?
   a. _____
   b. _____

9. A PJC is:
   a. a junctional complex that occurs later than the next expected complex of the underlying rhythm.
   b. any complex that occurs earlier than the next expected complex of a junctional dysrhythmia.
   c. a complex that occurs later than the next expected complex of a junctional dysrhythmia.
   d. a junctional complex that occurs earlier than the next expected complex of the underlying rhythm.

10. List three types of P waves that can be seen in a junctional dysrhythmia.
    a. _____
    b. _____
    c. _____

11. Where do the electrical impulses originate, which depolarize the atria forming the three types of P waves found in junctional dysrhythmias?
    a. _____
    b. _____
    c. _____

12. PJCs are usually followed by what kind of a pause?
    a. compensatory
    b. sinus
    c. junctional
    d. noncompensatory

13. Describe a wandering atrial pacemaker dysrhythmia, including measurements.

_____

_____

_____

14. What is the difference between a junctional tachycardia and an accelerated junctional dysrhythmia?

_____

_____

_____

RHYTHM STRIP REVIEW

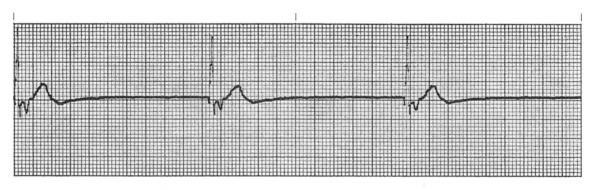

1. MEASURE: PR interval _____ Rhythm _____

   QRS complex _____ Heart rate _____

   INTERPRETATION: _____

2. MEASURE: PR interval _____ Rhythm _____

   QRS complex _____ Heart rate _____

   INTERPRETATION: _____

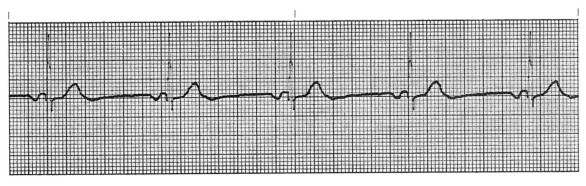

3. MEASURE: PR interval _____ Rhythm _____
                 QRS complex _____ Heart rate _____
    INTERPRETATION: _____

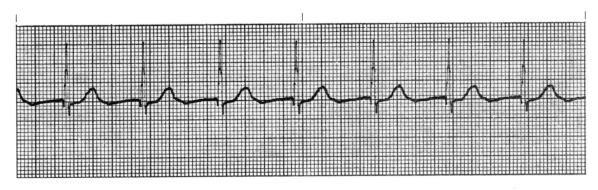

4. MEASURE: PR interval _____ Rhythm _____
                 QRS complex _____ Heart rate _____
    INTERPRETATION: _____

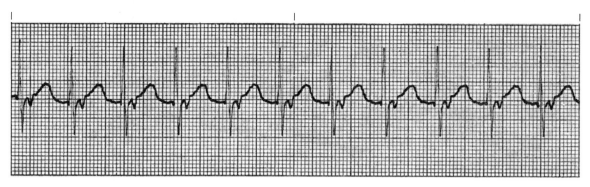

5. MEASURE: PR interval _____ Rhythm _____
QRS complex _____ Heart rate _____
INTERPRETATION: _____

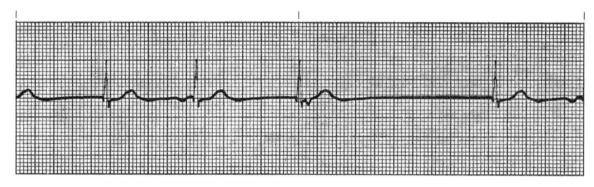

6. MEASURE: PR interval _____ Rhythm _____
QRS complex _____ Heart rate _____
INTERPRETATION: _____

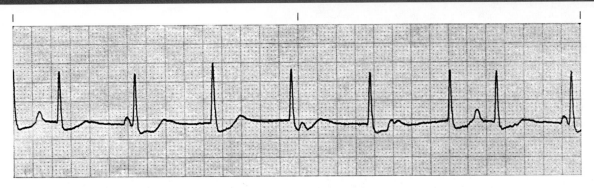

7. MEASURE: PR interval _____   Rhythm _____

               QRS complex _____   Heart rate _____

        INTERPRETATION: _____

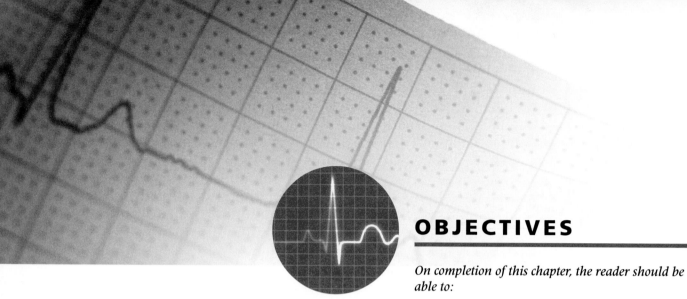

OBJECTIVES

On completion of this chapter, the reader should be able to:

1 Describe first-degree heart block, including measurements of the components.

2 Explain the appearance of second-degree heart block, type I, including measurements of the components.

3 Describe the appearance of second-degree heart block, type II, including measurements of the components.

4 Describe third-degree heart block, including the appearance and measurements of the components.

5 Explain the appearance of a bundle branch block, including measurements of the components.

6 Define the terms prolonged PR interval, progressive block, Wenckebach, complete AV dissociation.

HEART BLOCKS

OUTLINE

DEFINITIONS

AV Dissociation A dysrhythmia also known as third-degree heart block or complete heart block

Heart Block A partial or complete interruption in the normal cardiac electrical conduction system

Intermittent Heart Block An interruption of the electrical impulse that occurs suddenly and without warning, completely blocking the conduction of the impulse to the ventricles

Lethal Dysrhythmia A dysrhythmia that cannot sustain life; death producing

Mobitz I A dysrhythmia also known as second-degree heart block, type I or Wenckebach

Mobitz II A dysrhythmia also known as second-degree heart block, type II

Progressive Heart Block An interruption of the electrical impulse that becomes longer with each impulse, until it is completely blocked and does not reach the ventricles

"Rabbit Ears" An informal term used to describe the notched appearance of the widened QRS complexes in bundle branch blocks

HEART BLOCKS

Heart blocks occur when there is a *partial* or *complete interruption* in the cardiac electrical conduction system. This interruption occurs between the atria and the bundle of His, or in the ventricles between the AV junction and the Purkinje's fibers.

The appearance of the P wave and the QRS complex varies, depending on the type of heart block. The rate and the rhythm also may vary.

The location of the block and the resulting patient symptoms determine if the dysrhythmia is lethal.

FIRST-DEGREE HEART BLOCK

A *first-degree heart block* is caused by a delay in the conduction of an electrical impulse between the atria and the bundle of His. This delay occurs when there is a partial interruption or slowing in the conduction of an electrical impulse through the atrioventricular (AV) junctional area (Fig. 5-1).

Although all electrical impulses are eventually conducted to the ventricles, the interruption causes the impulse to be delayed. Therefore a first-degree heart block is **not** a true block, but simply a **delay** in the electrical conduction system. The delay is seen on the monitor screen or rhythm strip as a prolonged PR interval, greater than 0.20 second (Fig. 5-2).

A P wave occurs before every QRS complex; however, the PR interval is always greater than 0.20 second. The size and shape of both the P wave and QRS complex may vary, depending on the underlying rhythm. The P to P and the R to R intervals are usually regular, also depending on the underlying rhythm.

Because a first-degree heart block may be found in any rhythm that has a P wave before the QRS complex, the rate may be normal, bradycardic, or tachycardic. When describing a rhythm containing a first-degree heart block, identify the underlying rhythm first; for example, sinus bradycardia with a first-degree heart block (Fig. 5-3).

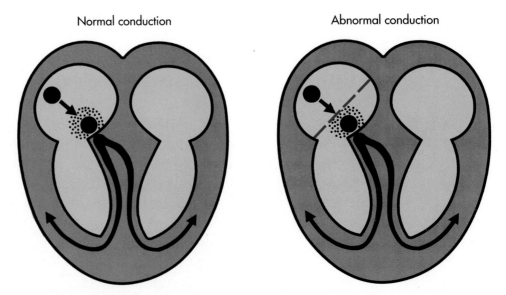

Normal conduction   Abnormal conduction

FIG. 5-1 *Left heart* shows normal electrical conduction pathway. *Right heart* shows conduction pathway of a first-degree heart block with a delay between atria and AV junction.

Although a first-degree heart block is not usually a serious dysrhythmia, it **is** important to assess the patient carefully when the block indicates a recent change in the patient's electrical conduction system. This change may **indicate** damage to the myocardium, which can lead to a more serious dysrhythmia.

First-degree heart block may be caused by myocardial infarction or drugs.

SECOND-DEGREE HEART BLOCKS

There are two types of second-degree heart blocks, type I and type II. Both occur when there is an interruption in the conduction of an electrical impulse through the AV Junctional area.

Second-Degree Heart Block, Type I

Second-degree heart block, type I (Wenckebach, Mobitz I) is a **progressive** heart block. This block occurs when the electrical impulse traveling from the atria is interrupted at the AV junction, slowing the conduction of the impulse to the ventricles.

The interruption becomes longer with each impulse, delaying the depolarization of the ventricles, until the interruption completely blocks the conduction of an

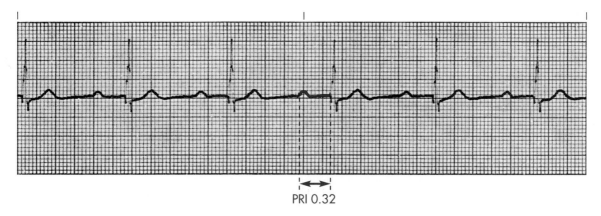

PRI 0.32

FIG. 5-2 PR interval greater than 0.20 second: The delay is seen on the monitor screen or rhythm strip as a prolonged PR interval.

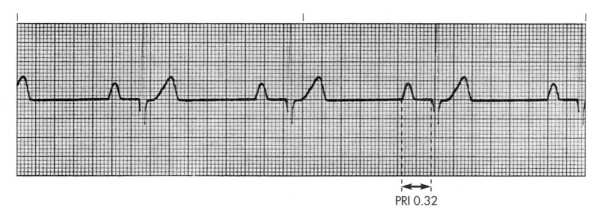

PRI 0.32

FIG. 5-3 Sinus bradycardia with first-degree heart block: PR interval, 0.32 second; heart rate, 40.

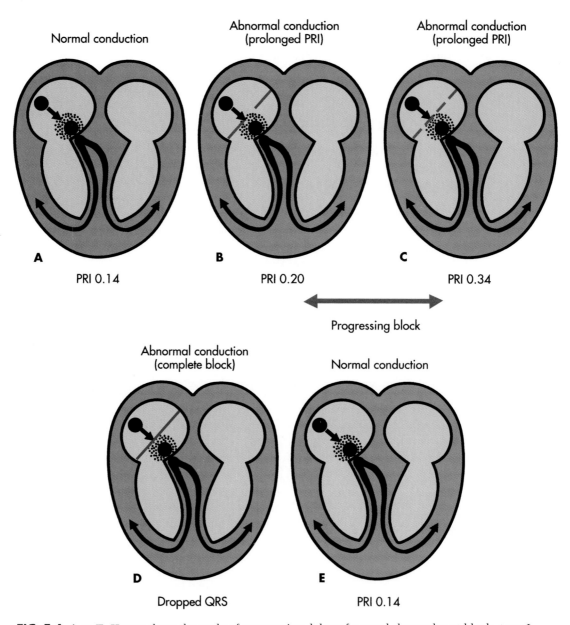

FIG. 5-4 A to **E,** Hearts show the cycle of progressive delay of second-degree heart block, type I (Wenckebach, Mobitz I).

electrical impulse to the ventricles. The cycle of **progressively delayed conduction** is then repeated (Fig. 5-4).

The delay is seen on the rhythm strip as PR intervals become longer with each QRS complex, until a *dropped,* or *absent,* QRS complex occurs (P wave is seen without a QRS complex). This pattern is repeated throughout the dysrhythmia.

A P wave occurs before every QRS complex, and the P waves are the same size and shape. A QRS complex follows each P wave until a QRS is dropped. The QRS complex is usually less than 0.12 second.

Although the PR interval becomes progressively longer, the R to R intervals usually become progressively shorter, until the QRS complex is dropped. The pattern then repeats itself. The P to P interval remains regular; however, the overall rhythm is irregular. The rate may vary (Fig. 5-5).

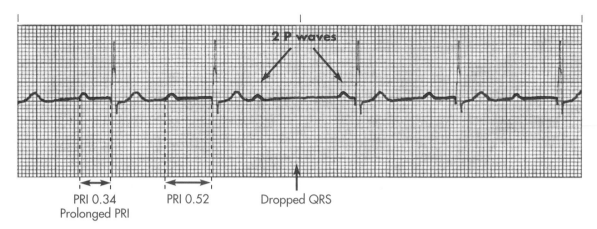

PRI 0.34   PRI 0.52   Dropped QRS
Prolonged PRI

FIG. 5-5 Second-degree heart block, type I (Wenckebach, Mobitz I): Atrial heart rate, 60; ventricular heart rate, 50.

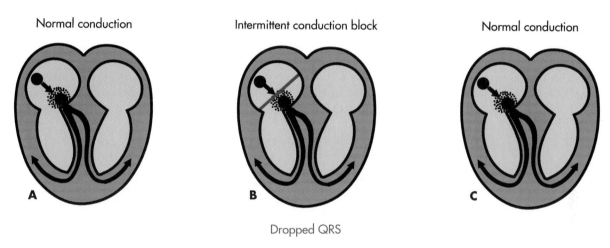

Normal conduction   Intermittent conduction block   Normal conduction

A   B   C

Dropped QRS

FIG. 5-6 A, Heart shows normal electrical conduction pathway. Hearts in **B** and **C** show conduction pathway of a second-degree heart block, type II (Mobitz II) with an intermittent interruption at the AV junction.

Although Wenckebach heart block (second-degree heart block, type I) is not a lethal dysrhythmia, the patient may become medically unstable because of a bradycardic rate, recent injury to the cardiac muscle, or prior illness. A Wenckebach heart block may be serious when it indicates a recent change in the electrical conduction system after an injury to the cardiac muscle. A Wenckebach heart block may be caused by infection, myocardial infarction, or drug toxicity.

As with any rhythm, **patient assessment** is necessary to determine the patient's tolerance of the dysrhythmia.

Second-Degree Heart Block, Type II

Second-degree heart block, type II (Mobitz II, classical) occurs when there is an **intermittent interruption** in the electrical conduction system near or below the AV junction. This interruption is **not** progressive but occurs **suddenly and without warning,** blocking the conduction of the impulse to the ventricles (Fig. 5-6).

The rhythm strip shows a P wave before every QRS complex, and all P waves are the same size and shape. A QRS complex follows every P wave until an interruption occurs and a QRS is dropped (absent). The PR intervals of the underlying rhythm usually remain the same length and may be either normal or prolonged.

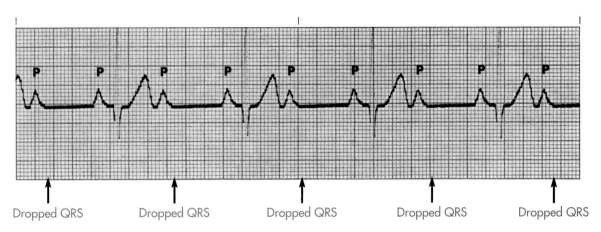

Dropped QRS   Dropped QRS   Dropped QRS   Dropped QRS   Dropped QRS

FIG. 5-7 Sinus rhythm with a second-degree heart block, type II (Mobitz II): Atrial heart rate, 90; ventricular heart rate, 40.

Although the QRS complex usually measures less than 0.12 second, the complex may be wider if the block occurs low in the bundle branches.

A Mobitz II heart block can occur in any rhythm that has a P wave followed by a QRS complex. The P to P intervals are usually regular, and the R to R intervals are usually regular until a QRS complex is dropped. The overall rhythm is usually irregular, and the heart rate varies, also depending on the underlying rhythm (Fig. 5-7).

When interpreting a dysrhythmia containing a second-degree heart block, type II, it is important to:

1. Identify the underlying rhythm, if possible.
2. Determine the ratio of P waves to each QRS complex. The number of P waves before each QRS complex helps to determine the severity of the block.

   Example: Two P waves before one QRS complex = 2:1 block (ratio)
   Three P waves before one QRS complex = 3:1 block (ratio)
   Four P waves before one QRS complex = 4:1 block (ratio)

   This ratio may be constant or may vary. Second-degree heart block, type II, becomes more serious as the ratio of P waves to QRS complexes increases or if the ratio varies.
3. Determine the frequency of occurrence. Second-degree heart block, type II, may occur in a pattern or at random. A second-degree heart block, type II, with no pattern (varying block) is more dangerous, because the lack of a pattern indicates the block is irregular and may progress to a more serious dysrhythmia (Fig. 5-8).

If a second-degree heart block (Mobitz II) ratio is a 3:1 or higher block, the dysrhythmia may be called an advanced AV block. This dysrhythmia is described in more detail in 12 Lead EKG textbooks and classes.

A second-degree heart block, type II, is a dangerous dysrhythmia because of the increased irritability of the myocardium, which may lead to a more serious dysrhythmia such as third-degree heart block. If the block is severe enough, the ventricular rate may become bradycardic. A ventricular rate of 40 electrical impulses per minute or less is usually not sufficient to maintain adequate circulation to the vital organs of the body. Frequent assessment is very important to determine the patient's tolerance of the dysrhythmia.

A second-degree heart block, type II, may be caused by myocardial infarction, heart disease, or drug toxicity.

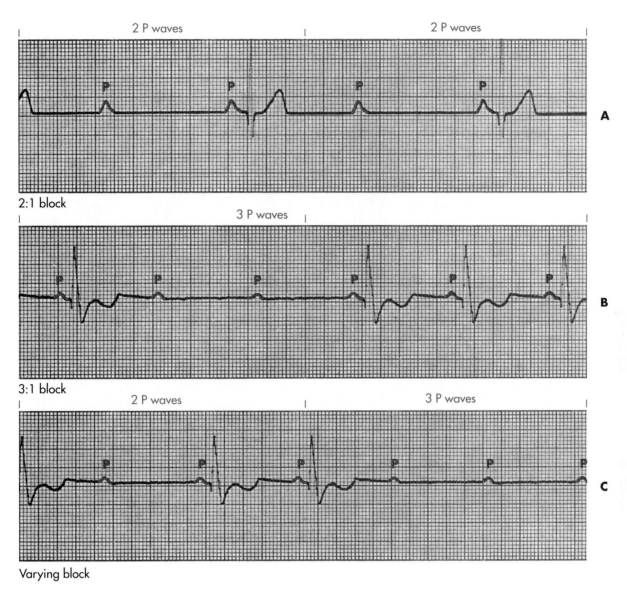

FIG. 5-8 A, Second-degree heart block, type II (Mobitz II) with a 2:1 block. **B,** Second-degree heart block, type II (Mobitz II) with a 3:1 block. **C,** Second-degree heart block, type II (Mobitz II) with a varying block.

THIRD-DEGREE HEART BLOCK

Third-degree heart block (complete heart block or complete AV dissociation) occurs when the electrical impulse is completely blocked between the atria and the ventricles. The interruption usually takes place between the AV junction and the bundle of His (Fig. 5-9).

The electrical impulse causes depolarization of the atria; however, the impulse is blocked before it can reach the ventricles. Because the electrical conduction system is completely interrupted, the ventricles must initiate their own impulses to cause cardiac muscle contraction. Both the atria and the ventricles function independently, as if they were two separate hearts (Fig. 5-10).

The rhythm strip shows both P waves and QRS complexes, as well as what appear to be PR intervals that are constantly changing in length. However, the PR intervals do **not** become progressively longer as they do in second-degree heart block, type I.

Normal conduction   Abnormal conduction

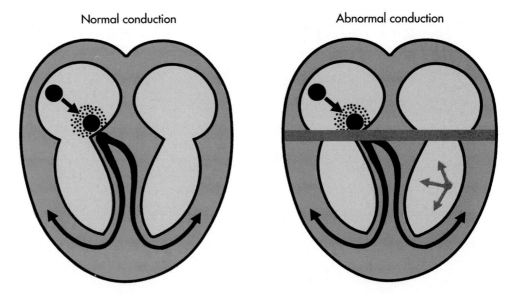

FIG. 5-9 *Left heart* shows normal electrical conduction pathway. *Right heart* shows conduction pathway of a third-degree heart block with a complete interruption between the atria and the ventricles.

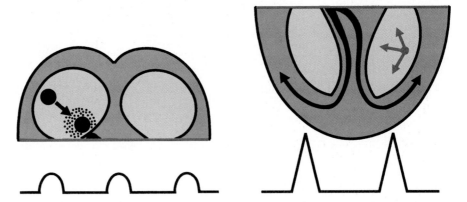

FIG. 5-10 Third-degree heart block with separate atrial and ventricular responses.

On closer inspection of the rhythm strip, one can see that no relationship exists between the P waves and the QRS complexes. Because the atria and the ventricles are each functioning independently, no true PR interval occurs (Fig. 5-11).

The P waves usually are the same size and shape, although some may be hidden in a QRS complex or in a T wave, changing their appearance. The QRS complexes are usually wide, longer than 0.12 second, and bizarre in appearance but are usually the same size and shape. Occasionally, the QRS complexes will measure less than 0.12 second, if the block occurs at the AV junction.

Because both the atria and the ventricles are generating their own impulses, each will depolarize at its own inherent heart rate, causing the P to P intervals to be equal and the R to R intervals to be equal. However, the P to P intervals are usually not equal to the R to R intervals (Fig. 5-12).

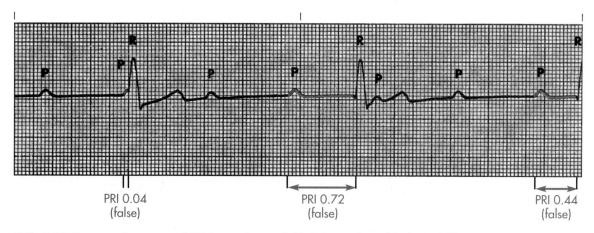

PRI 0.04
(false)

PRI 0.72
(false)

PRI 0.44
(false)

FIG. 5-11 Separate P waves and QRS complexes of third-degree heart block: Atrial heart rate, 70; ventricular heart rate, 20 to 30.

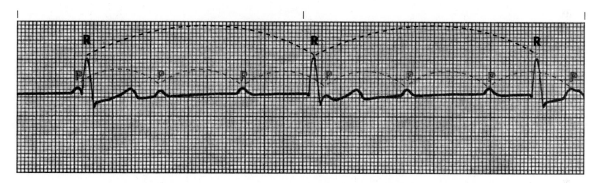

FIG. 5-12 Third-degree heart block: Atrial heart rate, 70; ventricular heart rate, 30.

The atrial heart rate is usually 60 to 100 electrical impulses per minute; the ventricular heart rate is usually 20 to 40 electrical impulses, however, these rates may vary.

Third-degree heart block is a **lethal** dysrhythmia because it may progress to asystole (no heart beat). It is also lethal because the ventricular rate is usually so slow and inefficient that the heart cannot maintain a cardiac output adequate to sustain life.

Third-degree block often is caused by a myocardial infarction or severe heart disease.

BUNDLE BRANCH BLOCK

A *bundle branch block* (BBB) occurs when there is an interruption in the cardiac electrical conduction system of either the right, the left, or both bundle branches. This interruption causes a delay in the conduction of the electrical impulse to the ventricle of the blocked bundle branch (Fig. 5-13, *A* to *D*).

The atria are usually depolarized in a normal manner. The electrical impulse then follows the normal conduction pathway until it reaches the interruption in the bundle branch. The interruption in the electrical conduction system forces the impulse to "detour" and take an alternate route.

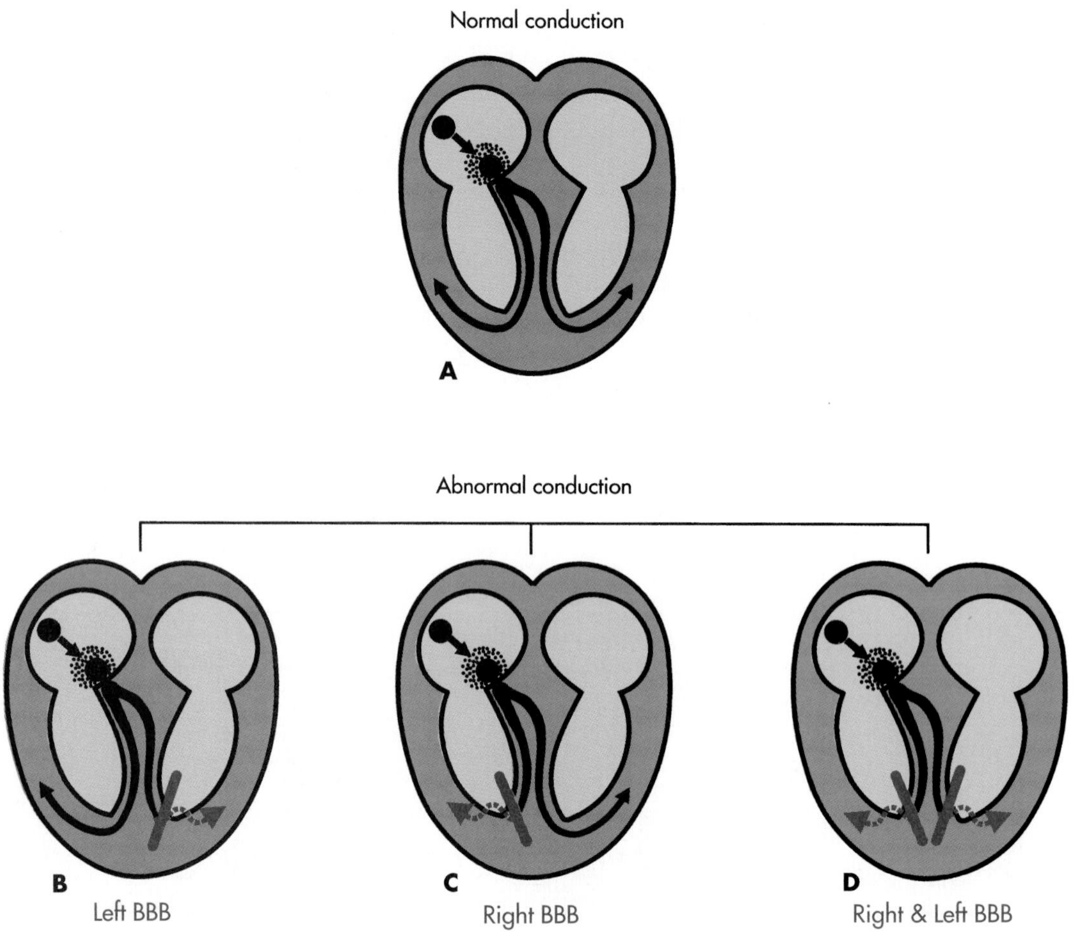

Normal conduction

Abnormal conduction

B	**C**	**D**
Left BBB	Right BBB	Right & Left BBB

FIG. 5-13 A, Heart shows normal electrical conduction pathway. Hearts in **B, C,** and **D** show, respectively, the delayed conduction pathway of a left bundle, right bundle, and both a left and right bundle branch block (BBB).

As with any detour, the alternate route takes more time to travel. This extra time causes the electrical impulse to reach the ventricle of the blocked bundle branch later than the ventricle of the normal bundle branch.

As a result, the blocked ventricle depolarizes slightly later than the normal ventricle, causing two separate depolarizations (Fig. 5-14). The two depolarizations are shown on the rhythm strip as a single notched or widened QRS complex. The notched QRS is frequently referred to as *rabbit ears.* The QRS complex is wider than normal, measuring more than 0.12 second (Fig. 5-15).

If both bundle branches are blocked, the electrical impulse must detour around both interruptions, causing the electrical impulse to reach both ventricles later than normal. The electrical impulse rarely reaches both ventricles at the same time.

A bundle branch block can occur in any rhythm. The presence of P waves and PR intervals is determined by the underlying rhythm. The rate and rhythm also may vary, depending on the underlying rhythm.

When interpreting a rhythm strip containing a BBB, you must first identify the underlying rhythm; for example, sinus rhythm with a bundle branch block (Fig. 5-16).

Widened QRS   "Rabbit ears"

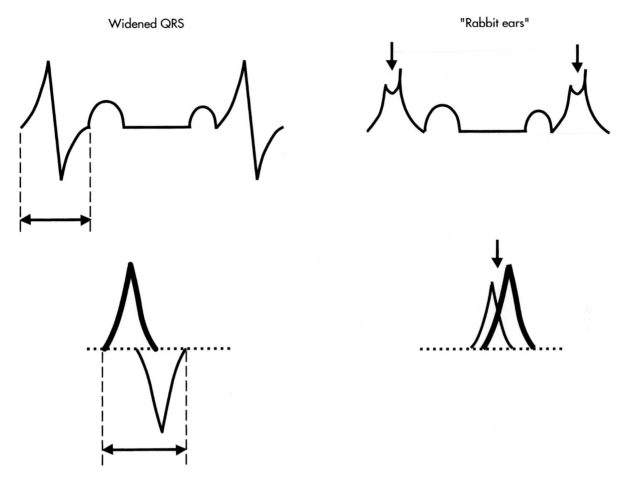

FIG. 5-14 Two types of ventricular depolarizations seen with a bundle branch block: either a widened QRS or "rabbit ears."

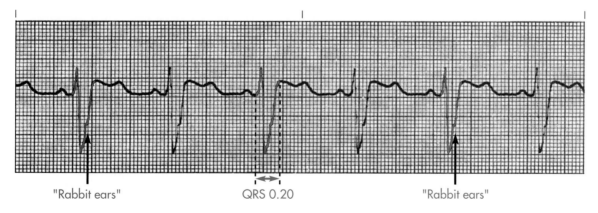

"Rabbit ears"   QRS 0.20   "Rabbit ears"

FIG. 5-15 Typical "rabbit ears" QRS seen with bundle branch block.

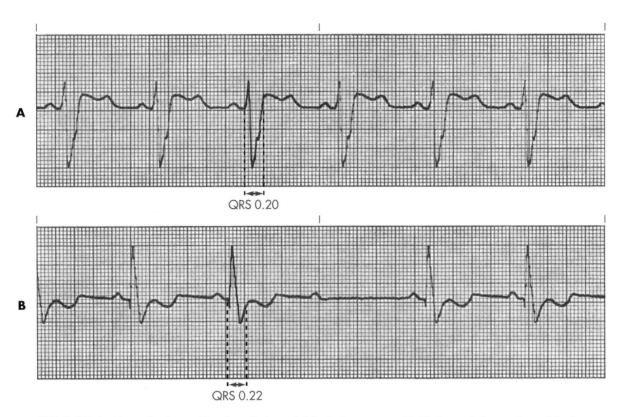

FIG. 5-16 A, Sinus rhythm with a bundle branch block; heart rate, 60. **B,** Second-degree heart block, type II (Mobitz II) and a bundle branch block. Overall heart rate, 40 to 50.

Although a BBB is not usually a serious dysrhythmia, it **is** important to assess the patient carefully when the block indicates a recent change in the patient's electrical conduction pathway. This change may indicate damage to the myocardium, which can lead to a more serious dysrhythmia.

A 12-Lead electrocardiogram (EKG, ECG) is necessary to determine the seriousness of the block, and if the block is in the right or left bundle branch.

Bundle branch blocks may be caused by heart disease or myocardial infarction.

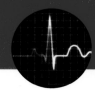

REVIEW QUESTIONS

TRUE   FALSE   1. Heart blocks occur when there is a partial or complete interruption in the cardiac electrical conduction system.

TRUE   FALSE   2. A first-degree heart block occurs when there is a partial or complete interruption anywhere in the ventricles.

TRUE   FALSE   3. A third-degree heart block may progress to a Mobitz II heart block.

TRUE   FALSE   4. A third-degree heart block exists when the atria and ventricles function independently.

5. In a bundle branch block, the two depolarizations are seen on the rhythm strip as a notched or widened:
   a. T wave
   b. PR interval
   c. QRS complex
   d. ST segment

6. A third-degree heart block is a lethal dysrhythmia because:
   a. the additional force of the ventricular contraction can cause cardiac exhaustion
   b. it can progress to asystole
   c. the electrical impulse cannot be transmitted to the Purkinje's fibers
   d. the atria do not depolarize

7. Second-degree heart block, type I is also known as:
   a. Mobitz II
   b. AV dissociation
   c. Wenckebach
   d. bundle branch block

8. In a first-degree heart block, the PR interval is greater than _____ second.

9. Complete heart block, or AV dissociation, is also known as

   _____.

10. In a second-degree heart block, type I, the PR intervals become progressively _____ , until a P wave is followed by a dropped or absent _____.

11. Explain why a second degree heart block, type II, is considered a dangerous dysrhythmia: _____

    _____

    _____

12. When identifying a second-degree heart block, type II, which three aspects of a rhythm are important to evaluate?
    a. _____
    b. _____
    c. _____

RHYTHM STRIP REVIEW

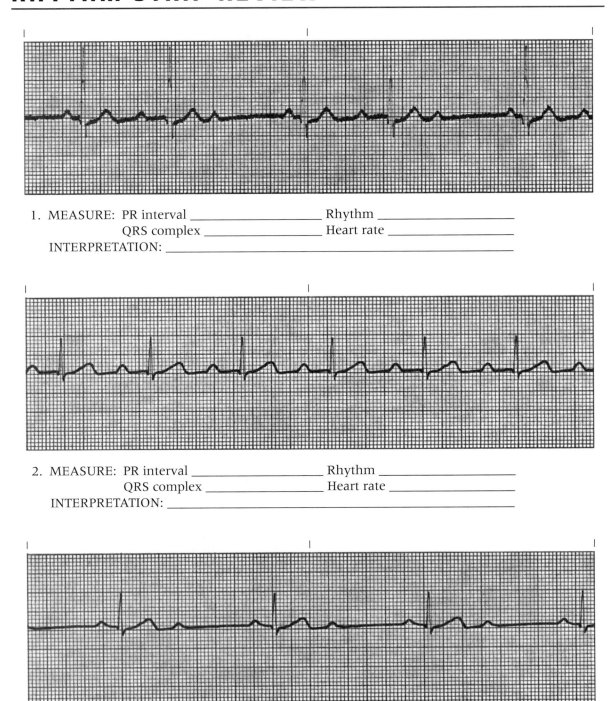

1. MEASURE: PR interval _____ Rhythm _____

                  QRS complex _____ Heart rate _____

    INTERPRETATION: _____

2. MEASURE: PR interval _____ Rhythm _____

                  QRS complex _____ Heart rate _____

    INTERPRETATION: _____

3. MEASURE: PR interval _____ Rhythm _____

                  QRS complex _____ Heart rate _____

    INTERPRETATION: _____

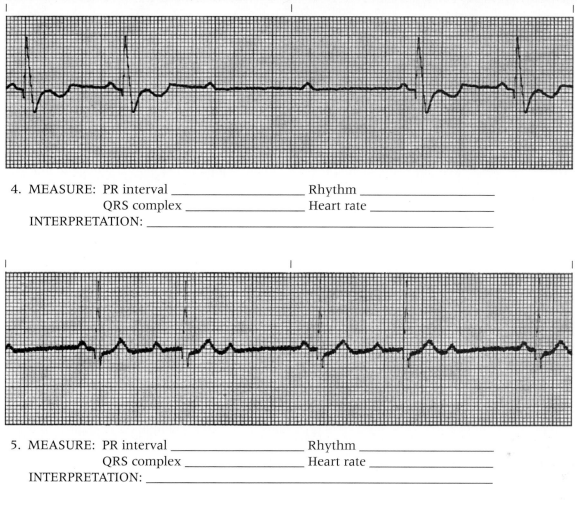

4. MEASURE: PR interval _____ Rhythm _____
                QRS complex _____ Heart rate _____
    INTERPRETATION: _____

5. MEASURE: PR interval _____ Rhythm _____
                QRS complex _____ Heart rate _____
    INTERPRETATION: _____

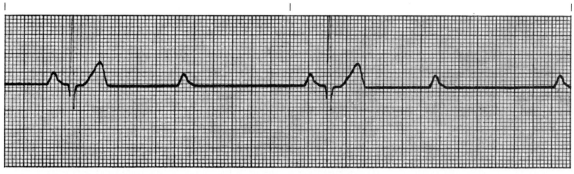

6. MEASURE: PR interval _____ Rhythm _____
                QRS complex _____ Heart rate _____
    INTERPRETATION: _____

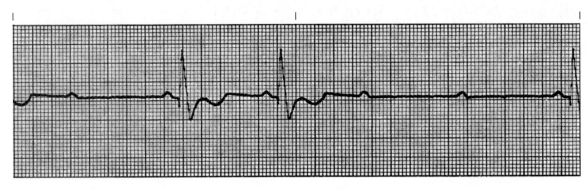

7. MEASURE: PR interval _____ Rhythm _____

QRS complex _____ Heart rate _____

INTERPRETATION: _____

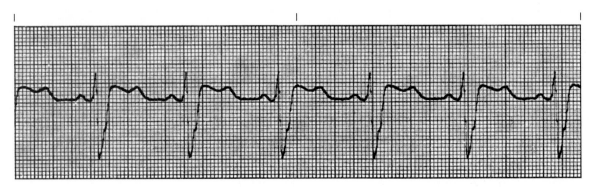

8. MEASURE: PR interval _____ Rhythm _____

QRS complex _____ Heart rate _____

INTERPRETATION: _____

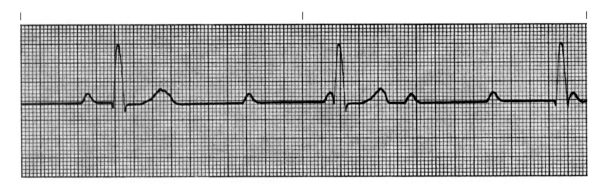

9. MEASURE: PR interval _____ Rhythm _____

QRS complex _____ Heart rate _____

INTERPRETATION: _____

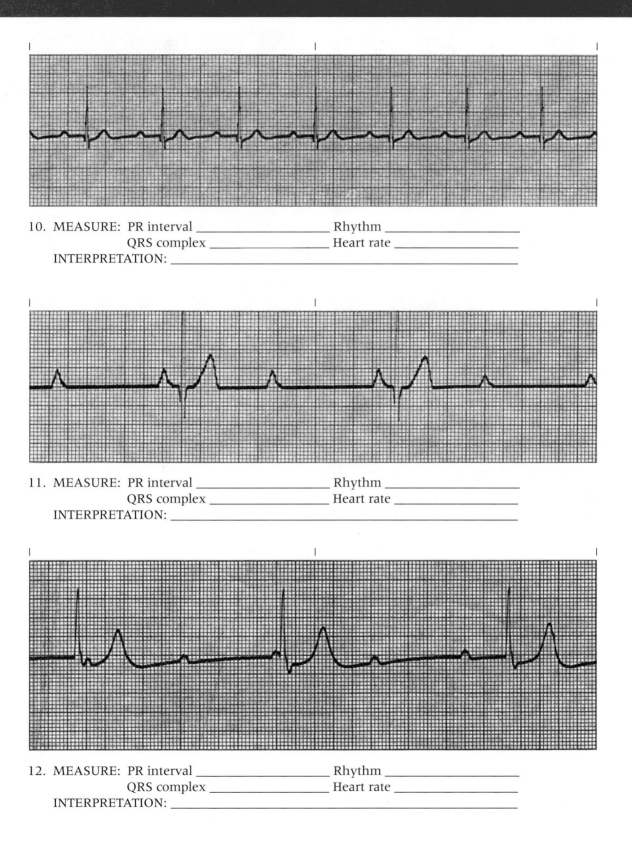

10. MEASURE: PR interval _____ Rhythm _____
    QRS complex _____ Heart rate _____
    INTERPRETATION: _____

11. MEASURE: PR interval _____ Rhythm _____
    QRS complex _____ Heart rate _____
    INTERPRETATION: _____

12. MEASURE: PR interval _____ Rhythm _____
    QRS complex _____ Heart rate _____
    INTERPRETATION: _____

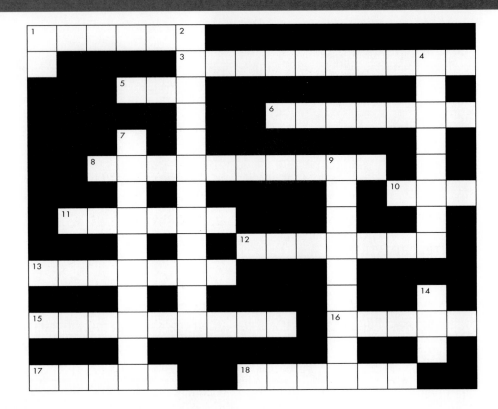

CROSSWORD PUZZLE CLUES

Across

1. Mobitz II is a _____-degree heart block.

3. Stops suddenly; intermittent conduction.

5. Bundle of _____.

6. Absent or _____ QRS complex.

8. Second-degree heart block, type I.

10. Prolonged _____; first-degree heart block.

11. Life threatening.

12. Pertaining to the heart.

15. Extended.

16. AV dissociation; _____-degree heart block.

17. Delay between atria and AV node; _____-degree heart block.

18. _____ branch.

Down

1. _____ node; primary cardiac pacemaker.

2. Comple AV _____; third-degree heart block.

4. The impulse that travels through the conduction pathway is an _____al impulse.

7. Lower heart chambers.

9. Led from place to place.

14. Ventricular depolarization; _____ complex.

```
R  N  J  K  U  H  Y  T  A  D  N  N  D  L  J  Z  J  P  K  Q  N
N  P  W  C  H  C  A  B  E  K  C  N  E  W  K  Y  W  A  I  J  O
F  Q  D  T  X  L  L  T  Q  P  P  U  H  Z  I  O  V  T  N  D  T
T  J  J  N  G  C  C  Z  T  R  S  Z  C  W  D  R  I  H  T  J  A
V  X  H  I  H  S  O  F  O  A  T  P  T  Q  Y  L  M  W  E  V  I
E  L  V  R  A  K  J  G  Z  C  R  S  O  I  E  D  I  A  R  I  C
N  X  K  H  S  B  R  Y  G  G  A  B  N  B  B  B  A  Y  U  N  O
T  E  R  X  F  E  G  O  P  U  E  T  B  C  L  O  P  S  P  T  S
R  H  M  D  S  V  C  G  N  C  H  E  R  M  O  O  M  Q  T  E  S
I  Z  D  S  C  D  E  O  H  O  H  L  A  I  F  M  C  C  I  R  I
C  W  I  D  N  Q  H  D  N  N  R  X  D  P  A  W  P  K  O  M  D
L  V  N  Y  D  F  B  D  J  D  W  A  Y  X  G  J  I  L  N  I  E
E  C  L  O  T  Q  M  A  H  U  X  G  C  N  T  B  B  Z  E  T  G
W  V  A  V  T  A  K  O  X  C  P  F  A  S  U  G  G  E  G  T  R
B  D  J  D  I  C  X  E  I  T  T  U  R  N  D  X  F  E  I  E  E
E  R  O  R  J  R  O  F  O  I  Z  I  D  E  Y  A  L  E  D  N  E
C  U  O  T  D  M  A  A  R  O  F  L  I  O  V  O  Z  X  J  T  G
L  P  N  Y  L  Z  O  T  N  N  E  L  A  H  T  E  L  L  R  O  Q
E  A  K  W  F  U  O  E  K  U  R  R  M  A  A  K  K  J  Z  K  Z
K  B  A  K  C  T  P  O  U  F  X  U  U  X  Z  V  J  G  L  S  R
U  K  J  Q  Y  K  O  Q  X  U  Z  Y  Y  Y  Q  K  O  K  Z  K  J
```

WORD PUZZLE

This word puzzle is designed to help familiarize you with some of the new terminology found in this chapter. Have fun finding all the words on this list. The words can be spelled forward (normally), backward, up, down, or diagonally in any direction. The words will always be in upper case and found in a straight line. Good luck.

ATRIA	HEART
BBB	INTERMITTENT
BLOCK	LETHAL
BRADYCARDIA	MOBITZ
BUNDLE	NOTCHED
COMPLETE	PATHWAYS
CONDUCTION	PROGRESSIVE
DEGREE	SECOND
DELAYED	THIRD
DISSOCIATION	VENTRICLE
FIRST	WENCKEBACH

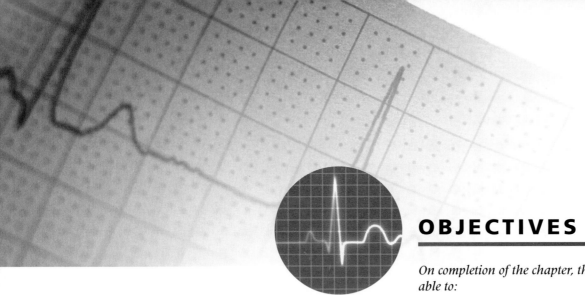

OBJECTIVES

On completion of the chapter, the reader should be able to:

1 Describe a premature ventricular contraction, including measurements of the components.

2 Define compensatory pause, unifocal and multifocal premature ventricular contractions, bigeminy, trigeminy, quadrigeminy, couplet, run of ventricular tachycardia, and R on T phenomenon.

3 Explain the difference between ventricular tachycardia and torsades de pointes.

4 Describe ventricular fibrillation, including coarse and fine fibrillation waves.

5 Describe an idioventricular rhythm.

6 Explain the difference between ventricular standstill and asystole, including measurements of the components.

VENTRICULAR DYSRHYTHMIAS

OUTLINE

DEFINITIONS

Asystole Complete lack of electrical activity in the heart; there is no pulse

Bigeminy of PVCs Every other QRS complex in a rhythm is a premature ventricular contraction (PVC)

Couplet (Pair) Two PVCs in a row

Inherent Heart Rate Normal rate at which electrical impulses are generated; the inherent heart rate for the ventricles is 20 to 40 impulses per minute

Multifocal PVCs PVCs that originate from different sites in the ventricles; the complexes vary in size and shape; also known as *multiform* or *polymorphic*

Quadrigeminy of PVCs Every fourth QRS complex in a rhythm is a PVC

PVC Premature ventricular contraction; a complex that originates from any site below the bundle of His and occurs earlier than expected

R on T Phenomenon This occurs when the R wave of a PVC falls on the T wave of the previous complex

Run of Ventricular Tachycardia Three or more PVCs in a row; also called *salvo* or *burst*

Salvo A run of ventricular tachycardia; may also be called a *burst* of PVCs

Trigeminy of PVCs Every third QRS complex in a rhythm is a PVC

Unifocal PVCs PVCs that originate from one site in the ventricles; the complexes look the same; also known as *uniform* or *monomorphic*

Ventricular Dysrhythmia A cardiac rhythm that is initiated from a pacemaker cell in the ventricles when the sinoatrial node, atrial sites, and the atrioventricular junction fail to initiate an electrical impulse

Vulnerable period (relative refractory period) Time during the cardiac cycle when cardiac cells have repolarized to the point that some cells can be stimulated to contract again, if the stimulus is strong enough

VENTRICULAR DYSRHYTHMIAS

When the sinoatrial (SA) node, the atria, and the atrioventricular (AV) junction fail to initiate an electrical impulse, the ventricles may become the pacemaker of the heart. The electrical stimulus can be initiated from any pacemaker cell in the ventricles, including the bundle branches, the Purkinje's fibers, or the ventricular muscle.

Because the electrical impulse begins in the lower portion of the heart, the impulse must take an alternate conduction pathway. The electrical impulse must travel in a retrograde (backward) direction to depolarize the atria **and** also in a forward direction to depolarize the ventricles (Fig. 6-1).

Because the atria depolarize at almost the same time as the ventricles, the P wave is usually hidden in the QRS complex and will not be seen (Fig. 6-2). The QRS complex is wide, bizarre in appearance, and measures greater than 0.12 second.

Abnormal conduction

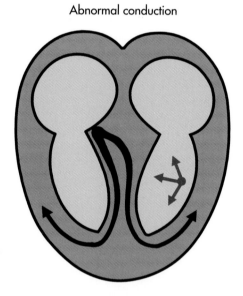

FIG. 6-1 Ventricular electrical conduction pathway.

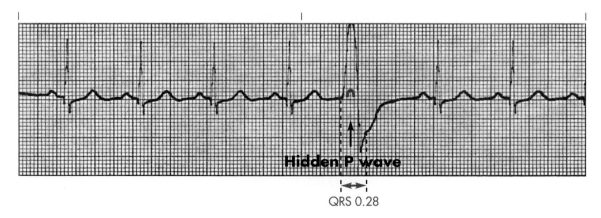

Hidden P wave

QRS 0.28

FIG. 6-2 Ventricular response with hidden P wave within QRS complex.

Because the ventricles are the least efficient pacemaker of the heart, they usually generate 20 to 40 electrical impulses per minute (inherent ventricular heart rate). However, many factors can affect the inherent heart rate. For example, poor cardiac output could cause a significant increase in the rate, as the heart beats faster in an attempt to improve the cardiac output.

Ventricular dysrhythmias are usually considered **life threatening.** However, as with any rhythm, **patient assessment** is essential to determine the patient's tolerance of the dysrhythmia.

PREMATURE VENTRICULAR CONTRACTION

A *premature ventricular contraction* (PVC) is an individual complex that originates from an area below the bundle of His and occurs earlier than the next expected complex of the underlying rhythm (Fig. 6-3). PVCs are very common and can occur in any cardiac rhythm.

Although PVCs are *individual* complexes and not rhythms, they are included in this chapter because they originate from the ventricles.

When the ventricles initiate a PVC, the atria may or may not depolarize. If the atria do not depolarize, a P wave will not be formed. When atrial depolarization does occur, the P wave is usually hidden in the QRS complex because the ventricles depolarize at about the same time.

The QRS complex has a wide and bizarre appearance, is greater than 0.12 second, and may deflect in the opposite direction of the QRS complexes in the underlying rhythm.

The T wave immediately following the PVC is usually deflected in the opposite direction of the QRS complex of the PVC. The ST segment of the PVC appears abnormal because of this opposite direction.

A premature ventricular contraction is usually followed by a complete compensatory pause. This pause allows the underlying rhythm to continue again at its normal rate, as if the PVC had never occurred (Fig. 6-4).

You can check the complete compensatory pause by measuring the R to R intervals before and after the PVC. Measure from the R wave of the complex before

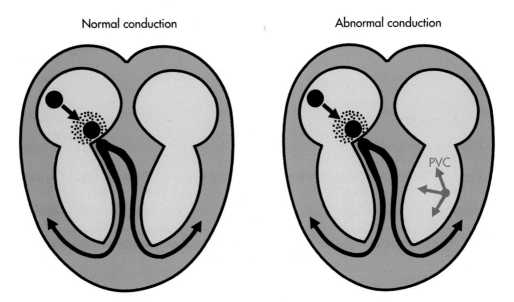

FIG. 6-3 *Left heart* shows normal electrical conduction pathway. *Right heart* shows conduction pathway of a premature ventricular contraction (PVC).

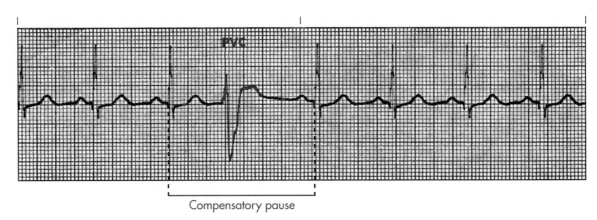

Compensatory pause

FIG. 6-4 Premature ventricular contraction with a complete compensatory pause.

the PVC to the R wave of the complex after the PVC. The distance will be equal to two times the R to R interval of the underlying rhythm (see Chapter 3).

The P to P and R to R intervals of the underlying rhythm vary, depending on that rhythm. A PVC, in even the most regular rhythm, may cause the P to P and R to R intervals to be irregular.

The rate of the rhythm also varies, depending on the underlying rhythm and the number of PVCs within that rhythm. When determining the rate of a rhythm that contains premature ventricular contractions, the PVCs are included in the total count of R waves.

Site of Origin

PVCs are further classified by the site of origin and the frequency of their occurrence.

1. *Unifocal* PVCs originate from a single site within the ventricles and therefore look alike (Fig. 6-5). The term *unifocal* is also known as *uniform* or *monomorphic*.
2. *Multifocal* PVCs originate from different ventricular sites and have varying sizes and shapes. These PVCs are more dangerous because they are the result of increased irritability within the ventricles (Fig. 6-6). The term *multifocal* is also known as *multiform* or *polymorphic*.

Frequency of Occurrence

The more frequently premature ventricular contractions occur, the more cardiac output can be decreased, since the ventricles may not have time to refill with an adequate amount of blood. The following are terms used to describe the frequency of PVCs.

1. *Quadrigeminy* occurs when every fourth QRS complex is a PVC (Fig. 6-7).
2. *Trigeminy* occurs when every third QRS complex is a PVC (Fig. 6-8, *A* and *B*).
3. *Bigeminy* occurs when every other QRS complex is a PVC. This rate of occurrence is more serious than quadrigeminy or trigeminy because it usually means a higher degree of irritability in the ventricular muscle (Fig. 6-9).

   NOTE: To identify bigeminy, trigeminy, and quadrigeminy in the clinical setting, there must be at least three episodes in a row on the monitor or rhythm strip.

4. *Couplet* (paired) describes two PVCs in a row that are not separated by a complex of the underlying rhythm (Fig. 6-10).

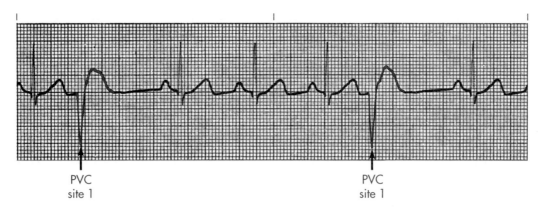

FIG. 6-5 Unifocal premature ventricular contractions.

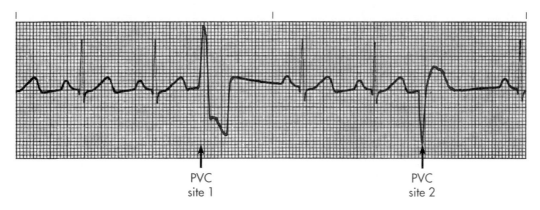

FIG. 6-6 Multifocal premature ventricular contractions.

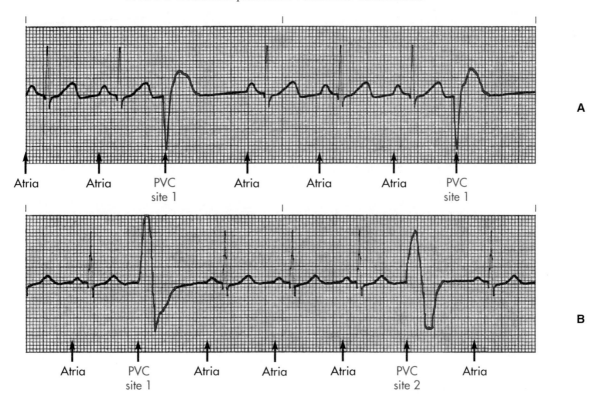

FIG. 6-7 Quadrigeminy. **A,** Sinus rhythm with unifocal quadrigeminy premature ventricular contractions; heart rate, 70. **B,** Sinus rhythm with multifocal quadrigeminy premature ventricular contractions; heart rate, 70.

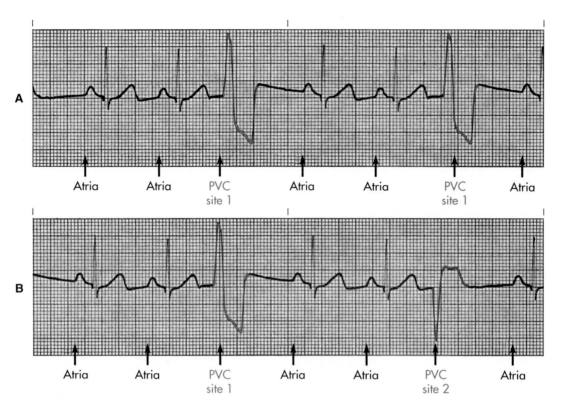

FIG. 6-8 Trigeminy. **A,** Sinus rhythm with an episode of unifocal trigeminy premature ventricular contractions; heart rate, 60-70. **B,** Sinus rhythm with an episode of multifocal trigeminy premature ventricular contractions; heart rate, 70.

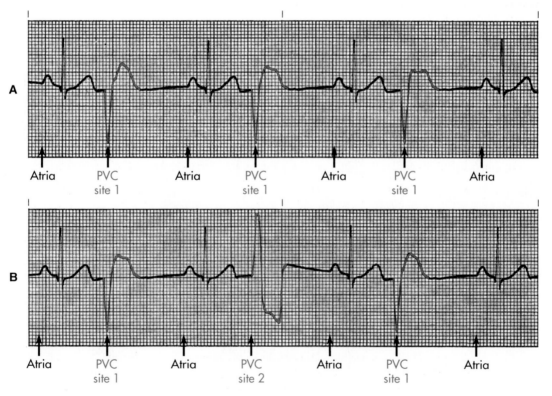

FIG. 6-9 Bigeminy. **A,** Sinus rhythm with an episode of unifocal bigeminy premature ventricular contractions; heart rate, 70. **B,** Sinus rhythm with multifocal bigeminy premature ventricular contractions; heart rate, 70.

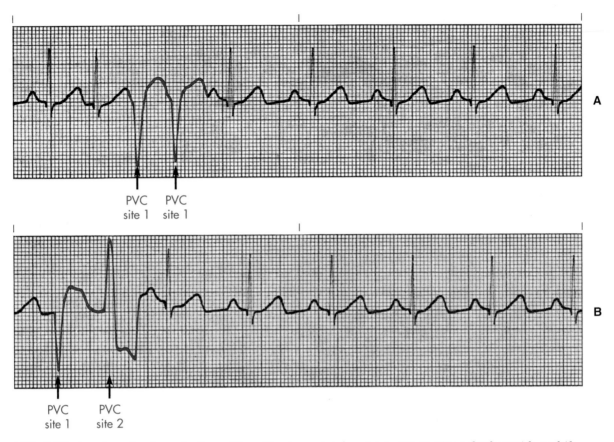

FIG. 6-10 Couplets. **A,** Sinus rhythm with unifocal couplet; heart rate, 90. **B,** Sinus rhythm with multifocal couplet; heart rate, 80.

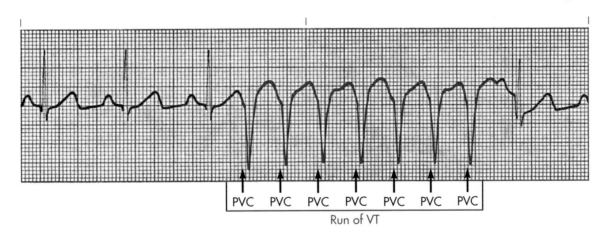

FIG. 6-11 Sinus rhythm with a run of ventricular tachycardia; heart rate, 110.

5. *Run of ventricular tachycardia* (run of VT) occurs when three or more PVCs occur in a row, not separated by a QRS complex of the underlying rhythm. A run of VT is of short duration, and the PVCs are usually all unifocal. Both couplets and runs of ventricular tachycardia indicate a high degree of irritability in the ventricles and may lead to a lethal dysrhythmia (Fig. 6-11). A run of VT may be called a *salvo* or *burst* of PVCs.

R on T Phenomenon

R on T phenomenon (R on T) is an additional term used to describe PVCs. It occurs when the R wave of the PVC falls on the T wave of the previous complex. R on T phenomenon may lead to a lethal dysrhythmia, such as ventricular tachycardia (V Tach), since the PVC occurs during the vulnerable period of ventricular repolarization (Fig. 6-12). This vulnerable period is also called the *relative refractory period,* and is the time during the cardiac cycle when cardiac cells have repolarized to the point that some cells can be stimulated to contract again, if the stimulus is strong enough (see Chapter 2).

Other Aspects

Patients with PVCs do not always require treatment. PVCs may be the heart's attempt to increase the cardiac rate to maintain adequate circulation and cardiac output, when the rate of the underlying rhythm is bradycardic. However, PVCs are usually considered dangerous, and patients may require immediate treatment, if one or more of the following occur:

1. More than six PVCs on a 1-minute rhythm strip
2. Multifocal PVCs
3. Couplets
4. Run of VT
5. R on T phenomenon
6. A patient who is medically unstable

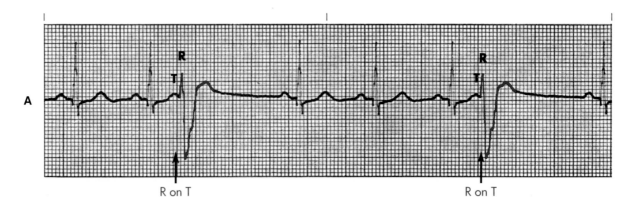

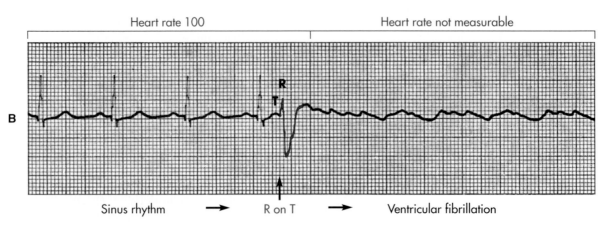

FIG. 6-12 R on T phenomenon. **A,** Sinus rhythm with unifocal premature ventricular contractions with R on T; heart rate, 80. **B,** Sinus rhythm; heart rate, 100, with an R on T premature ventricular contraction, progressing to ventricular fibrillation (heart rate not measurable).

When assessing the patient's condition, it is also important to remember that the patient's pulse may not match the heart rate seen on the monitor because of the following factors:

1. The ventricular muscle cells may not have repolarized enough to respond to the electrical impulse of the PVC and to contract effectively.
2. The PVC may not allow the ventricles to refill with enough blood to be felt as a pulse when the left ventricle contracts.

Because a PVC may or may not actually produce a pulse, it is **essential** to assess the patient and not rely on the monitor alone. This assessment will determine the patient's tolerance of the dysrhythmia and the possible need for immediate treatment.

PVCs can be caused by heart disease, myocardial infarction, or stimulants such as caffeine or nicotine. Stress and anxiety can also cause PVCs.

VENTRICULAR TACHYCARDIA

Ventricular tachycardia (VT, V Tach) is a dysrhythmia that usually originates from a single site in the ventricles at a rate of 101 to 250 electrical impulses per minute (Fig. 6-13). A ventricular tachycardia with a rate of 41 to 100 is considered a *slow ventricular tachycardia* or an accelerated idioventricular dysrhythmia. However, because the inherent rate of the ventricles is 20 to 40 electrical impulses per minute, any ventricular rate greater than 40 can be considered ventricular tachycardia.

P waves, if present, are from the underlying rhythm, not the ventricular tachycardia. PR intervals and P to P intervals are not measurable.

The QRS complex is wide, bizarre, and measures greater than 0.12 second. The R to R interval is usually regular, although it may be slightly irregular (Fig. 6-14).

This dysrhythmia starts suddenly and is frequently triggered by a PVC. Although the definition of ventricular tachycardia is more than three PVCs in a row, VT that lasts 30 seconds or less is usually called *unsustained VT* or a *run of VT,* while *sustained* (prolonged) ventricular tachycardia is longer than 30 seconds.

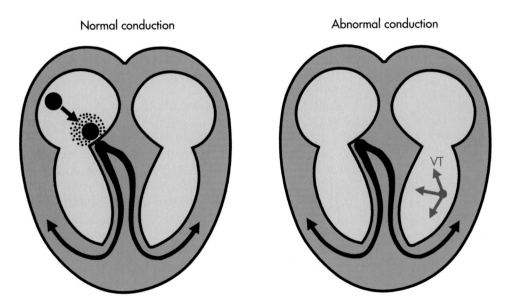

Normal conduction   Abnormal conduction

FIG. 6-13 *Left heart* shows normal electrical conduction pathway. *Right heart* shows conduction pathway of ventricular tachycardia.

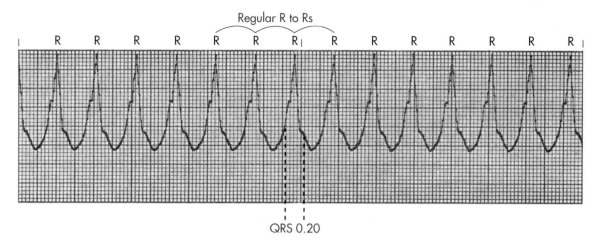

FIG. 6-14 Ventricular tachycardia with regular R to R intervals and QRS greater than 0.12 second; heart rate, 140 to 150.

Ventricular tachycardia is a **life-threatening** dysrhythmia. As the heart rate increases, the ventricles do not have time to completely empty and refill. Therefore cardiac output is decreased, and adequate amounts of blood are not circulated to vital organs, such as the heart and brain.

Patient symptoms vary, depending on the duration of the ventricular tachycardia. For example, with a run of VT, the patient may feel slightly weak or complain of occasional "palpitations" or a "racing heart." However, in *sustained VT* the patient's condition usually becomes unstable, leading to unresponsiveness and **loss of pulse,** requiring immediate treatment. Again, the patient **must** be assessed frequently to determine the patient's tolerance of the dysrhythmia and the appropriate treatment.

Ventricular tachycardia may be the result of increased irritability within the ventricles, which can be caused by myocardial infarction, advanced heart disease, severe ischemia, electrical shock, or drugs such as epinephrine or digitalis.

TORSADES DE POINTES

Torsades de pointes is a dysrhythmia that looks similar to ventricular tachycardia. The dysrhythmia originates from the ventricles, but it is unclear whether it is from a single site or multiple sites.

Unlike VT, the wave amplitude (height) of torsades de pointes begins close to the baseline, gradually increasing and decreasing in a repeating pattern. The rhythm resembles a twisting and turning motion along the baseline (Fig. 6-15). It is important to determine if the dysrhythmia is ventricular tachycardia or torsades de pointes because each of these dysrhythmias is treated differently (see Chapter 9).

This dysrhythmia usually starts suddenly and is frequently preceded by a prolonged QT interval; more than one half the R to R interval of that complex and the R wave of the following complex (see Chapter 2). P waves, if seen, are from the underlying rhythm, not the torsades de pointes. PR intervals and P to P intervals are not measurable. The QRS complex is wide, bizarre, and greater than 0.12 second. The R to R interval is usually regular, although it may be slightly irregular. The ventricular rate is often greater than 150 electrical impulses per minute.

The duration of the torsades de pointes will affect the patient's tolerance of the dysrhythmia. If the torsades de pointes lasts only a few seconds, the patient may complain of symptoms such as slight weakness, occasional palpitations, or a "rac-

Increasing amplitude   Decreasing amplitude

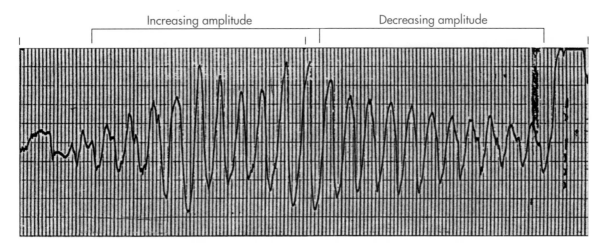

FIG. 6-15 Torsade de pointes; heart rate, 240 to 250.

ing heart." However, a torsades de pointes with a longer duration usually leads to an unstable condition, with signs and symptoms of poor cardiac output such as low blood pressure, unresponsiveness, and **loss of pulse.**

Torsades de pointes is a **life-threatening** dysrhythmia. As the heart rate increases, the ventricles do not have enough time to completely empty and refill. Therefore, good cardiac output is not maintained, and adequate amounts of blood and oxygen are **not** circulated to the vital organs, such as the heart and brain.

Patient assessment **must** be performed frequently to determine the patient's tolerance of the dysrhythmia and the proper treatment protocol.

Some common causes of torsades de pointes include myocardial infarction, severe heart disease, or drugs that prolong the QT interval, such as lidocaine or procainamide.

VENTRICULAR FIBRILLATION

Ventricular fibrillation (V Fib, VF) is a **lethal** dysrhythmia that originates from many different sites within the ventricles (Fig. 6-16). Because so many ventricular sites initiate electrical impulses, the cardiac cells do not have time to completely depolarize and repolarize. Therefore electrical impulses are not transmitted through **any** conduction pathway of the heart.

Neither the atria nor the ventricles depolarize; therefore P waves, QRS complexes, PR intervals, P to P intervals, and R to R intervals are **not** present. Only a chaotic, wavy line is seen on the monitor or rhythm strip. Because QRS complexes are not seen, it is impossible to measure a heart rate (Fig. 6-17).

The ventricles make ineffective quivering movements, not actual contractions. Consequently, blood is not being pumped throughout the body, and the patient **does not** have a pulse. Death will occur if treatment is not begun immediately.

Ventricular fibrillation is described as either coarse or fine. The *coarse V Fib* waves have a higher amplitude (height) and are more irregular than the *fine V Fib* waves. This difference indicates that a greater number of cardiac cells are able to respond to the electrical stimulation. Coarse V Fib may progress to fine V Fib, which responds less easily to treatment (Fig. 6-18).

Fine ventricular fibrillation waves have less amplitude, indicating fewer cardiac cells are able to respond to an electrical impulse (Fig. 6-19).

Normal conduction   Abnormal conduction

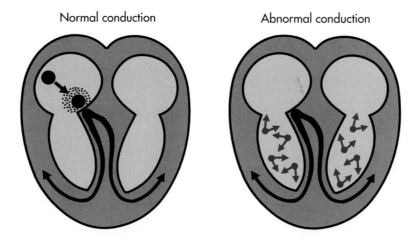

FIG. 6-16 *Left heart* shows normal electrical conduction pathway. *Right heart* shows conduction pathway of ventricular fibrillation.

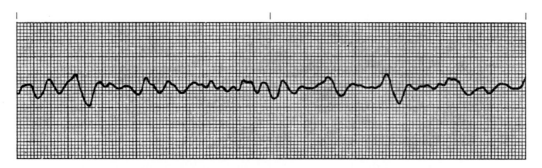

FIG. 6-17 Coarse ventricular fibrillation; heart rate, not measurable.

Coarse ventricular fibrillation   Fine ventricular fibrillation

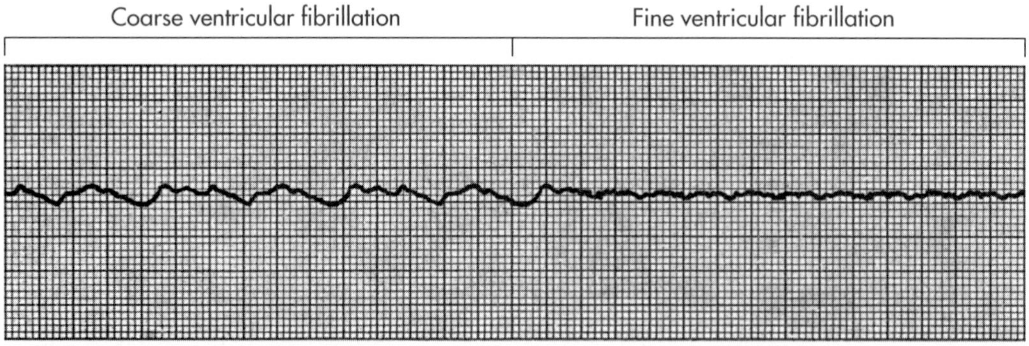

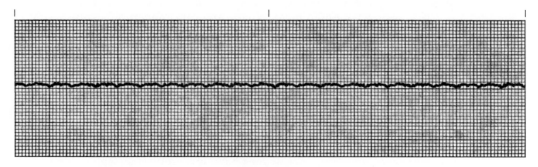

FIG. 6-18 Coarse ventricular fibrillation progressing to fine ventricular fibrillation; heart rate, not measurable.

FIG. 6-19 Fine ventricular fibrillation; heart rate, not measurable.

Ventricular fibrillation is usually the result of severe heart disease, electrical shock, or drug toxicity. Patients with this dysrhythmia **do not** have a pulse and require **immediate** treatment.

> NOTE OF CAUTION: Assessment of the patient before beginning treatment is very important, because loose leads or artifact can mimic this dysrhythmia on the monitor screen or rhythm strip.

IDIOVENTRICULAR/AGONAL DYSRHYTHMIA

Idioventricular dysrhythmia (agonal or dying heart) is a **lethal** dysrhythmia that usually originates from a single site in the ventricles.

The atria, AV junction, bundle of His, and bundle branches can no longer function as pacemakers. This is the **final attempt** of the cardiac conduction system to initiate an electrical impulse from the ventricular muscle. However, the cardiac muscle is so damaged that it **cannot** respond effectively (Fig. 6-20).

The atria do not depolarize. Therefore P waves, PR intervals, and P to P intervals are not present. Ventricular depolarization is slow and ineffective, causing the QRS complexes to be very wide and bizarre, measuring more than 0.12 second (Fig. 6-21, *A*). The R to R intervals may be irregular.

The ventricular rate of an idioventricular dysrhythmia is usually less than 40 electrical impulses per minute. (If the rate is 41 to 100 electrical impulses per minute, the dysrhythmia is known as *accelerated idioventricular dysrhythmia* or *slow ventricular tachycardia*.) When the ventricular rate becomes less than 20 electrical impulses per minute, the rhythm is known as *agonal* (dying heart) dysrhythmia (Fig. 6-21, *B*). As the ventricles weaken and their electrical impulses become slower, the QRS complexes progressively show less amplitude and become wider, until **all** cardiac electrical activity stops.

The heart muscle is so damaged that cardiac contractions are ineffective, and cardiac output is so poor that oxygen is not reaching the body cells in sufficient amounts to maintain life. Both idioventricular and agonal dysrhythmias are **lethal** dysrhythmias, and treatment **must** be started immediately.

These dysrhythmias are usually seen in the end stage of advanced heart disease.

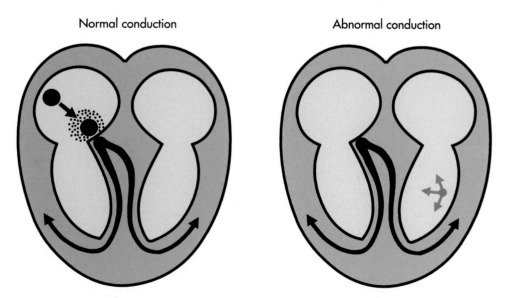

Normal conduction   Abnormal conduction

FIG. 6-20 *Left heart* shows normal electrical conduction pathway. *Right heart* shows conduction pathway of idioventricular/agonal dysrhythmia.

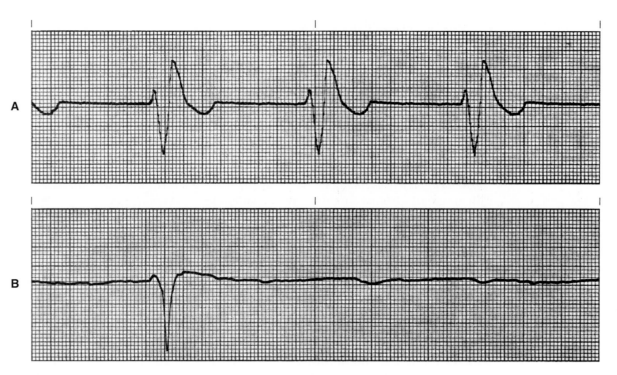

FIG. 6-21 A, Idioventricular rhythm; ventricular heart rate, 30. **B,** Agonal dysrhythmia; ventricular heart rate, 10.

VENTRICULAR STANDSTILL

Ventricular standstill occurs when only atrial depolarization exists and there is no ventricular depolarization (Fig. 6-22).

P waves are present, and the P to P intervals are regular. The ventricles do not depolarize; therefore QRS complexes, PR intervals, and R to R intervals are not present (Fig. 6-23).

The atrial heart rate usually varies from 60 to 100 electrical impulses per minute; however, the ventricular rate is 0. Because the ventricles do **not** depolarize, there is **no** ventricular contraction. Blood **does not** circulate to any part of the body. The patient **does not** have a pulse. This dysrhythmia is **lethal** and requires **immediate** treatment.

Ventricular standstill may be the result of third-degree heart block, massive myocardial infarction, or a ventricular rupture.

ASYSTOLE

Asystole occurs when there is a complete lack of electrical activity in both the atria and the ventricles. Therefore the atria and ventricles do not depolarize (Fig. 6-24).

No P waves, PR intervals, QRS complexes, P to P intervals, or R to R intervals exist. Asystole appears as a slightly wavy or straight line on the monitor screen or rhythm strip (Fig. 6-25). Because it may be difficult to distinguish asystole from very fine V Fib, two different leads should be used to confirm asystole, for example, Lead II and MCL I (see Chapter 2).

This dysrhythmia is **lethal.** The patient will **not** have a pulse, and **immediate** assessment and treatment are required.

Asystole usually follows untreated VT or V Fib. It may also be caused by massive myocardial infarction, advanced cardiac disease, or electrical shock.

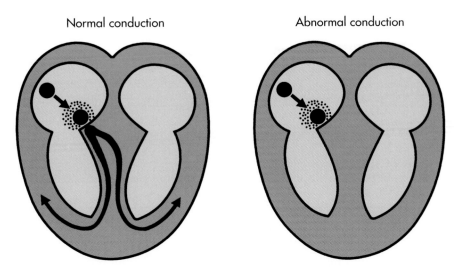

FIG. 6-22 *Left heart* shows normal electrical conduction pathway. *Right heart* shows conduction pathway of ventricular standstill.

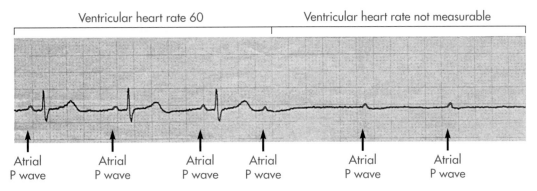

FIG. 6-23 Sinus rhythm changing into ventricular standstill; atrial heart rate, 80; ventricular heart rate, 60, going into atrial heart rate 40; ventricular heart rate, not measurable.

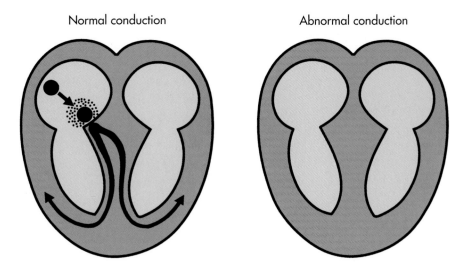

FIG. 6-24 *Left heart* shows normal electrical conduction pathway. *Right heart* shows conduction pathway of asystole.

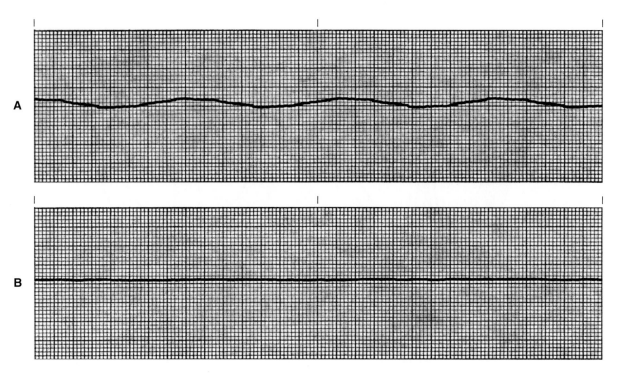

FIG. 6-25 Asystole. **A,** Lead II, slightly wavy line, possibly fine ventricular fibrillation. **B,** MCL I, straight line. Rhythm is asystole.

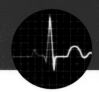

REVIEW QUESTIONS

TRUE FALSE   1. Ventricular tachycardia is a dysrhythmia that originates from many ventricular sites.

TRUE FALSE   2. Asystole occurs when there is no electrical activity in the atria or ventricles.

TRUE FALSE   3. PVCs are a common ventricular dysrhythmia and can occur in any cardiac rhythm.

TRUE FALSE   4. If two PVCs occur in a row, the dysrhythmia is called a run of VT.

TRUE FALSE   5. In ventricular fibrillation, the QRS complex usually measures greater than 0.12 second.

6. The heart rate of agonal dysrhythmia is usually less than _____ electrical impulses per minute.

7. Explain the difference between the appearance of ventricular tachycardia and torsades de pointes on the monitor or rhythm strip. _____ _____

8. Define the following terms:
   a. Multifocal PVCs _____
   b. Couplet _____
   c. Bigeminy _____

9. List three causes of ventricular fibrillation:
   a. _____
   b. _____
   c. _____

10. In an idioventricular dysrhythmia, the heart rate usually varies from:
    a. The heart rate cannot be measured
    b. 20 to 40 electrical impulses per minute
    c. 60 to 100 electrical impulses per minute
    d. 80 to 100 electrical impulses per minute

11. The QRS complex of a PVC usually measures:
    a. 0.04 to 0.08 second
    b. 0.04 to 0.12 second
    c. Less than 0.12 second
    d. Greater than 0.12 second

12. The rate of a rhythm containing a PVC varies, depending on the underlying rhythm and the:
    a. Cause of the PVC in the underlying rhythm
    b. Site of origin of the PVC
    c. Width of the QRS complex
    d. Number of PVCs in the underlying rhythm

RHYTHM STRIP REVIEW

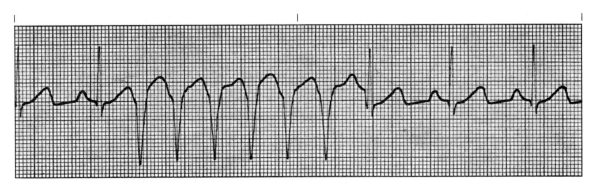

1. MEASURE: PR interval _____ Rhythm _____
   QRS complex _____ Heart rate _____
   INTERPRETATION: _____

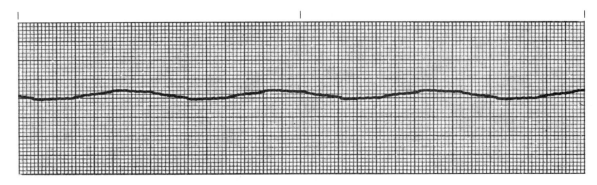

2. MEASURE: PR interval _____ Rhythm _____
   QRS complex _____ Heart rate _____
   INTERPRETATION: _____

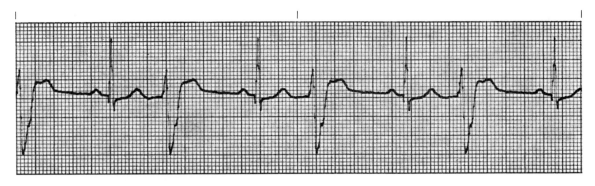

3. MEASURE: PR interval _____ Rhythm _____
   QRS complex _____ Heart rate _____
   INTERPRETATION: _____

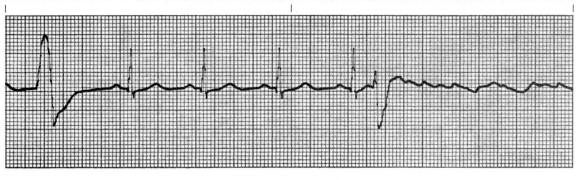

4. MEASURE: PR interval _____ Rhythm _____
                 QRS complex _____ Heart rate _____
INTERPRETATION: _____

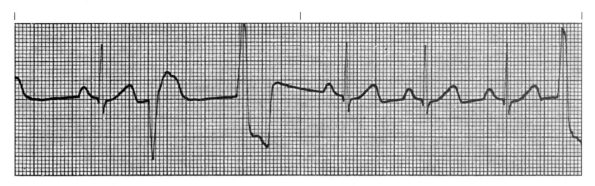

5. MEASURE: PR interval _____ Rhythm _____
                 QRS complex _____ Heart rate _____
INTERPRETATION: _____

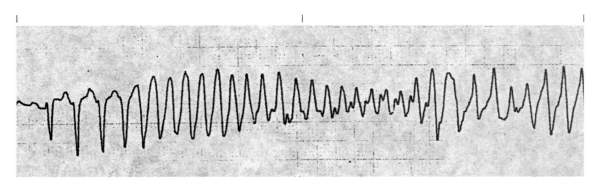

6. MEASURE: PR interval _____ Rhythm _____
                 QRS complex _____ Heart rate _____
INTERPRETATION: _____

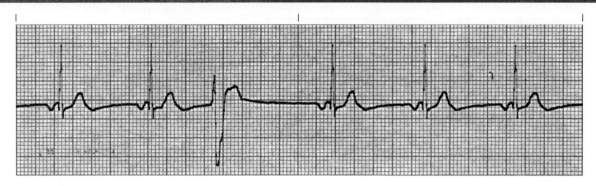

7. MEASURE: PR interval _____ Rhythm _____

                QRS complex _____ Heart rate _____

INTERPRETATION: _____

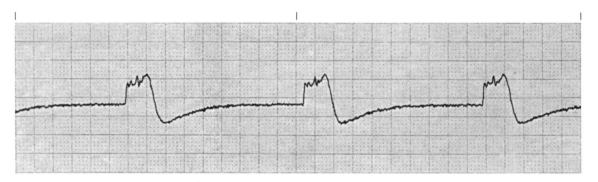

8. MEASURE: PR interval _____ Rhythm _____

                QRS complex _____ Heart rate _____

INTERPRETATION: _____

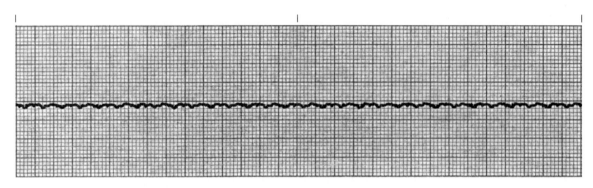

9. MEASURE: PR interval _____ Rhythm _____

                QRS complex _____ Heart rate _____

INTERPRETATION: _____

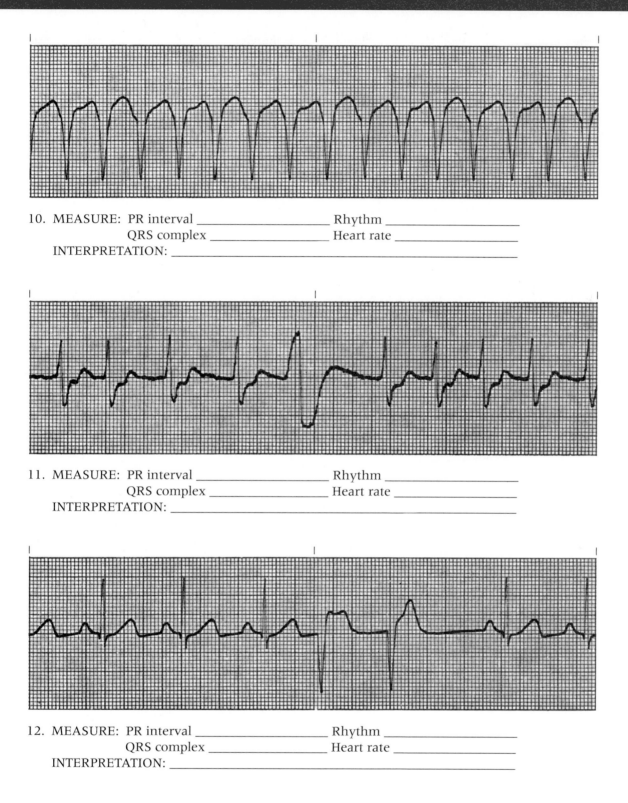

10. MEASURE: PR interval _____ Rhythm _____
                  QRS complex _____ Heart rate _____
     INTERPRETATION: _____

11. MEASURE: PR interval _____ Rhythm _____
                  QRS complex _____ Heart rate _____
     INTERPRETATION: _____

12. MEASURE: PR interval _____ Rhythm _____
                  QRS complex _____ Heart rate _____
     INTERPRETATION: _____

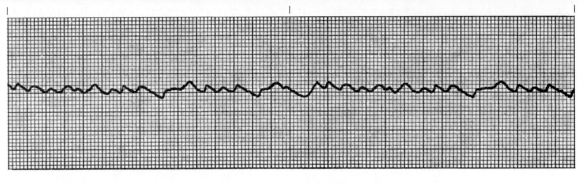

13. MEASURE: PR interval _____ Rhythm _____

                 QRS complex _____ Heart rate _____

        INTERPRETATION: _____

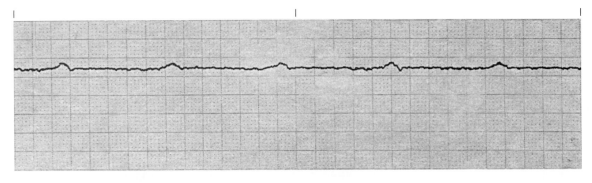

14. MEASURE: PR interval _____ Rhythm _____

                 QRS complex _____ Heart rate _____

        INTERPRETATION: _____

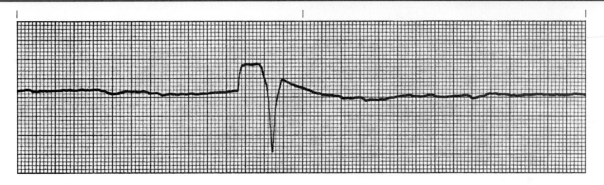

15. MEASURE: PR interval _____ Rhythm _____
                QRS complex _____ Heart rate _____
      INTERPRETATION: _____

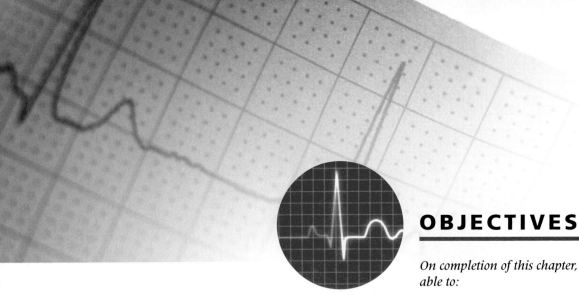

OBJECTIVES

On completion of this chapter, the reader should be able to:

1 Describe an escape beat and an escape rhythm, including measurements of all components.

2 Describe an aberrantly conducted complex.

3 Explain pulseless electrical activity.

4 Explain the difference between permanent and temporary pacemakers and the indications for the use of each type.

5 Explain the differences between atrial, ventricular, and sequential pacemakers.

6 Define capture and pacing and give examples of 50% pacing and 75% capture.

7 Describe an automatic implantable cardioverter defibrillator and its use.

8 Describe an automated external defibrillator and its use.

"FUNNY LOOKING" BEATS (FLBs)

OUTLINE

DEFINITIONS

AED Automated external defibrillator; a temporary device that determines the patient's cardiac rhythm and defibrillates the heart, if necessary

AICD Automatic implantable cardioverter defibrillator; a surgically implanted device that delivers programmed electrical impulses when the heart rate becomes too rapid

Capture The ability of the cardiac muscle cells to conduct the electrical impulses generated by a mechanical pacemaker

Cardiac Tamponade Blood or extra fluid in the pericardial sac

Defibrillation Procedure that uses measured electrical current to correct V Fib and pulseless V Tach

Escape Beat An electrical impulse that "escapes" from a site other than the sinoatrial node and causes ventricular depolarization

"Funny Looking" Beats Informal term for complexes that do not follow the usual patterns

Mechanical Pacemaker Small, battery-operated device that initiates electrical impulses in the heart; may be temporary or permanent

Pacing The percentage of complexes generated by a mechanical pacemaker, as seen on a monitor or rhythm strip

Pulseless Electrical Activity Complex formations are seen on a monitor, but the heart muscle is not contracting

Shock Informal term used to mean defibrillation

"FUNNY LOOKING" BEATS

Some complexes and wave formations do not fall into any of the specific patterns discussed in the previous chapters. In many parts of the United States, the slang expression for these complexes is *"funny looking beats"* or *FLBs.*

ESCAPE BEATS

When the cardiac electrical conduction system is interrupted for a brief period of time (sinus arrest) or when the heart rate is bradycardic, an impulse may "escape" from a site other than the sinoatrial (SA) node and cause depolarization of the myocardium. This electrical impulse is called an *escape beat* (Fig. 7-1).

An escape beat is one way the heart tries to maintain a normal rate or rhythm. For example, if the inherent heart rate of the SA node falls below 60, an electrical impulse may be initiated from outside the SA node. This escape beat is the heart's attempt to maintain normal cardiac output by increasing the heart rate. The escape beat will usually occur later than the next expected complex of the underlying rhythm, but it may be premature. The complex that ends a sinus arrest or sinus exit block is an example of an escape beat.

An escape beat may originate from the atria, the atrioventricular (AV) junction, or the ventricles and is named by the approximate point of origin. The rate of a rhythm containing an escape beat will vary, depending on the underlying rhythm and the number of escape beats.

Atrial escape beats can originate from anywhere in the atria, except the SA node, and usually meet the same criteria as other atrial complexes: an upright P wave before the QRS complex, a PR interval of 0.12 to 0.20 second, and a QRS complex of less than 0.12 second. An atrial complex that ends a sinus arrest or sinus exit block is usually the only atrial complex referred to as an *escape beat* (Fig. 7-2, *A*).

If the SA node and atria fail to generate an electrical impulse or if the impulse is not conducted, the AV junctional area can initiate an electrical impulse that "escapes" to increase the heart rate. This impulse is a *junctional escape beat* and will have the same characteristics as all junctional complexes. The P wave is either inverted, hidden, or retrograde, and the QRS complex is usually less than 0.12 second (Fig. 7-2, *B*).

If the SA node, the atria, and the AV junction fail to generate an electrical impulse or the heart rate falls below the junctional inherent rate of 40, a *ventricular escape beat* may be initiated from anywhere in the ventricles. As with all other ventricular complexes, the QRS complex of a ventricular escape beat is greater than 0.12 second and a P wave is usually not seen.

An escape beat can either remain a single complex or progress to an escape rhythm, if the myocardial pacemaker cells do not initiate enough electrical impulses to maintain an adequate cardiac output. Junctional tachycardia and idioventricular dysrhythmias are examples of escape rhythms.

ABERRANTLY CONDUCTED COMPLEXES

An *aberrantly conducted complex* is formed when an electrical impulse is generated above the bundle of His and travels through the bundle branches in an abnormal manner. This causes one ventricle to repolarize at a slower rate than the other. One ventricle is then able to accept an electrical impulse causing depolarization earlier than the other ventricle, resulting in a QRS complex that resembles a bundle branch block.

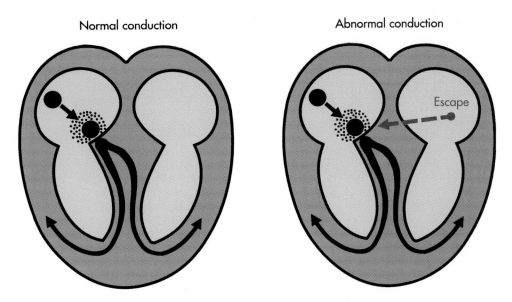

Normal conduction   Abnormal conduction

FIG. 7-1 *Left heart* shows normal electrical conduction pathway. *Right heart* shows conduction pathway of an atrial escape beat.

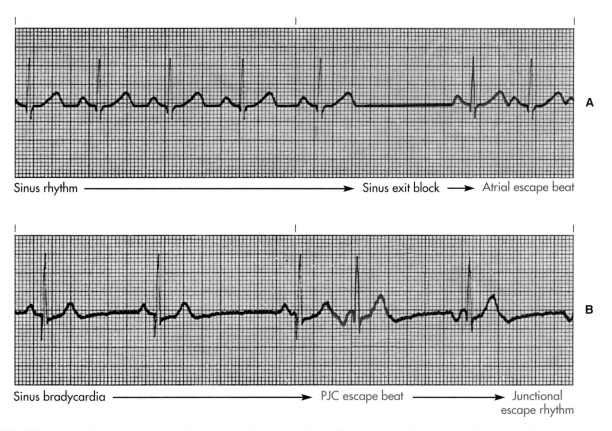

Sinus rhythm ⟶ Sinus exit block ⟶ Atrial escape beat

A

Sinus bradycardia ⟶ PJC escape beat ⟶ Junctional escape rhythm

B

FIG. 7-2 Escape beats and escape rhythm. **A,** Sinus rhythm with sinus exit block ended by an atrial escape beat. **B,** Sinus bradycardia with premature junctional contraction (PJC) escape beat beginning a junctional escape rhythm.

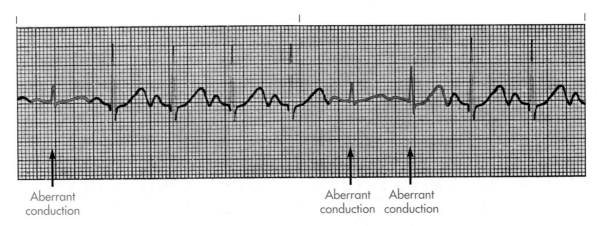

Aberrant
conduction

Aberrant
conduction

Aberrant
conduction

FIG. 7-3 Aberrantly conducted complexes. Sinus rhythm with three aberrantly conducted complexes; heart rate, 90.

Aberrantly conducted complexes are individual complexes that appear different than the complexes of the underlying rhythm because they do not follow the same electrical conduction pathway as the underlying rhythm (Fig. 7-3).

Examples of aberrantly conducted complexes include the following:

1. An aberrantly conducted complex that has a negative QRS complex when the underlying rhythm has a positive QRS complex.
2. The QRS of the aberrantly conducted complex may be wider, narrower, or shorter than the complexes of the underlying rhythm.

Aberrantly conducted complexes can originate from anywhere in the atria, the AV junction, or the ventricles. The origin of the aberrantly conducted complex will determine its size and shape. Because most aberrant complexes have a wide QRS complex, they may be hard to distinguish from a bundle branch block. However, aberrantly conducted complexes usually occur as individual complexes, not entire rhythms.

The presence of P waves, PR intervals, and QRS complexes in the underlying rhythm varies. The rate and regularity of the rhythm containing the aberrantly conducted complex also vary, depending on the underlying rhythm.

PULSELESS ELECTRICAL ACTIVITY

Pulseless electrical activity (PEA) is the current term used to describe any dysrhythmia that shows the conduction of electrical impulses, without contraction of the myocardium. Electrical depolarization of cardiac cells appears to occur throughout the heart, but the patient **does not** have a pulse or blood pressure. Electromechanical dissociation (EMD) is an older term for PEA dysrhythmia.

Almost any cardiac rhythm may be seen on the monitor screen or rhythm strip. The rhythm usually appears bradycardic and may have either wide or narrow QRS complexes (Fig. 7-4).

Because the patient does not have a pulse and cardiac output has ceased, this dysrhythmia is **lethal,** and treatment **must** be started immediately. Patient assessment is the **only** means of determining the presence or absence of a pulse. The patient, **not** the monitor, must be treated.

Some types of pulseless electrical activity include idioventricular dysrhythmias, ventricular escape rhythms, and bradyasystolic (bradycardic rhythm without a pulse) dysrhythmias. These dysrhythmias all show complexes on the mon-

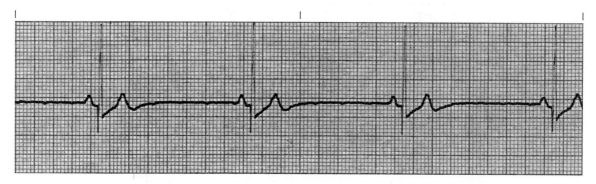

FIG. 7-4 Pulseless electrical activity. Rhythm strip shows sinus bradycardia (heart rate, 40), but the patient does not have a pulse.

itor screen indicating electrical activity. However, because there is **no mechanical** cardiac activity, blood is not being circulated and the patient does not have a pulse.

PEA may be caused by hypovolemia (loss of blood volume), hypoxia (decrease in oxygen), cardiac tamponade (blood or excess fluid in pericardial sac), or tension pneumothorax (air in the pleural cavity that prevents one lung from expanding). PEA may also occur when the cardiac muscle is too damaged to contract, although electrical impulses are still being conducted by the electrical conduction pathways.

NOTE: Remember, although pulseless electrical activity mimics other rhythms that would ordinarily have a pulse, there is <u>**NO pulse**</u> with PEA! You **must** assess the patient to determine the presence of a PEA dysrhythmia.

PACEMAKER RHYTHMS

Many dysrhythmias have bradycardic rates that are too slow to maintain a normal cardiac output. Other dysrhythmias may be too rapid to allow complete filling of the ventricles before each contraction, resulting in poor cardiac output and decreased circulation to the vital organs of the body. These are **lethal** dysrhythmias. Although many patients with these dysrhythmias respond to drug therapy, others will require assistance from an artificial pacemaker.

Pacemakers are small, battery-operated devices that initiate electrical impulses in the myocardium. The two main parts of a pacemaker are the generator and the leadwires (Fig. 7-5). The *generator* is a small box that initiates and controls the rate and strength of each electrical impulse. The *leadwire* has an electrode at its tip that transmits the electrical impulse from the generator to the myocardium.

TEMPORARY PACEMAKERS

Pacemakers may be either temporary or permanent. *Temporary pacemakers* are used to maintain a patient's heart rate in an emergency situation or until a permanent pacemaker can be surgically implanted.

There are two types of temporary pacemakers. Although the generator remains outside the patient's body with both types of pacemakers, the electrical impulse used to stimulate the cardiac muscle is delivered by two different means.

A method for delivery of the electrical impulse that has been used for many years is *transvenous* (through a vein). The leadwire is inserted through the skin and threaded through a large vein into the right atrium. The electrical impulse stimulates

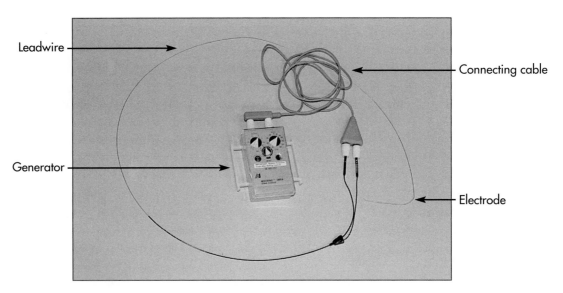

FIG. 7-5 External pacemaker generator, connecting cable, leadwire, and electrode.

the atrium and is then conducted through the cardiac electrical conduction pathway, causing depolarization (Fig. 7-6, *A*).

Another method is *transdermal* or *transcutaneous* (through the skin). This method uses two large pads as electrodes to conduct the electrical impulses. There are two leadwires, each connected to a pad. One pad is placed on the front of the patient's chest and the other pad on the patient's back (Fig. 7-6, *B*). The electrical impulses are then conducted through the body and heart, stimulating the entire cardiac muscle and causing depolarization of the cardiac cells to occur in a normal manner. Transdermal (transcutaneous) pacing has a great advantage. It is quickly and easily positioned and does not require piercing the patient's skin to position the electrodes.

All pacemakers can be preset to initiate electrical impulses in one of two ways:

1. Fixed—set to generate impulses at a constant rate, usually 72 to 80 impulses per minute.
2. Demand—set to generate electrical impulses only when the patient's heart rate falls below a predetermined rate, usually less than 70 beats per minute.

   NOTE: The terms *fire* and *pace* are often used in a clinical setting to mean the initiation of an electrical impulse from an artificial pacemaker.

PERMANENT PACEMAKERS

A *permanent pacemaker* is necessary when the patient's heart is unable to maintain a normal heart rate or a normal cardiac output, even with the aid of medications.

The generator of a permanent pacemaker is surgically implanted under the patient's skin, usually in the upper left chest or upper abdominal area. The leadwire is then inserted into the heart through a large vein (Fig. 7-7).

There are three main types of permanent pacemakers: atrial, ventricular, and sequential.

Atrial Pacemakers

The leadwire and electrode of an *atrial pacemaker* are inserted into the right atrium. The electrical impulse that is generated by the pacemaker stimulates the atria, then

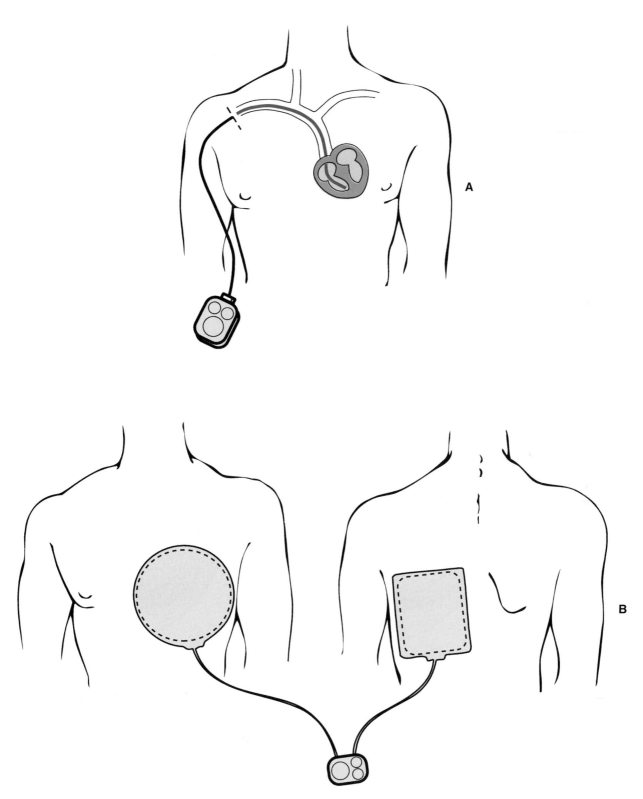

FIG. 7-6 **A,** Temporary transvenous pacemaker placement. **B,** Temporary transcutaneous (transdermal) pacemaker placement.

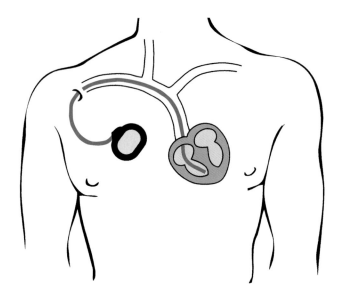

FIG. 7-7 Permanent pacemaker placement.

Normal conduction   Abnormal conduction

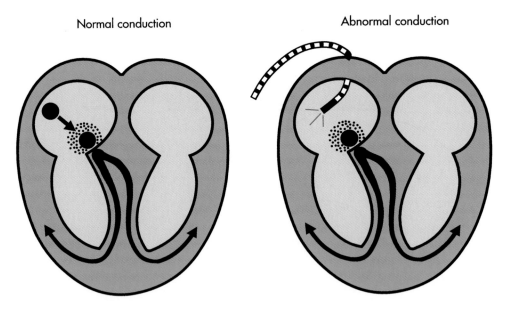

FIG. 7-8 *Left heart* shows normal electrical conduction pathway. *Right heart* shows conduction pathway of atrial pacemaker.

follows the normal electrical conduction pathway through the heart to the ventricles (Fig. 7-8).

The discharge of electrical energy from the pacemaker is represented on the rhythm strip by a vertical line, called a *pacer spike,* or *spike.* The pacer spike is usually followed by a P wave and a QRS complex, although the P wave may not be seen unless the electrode is positioned high in the right atrium (Fig. 7-9). The P wave that follows a pacer spike is usually not measured.

An atrial pacemaker can only be used if the AV junction and ventricular electrical conduction pathways are functioning. Atrial pacemakers are rarely used today because they are less efficient than ventricular or sequential pacemakers.

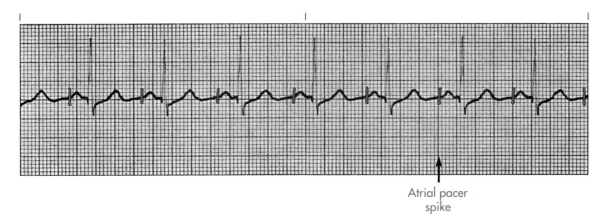

FIG. 7-9 Atrial pacemaker rhythm showing pacer spike.

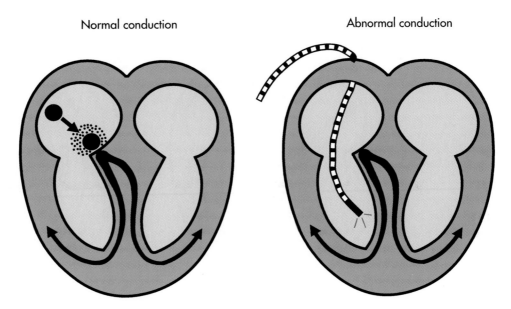

FIG. 7-10 *Left heart* shows normal electrical conduction pathway. *Right heart* shows conduction pathway of ventricular pacemaker.

Ventricular Pacemakers

With *ventricular pacemakers,* the leadwire and electrode may be placed in either the right atrium or the right ventricle (Fig. 7-10). The pacemaker impulse causes the depolarization of the ventricular muscle. The atria may not depolarize if they are extensively damaged.

A pacer spike, immediately followed by a QRS complex, will appear on the monitor screen or rhythm strip. Because the electrode is usually positioned low in the right ventricle, depolarization may not occur in a normal manner and the QRS is usually greater than 0.12 second (Fig. 7-11).

Sequential Pacemakers

One of the most commonly used type of pacemaker is the *sequential pacemaker.* The other two types of permanent pacemakers initiate depolarization of **either** the atria **or** the ventricles; however, the sequential pacemaker stimulates the depolarization of **both** the atria **and** the ventricles.

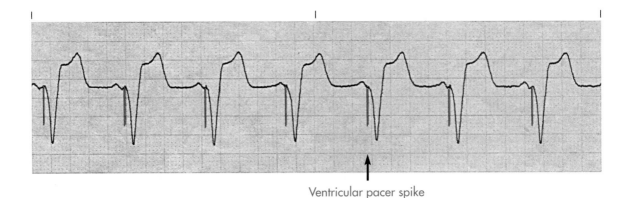

Ventricular pacer spike

FIG. 7-11 Ventricular pacemaker rhythm with pacer spikes.

Normal conduction   Abnormal conduction

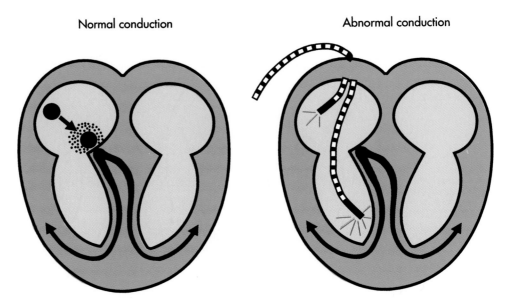

FIG. 7-12 *Left heart* shows normal electrical conduction pathway. *Right heart* shows conduction pathway of sequential pacemaker.

One type of sequential pacemaker has a leadwire with two electrodes, one positioned in the right atrium and one positioned in the right ventricle. The use of two electrodes allows the atria and the ventricles to depolarize in a normal sequential manner (Fig. 7-12).

The rhythm strip of a sequential pacemaker usually shows two pacer spikes before each QRS complex (Fig. 7-13). The spikes may occur so closely together that they appear as one long spike. The first spike represents the firing of the atrial electrode, and the second spike represents the firing of the ventricular electrode. A P wave may be seen, and the QRS is typically greater than 0.12 second.

CAPTURE AND PACING

When interpreting a pacemaker rhythm, the percentage of capture and the percentage of pacing must be determined.

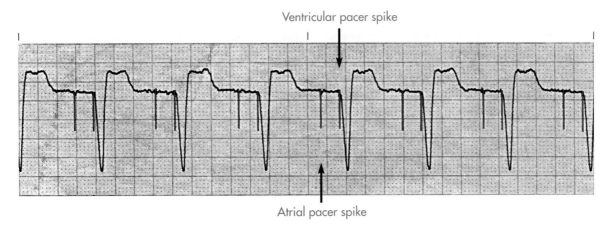

FIG. 7-13 Sequential pacemaker rhythm with two pacer spikes before each QRS complex.

Capture refers to the cardiac cell's ability to depolarize in response to the electrical impulse generated by a mechanical pacemaker. This depolarization is indicated by a P wave or QRS complex after **every** pacer spike. The presence of a QRS complex after a pacer spike **does not** always indicate the **contraction** of the myocardium, only the **conduction** of an electrical impulse through the cardiac muscle. The patient **must** be assessed to determine the presence of a pulse and adequate cardiac output.

The *percentage of capture* is determined by the number of pacer spikes that are followed by a complex in relationship to the total number of pacer spikes on the entire rhythm strip. For example, the rhythm strip will show 100% capture if every pacer spike is followed by a P wave or QRS complex (Fig. 7-14, *A*). If only 9 of 10 pacer spikes are followed by a complex, the rhythm strip will show 90% capture.

Loss of capture occurs when a QRS complex does not follow a pacer spike (Fig. 7-14, *B*). Loss of capture indicates that the electrical impulse generated by the artificial pacemaker has not been conducted and the cardiac cells have not depolarized. This situation may simply indicate that the voltage of the pacemaker electrical impulse needs to be increased. However, loss of capture may indicate that the myocardium is so damaged, it is unable to respond to every electrical impulse.

Pacing refers to the percentage of complexes generated by the mechanical pacemaker. For example, if every QRS complex is preceded by a pacer spike, the rhythm is 100% paced (Fig. 7-15, *A*). If a pacer spike occurs before only half of the QRS complexes, the strip is 50% paced (Fig. 7-15, *B*). QRS complexes that do not have a pacer spike are initiated by the patient's heart, not the mechanical pacemaker. These QRS complexes may appear normal or bizarre, depending on whether they follow the normal cardiac electrical conduction pathway.

The *percentage of pacing* depends on the pacemaking ability of the patient's own heart, as well as the type of pacemaker in use (demand or fixed-rate pacemaker).

The percentage of capture should **always** be 100%, regardless of the percent of pacing. For example, every pacer spike should be **followed** by a QRS complex. However, every QRS complex does **not** have to be **preceded** by a pacer spike. QRS complexes that appear without a pacer spike indicate that the patient's heart, not the mechanical pacemaker, has initiated the electrical impulse.

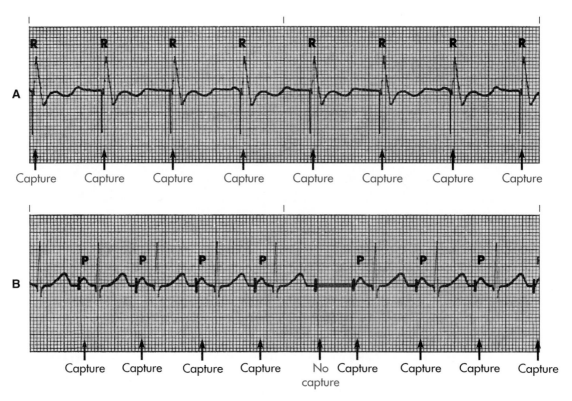

FIG. 7-14 Pacemaker capture. **A,** Ventricular pacemaker with 100% capture. **B,** Loss of capture; atrial pacemaker with 90% capture.

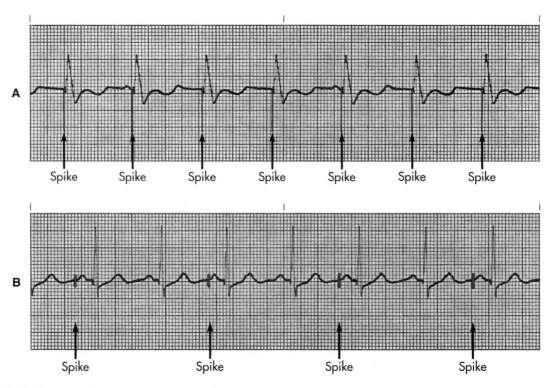

FIG. 7-15 Pacemaker pacing. **A,** Ventricular pacemaker with 100% pacing. **B,** Atrial pacemaker with 50% pacing.

AUTOMATIC IMPLANTABLE CARDIOVERTER DEFIBRILLATOR

Some potentially lethal dysrhythmias do not respond to mechanical pacing alone but also require defibrillation for immediate treatment. An *automatic implantable cardioverter defibrillator (AICD)* is one type of pacemaker/defibrillator available for this use. Although some AICDs do not pace the heart, they can all identify and treat some rapid lethal dysrhythmias, such as ventricular tachycardia.

The AICD unit is surgically implanted under the skin (similar to a pacemaker). Pads containing electrodes are sewn to the front and back of the heart muscle (Fig. 7-16, *A*), with electrodes or sensing units inserted into the ventricles (Fig. 7-16, *B*). The newest AICD offers the option of electrodes that can be inserted into the heart chambers through transvenous placement, instead of pads that require major surgery.

The AICD can be programmed to initiate low-voltage electrical impulses when the heart rate becomes rapid (more than 150). The impulse from the AICD attempts to force the heart into a normal rate. If the first electrical impulse from the AICD is not strong enough, the AICD may be programmed to increase the voltage and initiate an additional one to two impulses, raising the voltage slightly each time. The patient usually does not feel these mild electrical impulses.

If the patient's heart rate continues to increase, or if the rhythm becomes ventricular fibrillation or ventricular tachycardia, the AICD will deliver an electrical impulse that is strong enough for cardiac defibrillation ("shock"). This defibrillation is an attempt to allow the SA node to again initiate electrical impulses at a normal rate.

The AICD will continue to defibrillate the patient until the heart has recovered its normal rate or until the AICD is turned off by medical personnel.

The patient may complain of a feeling of being "kicked" in the chest while defibrillation is occurring. Anyone touching the patient while the AICD is defibrillating may feel a mild tingling sensation. The patient may "jump" or "jerk" slightly as an effect of the defibrillation.

On the monitor screen or rhythm strip, the firing of the AICD appears similar to a pacing spike, but it may have a greater amplitude.

Some of the newer models of AICDs can also temporarily pace bradycardic dysrhythmias that may occur after defibrillation.

AUTOMATED EXTERNAL DEFIBRILLATOR

The *automated external defibrillator (AED)* is a fairly new device that can increase the survival rate of people who have a cardiac arrest in the community. The AED provides a method of immediate treatment by trained nonmedical rescuers, before the arrival of 911 (emergency medical personnel). The AED senses and evaluates the patient's heart rhythm and rate. Then the machine either delivers the defibrillation or instructs the rescuer on what steps to take (Fig. 7-17).

Before attaching the AED, it is important to be sure that the patient is on a dry surface and not touching any metal objects. This is also an important precaution for the rescuer. If the patient is wearing a medication patch, such as nitroglycerin, remove it and wipe any moisture or medication from the chest.

The AED has two electrode pads and cables that are similar in appearance to telemetry electrodes and leadwires. The first electrode is attached to the skin, just below the collarbone on the patient's upper right chest. The second electrode is placed on the skin slightly beneath the left nipple. In a woman, the second electrode is placed beneath the left breast. Turn on the machine and ask everyone to

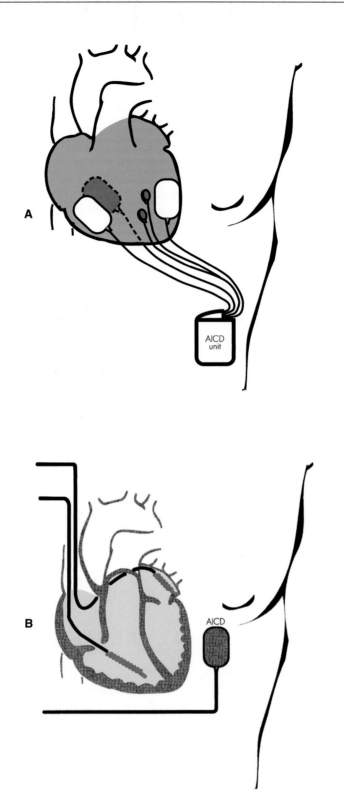

FIG. 7-16 AICD units. **A,** Electrode pads sewn onto heart muscle. **B,** Electrodes inserted into ventricles.

stand back from the patient. The device will then analyze the patient's cardiac rhythm and provide defibrillation, if needed. **Do not** let anyone **touch** the patient while the machine analyzes or defibrillates the patient.

The machine will then analyze the cardiac rhythm again and provide additional defibrillations, if necessary. The AED will also instruct the rescuer when to begin cardiopulmonary resuscitation (CPR), if required.

When the 911 medical personnel arrive, tell them how long the AED has been in use, if defibrillation was given (and how many times), and/or the length of time that CPR has been performed.

The AED has been used successfully in identifying and defibrillating rapid lethal dysrhythmias, such as ventricular fibrillation and pulseless ventricular tachycardia.

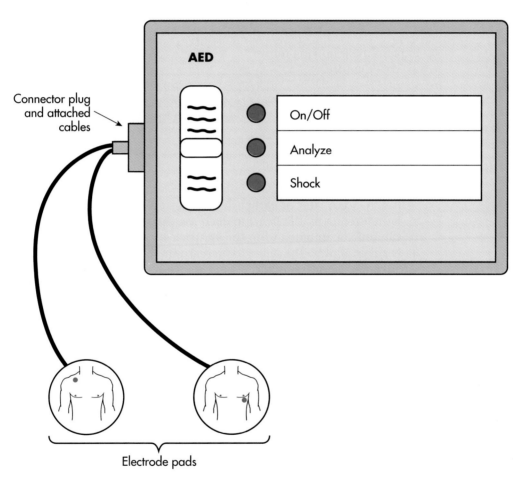

FIG. 7-17 AED unit.

REVIEW QUESTIONS

TRUE FALSE   1. Sequential pacemakers are used to stimulate either the atria or the ventricles.

TRUE FALSE   2. Escape beats are usually named for the approximate point of origin.

TRUE FALSE   3. The AED can only be used by trained medical personnel.

TRUE FALSE   4. PEA can only be identified on a 12-Lead electrocardiogram.

TRUE FALSE   5. The two types of pacemakers are permanent and implanted.

6. List the main parts of a mechanical pacemaker.
   a. _____
   b. _____
   c. _____

7. Explain the following terms:
   a. 75% Capture: _____
   _____
   _____

   b. 50% Paced: _____
   _____
   _____

8. An escape beat:
   a. occurs when a pacemaker fails and the next lower pacemaker "kicks in." It may occur later or earlier than expected.
   b. is an attempt by the heart to decrease the rate of a tachycardia.
   c. can only be initiated from the ventricles.
   d. is an attempt by the heart to increase the heart rate and maintain adequate cardiac output.
   (1) a, b, and c
   (2) b, c, and d
   (3) a and d
   (4) b and d

9. An AICD can automatically:
   a. decrease PJCs.
   b. control quadrigeminy PVCs.
   c. Identify and treat PEA.
   d. Recognize and defibrillate ventricular tachycardia.

10. An AED:
   a. is a device that can automatically sense the patient's rhythm and defibrillate, if necessary.
   b. should not be used if the patient is on wet ground or a rescuer is touching the patient.
   c. will instruct the rescuer when to begin CPR, if needed.
   d. all of the above.

11. An escape rhythm:
   a. may be the heart's attempt to increase the heart rate and improve cardiac output.
   b. is never from the junctional area.
   c. may be generated by any part of the heart, except the SA node.
   d. is the heart's attempt to slow ventricular tachycardia.
   (1) a and b
   (2) b and c
   (3) a and c
   (4) b and d

12. Define an aberrantly conducted complex.

   _____

   _____

13. List the three types of permanent artificial pacemakers and the area of the heart stimulated by each.
   a. _____
   b. _____
   c. _____

14. List two ways temporary pacemakers can be applied to a patient.
   a. _____
   b. _____

15. List two ways the heart rate can be set on pacemaker generators.
   a. _____
   b. _____

RHYTHM STRIP REVIEW

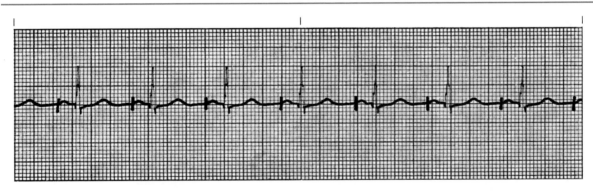

1. MEASURE: PR interval _____ Rhythm _____

   QRS complex _____ Heart rate _____

   INTERPRETATION: _____

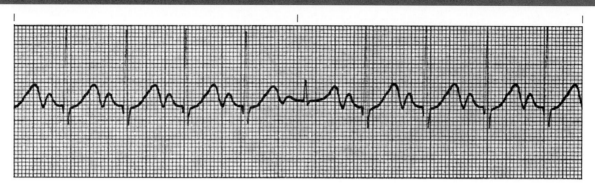

2. MEASURE: PR interval _____ Rhythm _____

               QRS complex _____ Heart rate _____

     INTERPRETATION: _____

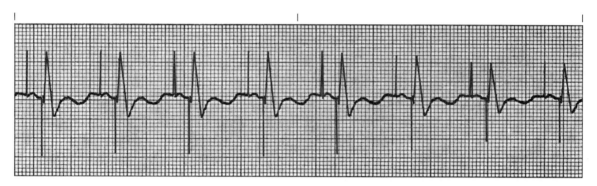

3. MEASURE: PR interval _____ Rhythm _____

               QRS complex _____ Heart rate _____

     INTERPRETATION: _____

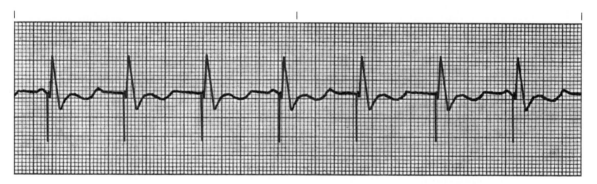

4. MEASURE: PR interval _____ Rhythm _____

               QRS complex _____ Heart rate _____

     INTERPRETATION: _____

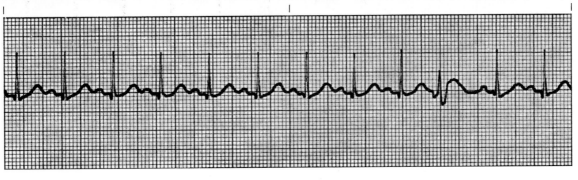

5. MEASURE: PR interval _____ Rhythm _____

QRS complex _____ Heart rate _____

INTERPRETATION: _____

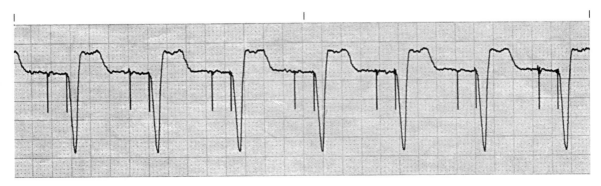

6. MEASURE: PR interval _____ Rhythm _____

QRS complex _____ Heart rate _____

INTERPRETATION: _____

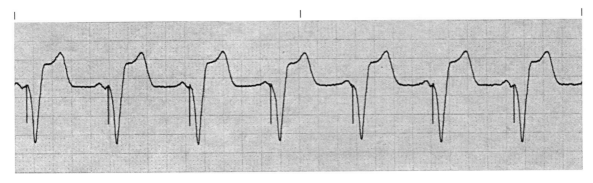

7. MEASURE: PR interval _____ Rhythm _____

QRS complex _____ Heart rate _____

INTERPRETATION: _____

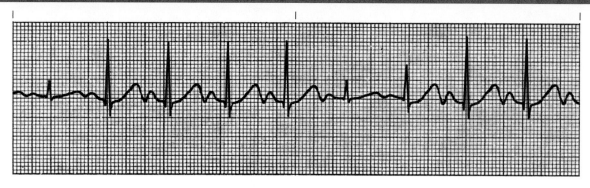

8. MEASURE: PR interval _____ Rhythm _____
QRS complex _____ Heart rate _____
INTERPRETATION: _____

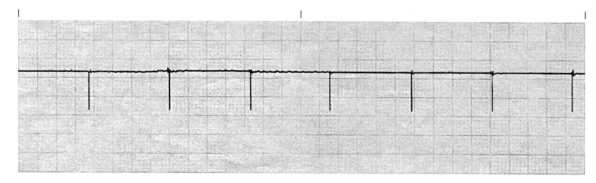

9. MEASURE: PR interval _____ Rhythm _____
QRS complex _____ Heart rate _____
INTERPRETATION: _____

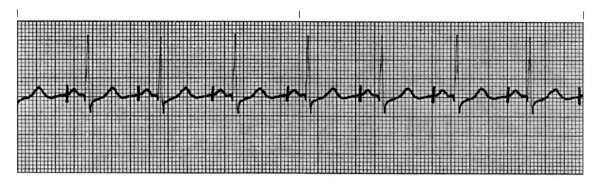

10. MEASURE: PR interval _____ Rhythm _____
QRS complex _____ Heart rate _____
INTERPRETATION: _____

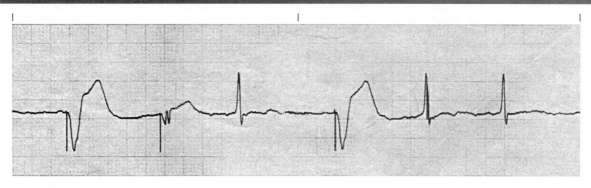

11. MEASURE: PR interval _____ Rhythm _____
    QRS complex _____ Heart rate _____
    INTERPRETATION: _____

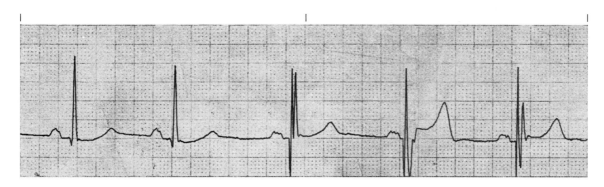

12. MEASURE: PR interval _____ Rhythm _____
    QRS complex _____ Heart rate _____
    INTERPRETATION: _____

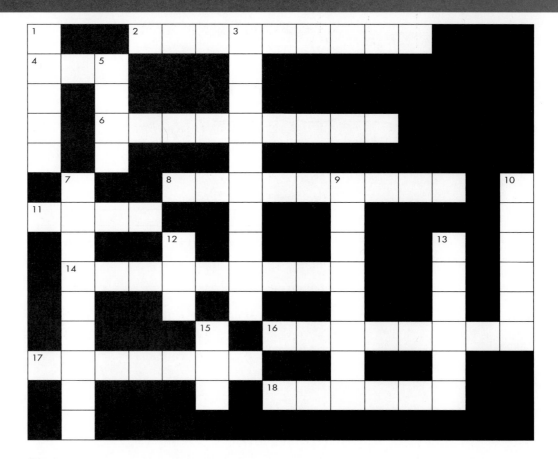

CROSSWORD PUZZLE CLUES

Across

2. Without a heartbeat

4. Lethal dysrhythmia

6. Moves from one place to another; transmitted

8. Mechanical pacemaker part; controls rate, and strength of impulses

11. Pulse or heart _____

14. _____ of the heart; SA node

16. _____ connect electrodes to a pacemaker

17. A complex appearing directly after a pacer spike indicates _____

18. May cause death

Down

1. Pacer _____ ; vertical line on monitor or rhythm strip

3. _____ pacemaker; stimulates both atria and ventricles

5. Defibrillator implanted under the skin

7. Not permanent

9. Single, abnormally conducted complex

10. Run away; get out of

12. Device that automatically defibrillates when necessary; used by trained nonmedical personnel

13. Pertaining to upper heart chambers

15. Complex showing depolarization of ventricles

```
G A U V H Y L X T H A P V C P N Q X H
E R J S E Q U E N T I A L P U V K K U
M A L G S B M Q E U H N Q B L G F I H
A L G H P P T T N F P X Q R S U D T U
L U R D O W U H A Y S P I K E D A U O
F C W R R B A G M H H I V N L K X L I
H I A W Z S R V R R P R K Z E I M G L
H R H D A C A B E R R A N T S L E Z W
Y T D E E T A E P C F E I V S G Y H Z
V N C F L C R P D B S C G C Z E S W U
N E V B O H A I T C E P E Y D L C G I
H V L R J Z J P A U I A N R O S T B H
I O T I U D P P S L R C E L U U B A Y
I V I L P D E O N O X E R J D Z W M X
M D F L D M R S T O K M A O W B E X Y
J Y Q A I W C V G G N A T N F Z C U W
U I W T L F E M K F F K O J C J F B F
O F L O P G N E L F K E R J Y K A X U
X Z X R H Y T H M Z F R N X Z U H N N
```

WORD PUZZLE

This word puzzle is designed to help familiarize you with some of the new terminology found in this chapter. Have fun finding all the words on this list. The words can be spelled forward (normally), backward, up, down, or diagonally in any direction. The words will always be in upper case and found in a straight line. Some phrases will not have any spaces between words; for example, P wave will appear as PWAVE. Good luck.

ABERRANT
AED
AICD
ATRIAL
CAPTURE
ESCAPE
GENERATOR
PACED
PACEMAKER
PEA

PERCENT
PERMANENT
PULSELESS
PWAVE
QRS
RHYTHM
SEQUENTIAL
SPIKE
TEMPORARY
VENTRICULAR

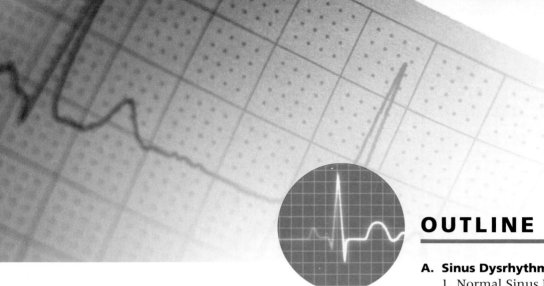

OUTLINE

CHAPTER 8

DYSRHYTHMIA REVIEW

This chapter is designed as a review of all the dysrhythmias discussed in Chapters 3 through 7. Each dysrhythmia is presented with a rhythm strip followed by the criteria for that dysrhythmia.

SINUS DYSRHYTHMIAS (Chapter 3)

NORMAL SINUS RHYTHM, p 49

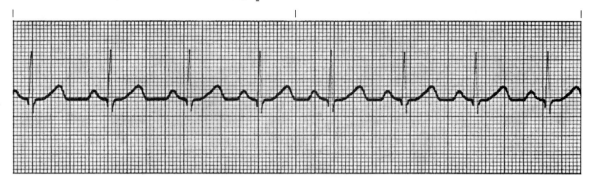

1. Site of origin: SA node
2. P wave: before every QRS; same size and shape
3. PR interval: 0.12 to 0.20 second
4. QRS: same size and shape; less than 0.12 second
5. Rhythm: (a) P to P interval: regular; (b) R to R interval: regular
6. Rate: 60 to 100

SINUS BRADYCARDIA, p 50

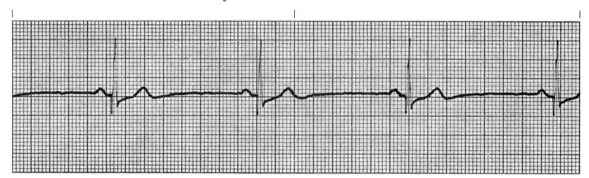

1. Site of origin: SA node
2. P wave: before every QRS; same size and shape
3. PR interval: 0.12 to 0.20 second
4. QRS: same size and shape; less than 0.12 second
5. Rhythm: (a) P to P interval: regular; (b) R to R interval: regular
6. Rate: less than 60

SINUS TACHYCARDIA, p 50

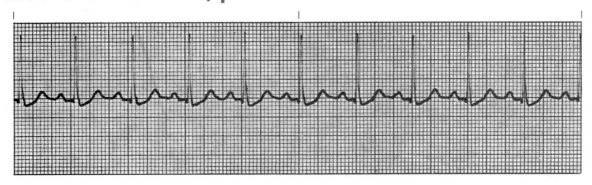

1. Site of origin: SA node
2. P wave: before every QRS; same size and shape
3. PR interval: 0.12 to 0.20 second
4. QRS: same size and shape; less than 0.12 second
5. Rhythm: (a) P to P interval: regular; (b) R to R interval: regular
6. Rate: 101 to 150

SINUS ARRHYTHMIA, p 52

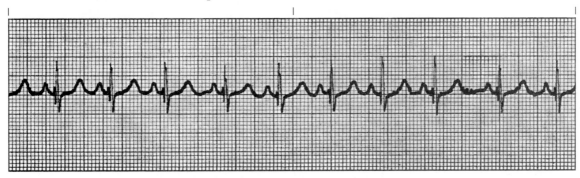

1. Site of origin: SA node
2. P wave: before every QRS; same size and shape
3. PR interval: 0.12 to 0.20 second
4. QRS: same size and shape; less than 0.12 second
5. Rhythm: (a) P to P interval: irregular; (b) R to R interval: irregular; (c) the longest R to R interval will be less than twice the length of remaining R to R intervals
6. Rate: overall rate varies with respirations; usually 60 to 100
   a. Increases as patient inhales
   b. Decreases as patient exhales

SINUS EXIT BLOCK AND SINUS ARREST, p 52

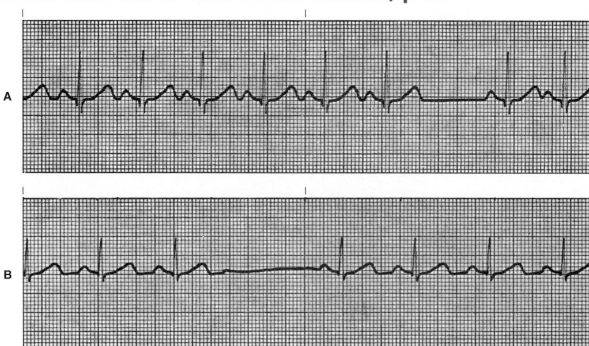

1. Site of origin: SA node fails to fire for at least two cardiac cycles
2. P wave: before every QRS; same size and shape
3. PR interval: varies slightly within normal limits of 0.12 to 0.20 second
4. QRS: same size and shape; less than 0.12 second
5. Rhythm: (a) P to P interval: regular, except during pause; (b) R to R interval: regular, except during pause
6. Rate: varies according to underlying rhythm
7. Pause: (a) **Sinus exit block:** the distance from the last normal beat to the next beat is equal to exactly two or more previous cardiac cycles; able to divide pause equally; (b) **Sinus arrest:** equal to more than two previous cardiac cycles; not able to divide pause equally

ATRIAL DYSRHYTHMIAS (Chapter 3)

PREMATURE ATRIAL CONTRACTION, p 54

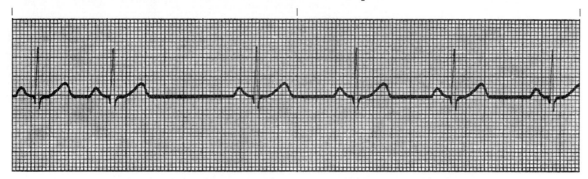

1. Site of origin: atria
2. P wave: before every QRS; may be buried in preceding T wave; may vary in size and shape
3. PR interval: varies within normal limits of 0.12 to 0.20 second
4. QRS: same size and shape; less than 0.12 second
5. Rhythm: (a) P to P interval: varies according to the underlying rhythm and the number of PACs; (b) R to R interval: varies according to the underlying rhythm and the number of PACs
6. Rate: varies according to the underlying rhythm and the number of PACs
7. Occurs: premature; usually followed by a noncompensatory pause

PAROXYSMAL ATRIAL TACHYCARDIA/PAROXYSMAL SUPRAVENTRICULAR TACHYCARDIA, p 56

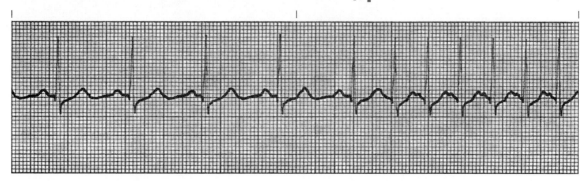

1. Site of origin: atria
2. P wave: before every QRS; may be buried in preceding T wave; same size and shape
3. PR interval: 0.12 to 0.20 second
4. QRS: same size and shape; less than 0.12 second
5. Rhythm: (a) P to P interval: regular; (b) R to R interval: regular
6. Rate: 151 to 250
7. Onset: starts suddenly; onset must be observed

SUPRAVENTRICULAR TACHYCARDIA, p 57

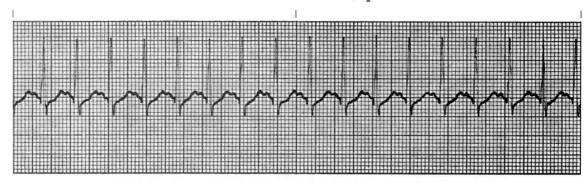

1. Site of origin: above bundle of His
2. P wave: (a) atrial: before every QRS or buried in preceding T wave; same size and shape; (b) junctional: inverted, hidden, or retrograde; same size and shape
3. PR interval: normal to not measurable
4. QRS: same size and shape; less than 0.12 second
5. Rhythm: (a) P to P interval: regular, if present; (b) R to R interval: regular
6. Rate: 151 to 250
7. Onset: starts suddenly; onset is not observed

ATRIAL FLUTTER, p 58

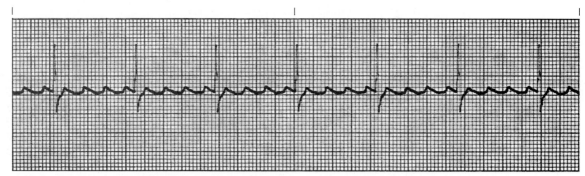

1. Site of origin: one atrial site
2. P wave: not present; T waves may be hidden in the flutter waves
3. Flutter waves: "saw-toothed" in shape; size may vary
4. PR interval: cannot be measured
5. QRS: same size and shape; less than 0.12 second
6. Rhythm: (a) P to P interval: not present; (b) F to F interval: regular; (c) R to R interval: regular, except in varying block
7. Rate:
   a. Atrial: 250 to 350
   b. Ventricular: usually 60 to 100 but may vary
      (1) Less than 60; slow ventricular response
      (2) 101 to 150; rapid ventricular response
8. Ratio of block:
   a. Two F waves to 1 QRS = 2:1 block (ratio)
   b. Three F waves to 1 QRS = 3:1 block (ratio)
   c. Four F waves to 1 QRS = 4:1 block (ratio)
   d. Varying number of F waves to 1 QRS = varying block

This strip shows a 4:1 block.

ATRIAL FIBRILLATION, p 61

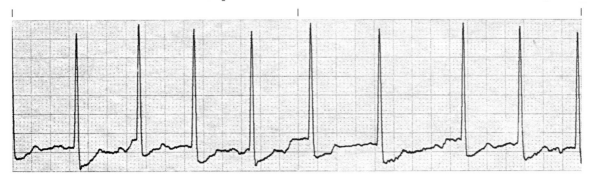

1. Site of origin: atria
2. P wave: no distinctive P wave
3. PR interval: cannot be measured
4. QRS: same size and shape; less than 0.12 second
5. Rhythm: (a) P to P interval: cannot be measured; (b) R to R interval: irregular
6. Rate:
   a. Atrial: 350 to 500 or more
   b. Ventricular:
      (1) Less than 60; slow ventricular response
      (2) 60 to 100; controlled A Fib
      (3) 101 to 150; rapid ventricular response
      (4) Greater than 150; uncontrolled A Fib

WOLFF-PARKINSON-WHITE SYNDROME, p 63

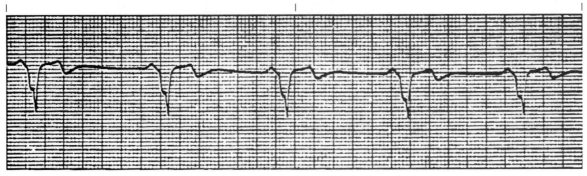

1. Site of origin: accessory pathway (Bundle of Kent)
   a. Atria to ventricle (antegrade)
   b. Ventricle to atria (retrograde)
   c. Both a and b in a continuous cycle
2. P wave: present, unless rhythm is an SVT, atrial flutter or atrial fibrillation
3. PR interval: less than 0.12 second, if P waves are present
4. QRS: (a) can be greater than 0.12 second; (b) slurring (curving of QRS complex); (c) may contain a delta wave
5. Rhythm: (a) P to P interval: varies according to the underlying rhythm; (b) R to R interval: varies according to the underlying rhythm
6. Rate:
   a. Varies according to the underlying rhythm
   b. Associated with SVT, including atrial flutter and atrial fibrillation, with uncontrolled ventricular response
   c. Ventricular rates of 200 to 300 can occur and become lethal

JUNCTIONAL DYSRHYTHMIAS (Chapter 4)

JUNCTIONAL DYSRHYTHMIA, p 78

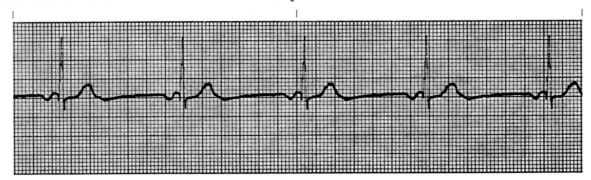

1. Site of origin: AV junction
2. P wave: inverted, buried, or retrograde; same size and shape, if present
3. PR interval: usually less than 0.12 second, if inverted P wave is present before the QRS
4. QRS: same size and shape; less than 0.12 second
5. Rhythm: (a) P to P interval: regular if present; (b) R to R interval: regular
6. Rate: 40 to 60

JUNCTIONAL BRADYCARDIA, p 83

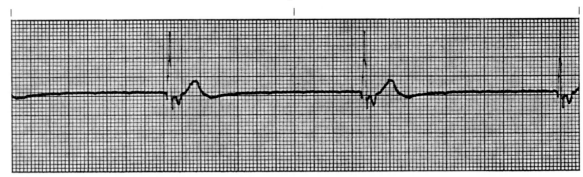

1. Site of origin: AV junction
2. P wave: inverted, buried, or retrograde; same size and shape, if present
3. PR interval: usually less than 0.12 second, if inverted P wave is present before the QRS
4. QRS: same size and shape, less than 0.12 second
5. Rhythm: (a) P to P interval: regular, if present; (b) R to R interval: regular
6. Rate: less than 40

ACCELERATED JUNCTIONAL DYSRHYTHMIA/JUNCTIONAL TACHYCARDIA, p 83

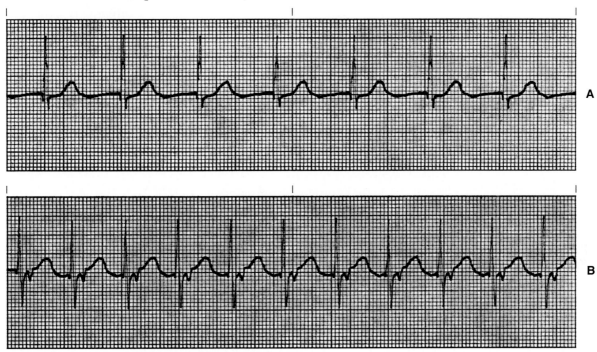

1. Site of origin: AV junction
2. P wave: inverted, buried, or retrograde; same size and shape, if present
3. PR interval: usually less than 0.12 second, if inverted P wave is present before the QRS
4. QRS: same size and shape, less than 0.12 second
5. Rhythm: (a) P to P interval: regular, if present; (b) R to R interval: regular
6. Rate:
   a. Accelerated junctional rhythm 61 to 100
   b. Junctional tachycardia 101 to 150

PREMATURE JUNCTIONAL CONTRACTION, p 84

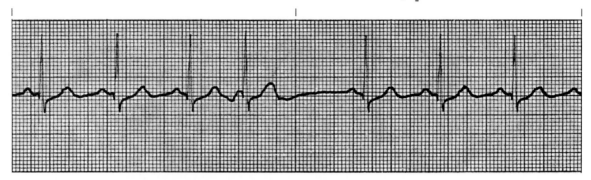

1. Site of origin: AV junction
2. P wave: inverted, buried, or retrograde
3. PR interval: usually less than 0.12 second, if inverted P wave is present before the QRS
4. QRS: less than 0.12 second
5. Rhythm: (a) P to P interval: varies according to the underlying rhythm and number of PJCs; (b) R to R interval: varies according to the underlying rhythm and number of PJCs
6. Rate: varies according to underlying rhythm and number of PJCs
7. Occurs: prematurely; usually followed by a compensatory pause

WANDERING JUNCTIONAL PACEMAKER, p 85

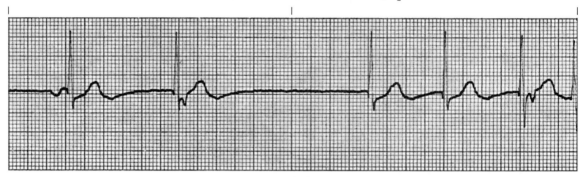

1. Site of origin: at least three junctional sites
2. P wave: inverted, buried, or retrograde; varies in size and shape, if present
3. PR interval: usually less than 0.12 second, if inverted P wave is present before the QRS
4. QRS: less than 0.12 second; size and shape may vary
5. Rhythm: (a) P to P interval: irregular, if present; (b) R to R interval: irregular
6. Rate: varies, usually 40 to 60

WANDERING ATRIAL PACEMAKER, p 86

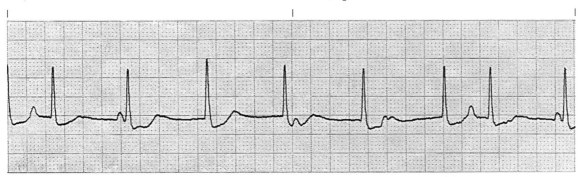

1. Site of origin: must be combination of three or more sites from above bundle of His
2. P wave: varies according to site of origin
3. PR interval: varies, if present
4. QRS: varies according to site of origin; may be greater than 0.12 second
5. Rhythm: (a) P to P interval: irregular; (b) R to R interval: irregular
6. Rate: varies, usually 60-100

HEART BLOCKS (Chapter 5)

FIRST-DEGREE HEART BLOCK, p 96

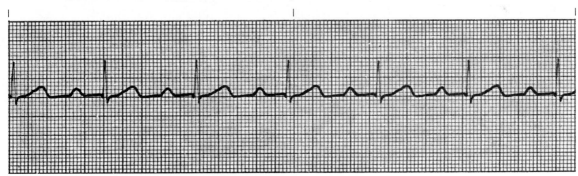

1. Site of origin: atria
2. Site of delay: between atria and bundle of His
3. P wave: before every QRS; same size and shape
4. PR interval: greater than 0.20 second
5. QRS: same size and shape; usually less than 0.12 second
6. Rhythm: (a) P to P interval: varies according to underlying rhythm; (b) R to R interval: varies according to underlying rhythm
7. Rate: varies according to underlying rhythm

SECOND-DEGREE HEART BLOCK, TYPE I (WENCKEBACH, MOBITZ I), p 97

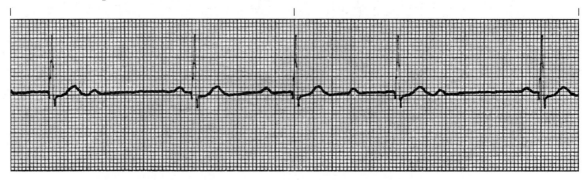

1. Site of origin: atria
2. Site of block: AV junction; progressive
3. P wave: at least one for every QRS; same size and shape
4. PR interval: becomes progressively longer, until QRS is dropped
5. QRS: same size and shape; less than 0.12 second
6. Rhythm: (a) P to P interval: regular; (b) R to R interval: irregular
7. Rate: varies

SECOND-DEGREE HEART BLOCK, TYPE II (MOBITZ II), p 99

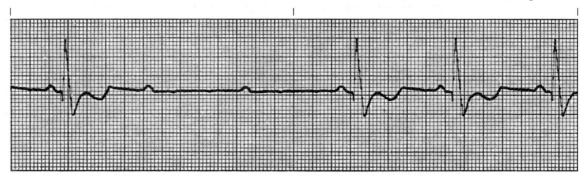

1. Site of origin: atria
2. Site of block: AV junction; intermittent block
3. P wave: at least one for every QRS; same size and shape
4. PR interval: equal throughout; may be normal or prolonged
5. QRS: same size and shape; usually less than 0.12 second
6. Rhythm: (a) P to P interval: varies according to underlying rhythm; (b) R to R interval: irregular
7. Rate: varies according to underlying rhythm
8. Ratio of block:
   a. 2 P waves to 1 QRS = 2:1 block
   b. 3 P waves to 1 QRS = 3:1 block
   c. 4 P waves to 1 QRS = 4:1 block
   d. Varying number of P waves to 1 QRS = varying block

   This strip shows a 3:1 block

THIRD-DEGREE HEART BLOCK (COMPLETE HEART BLOCK, COMPLETE AV DISSOCIATION), p 101

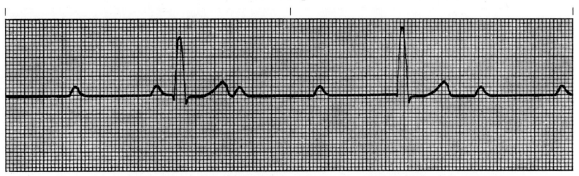

1. Site of origin: atria and ventricles
2. Site of block: between atria and ventricles
3. P wave: no relationship to QRS; same size and shape
4. PR interval: appears to vary; no true PR interval
5. QRS: same size and shape; usually wide, bizarre, and greater than 0.12 second
6. Rhythm: (a) P to P interval: regular; (b) R to R interval: regular
7. Rate:
   a. Atrial: usually 60 to 100
   b. Ventricular: usually 20 to 40

BUNDLE BRANCH BLOCK, p 103

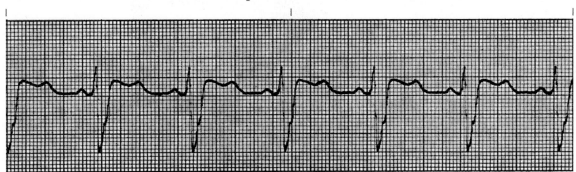

1. Site of origin: usually atria
2. Site of block: bundle branch (right, left, or both)
3. P wave: varies according to underlying rhythm
4. PR interval: varies according to underlying rhythm
5. QRS: usually same size and shape; notched appearance; usually greater than 0.12 second
6. Rhythm: (a) P to P interval: varies according to the underlying rhythm; (b) R to R interval: varies according to the underlying rhythm
7. Rate: varies according to the underlying rhythm

VENTRICULAR DYSRHYTHMIAS (Chapter 6)

PREMATURE VENTRICULAR CONTRACTION, p 117

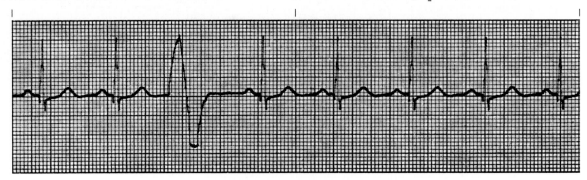

1. Site of origin: ventricles
2. P waves: not present, or hidden in PVC
3. PR interval: not measurable
4. QRS: may vary in size and shape; wide, bizarre, greater than 0.12 second
5. Rhythm: (a) P to P interval: not measurable in PVC; varies according to underlying rhythm and number of PVCs; (b) R to R interval: varies according to the underlying rhythm and number of PVCs
6. Rate: varies according to the underlying rhythm and number of PVCs
7. Occurs: premature; followed by a compensatory pause
8. T wave: deflected in the opposite direction of the QRS

NOTE: The following are types of PVCs (see pp 118-122).

UNIFOCAL PVCS

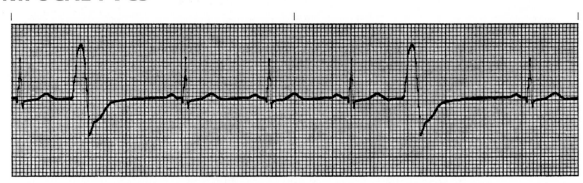

1. Site of origin: one ventricular site
2. QRS: same size and shape
3. Other characteristics: same as PVC

MULTIFOCAL PVCS

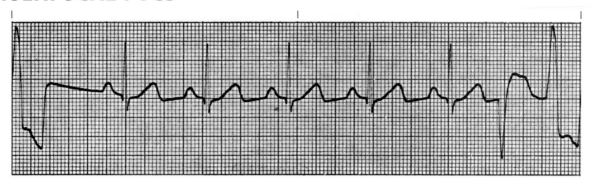

1. Site of origin: two or more ventricular sites
2. QRS: varies in size and shape
3. Other characteristics: same as PVC

QUADRIGEMINY

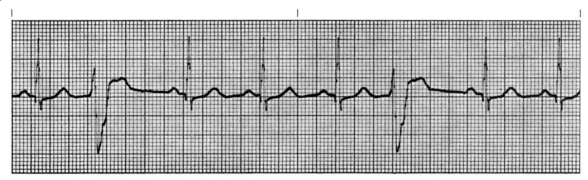

1. Site of origin: one or more ventricular sites
2. QRS: unifocal or multifocal
3. Occurs: every fourth complex is a PVC
4. Other characteristics: same as PVC

TRIGEMINY

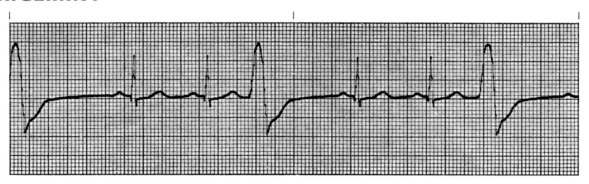

1. Site of origin: one or more ventricular sites
2. QRS: unifocal or multifocal
3. Occurs: every third complex is a PVC
4. Other characteristics: same as PVC

BIGEMINY

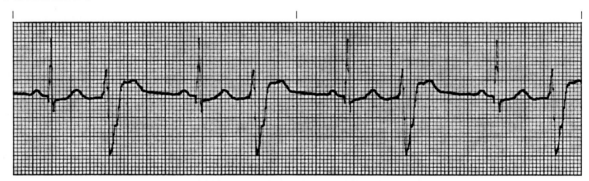

1. Site of origin: one or more ventricular sites
2. QRS: unifocal or multifocal
3. Occurs: every other complex is a PVC
4. Other characteristics: same as PVC

COUPLET

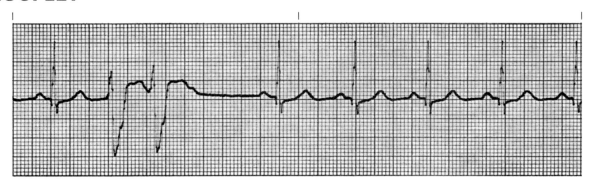

1. Site of origin: one or more ventricular sites
2. QRS: unifocal or multifocal
3. Occurs: two PVCs in a row
4. Other characteristics: same as PVC

R ON T PHENOMENON

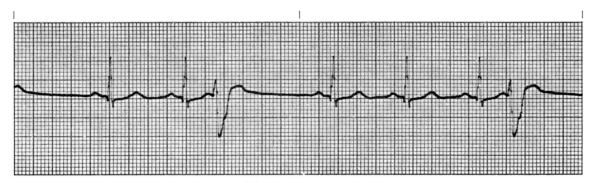

1. Site of origin: one or more ventricular sites
2. QRS: unifocal or multifocal
3. Occurs: R wave of PVC falls on the T wave of the preceding QRS
4. Other characteristics: same as PVC

RUN OF VENTRICULAR TACHYCARDIA (UNSUSTAINED VENTRICULAR TACHYCARDIA)

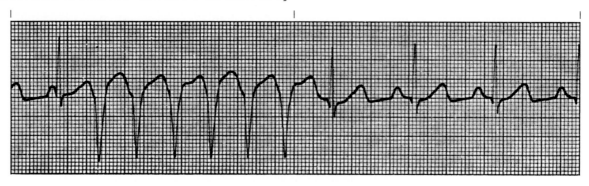

1. Site of origin: one or more ventricular sites
2. QRS: usually unifocal
3. Occurs: three or more PVCs in a row
4. Duration: less than 30 seconds
5. Other characteristics: same as PVC

VENTRICULAR TACHYCARDIA (SUSTAINED VENTRICULAR TACHYCARDIA), p 123

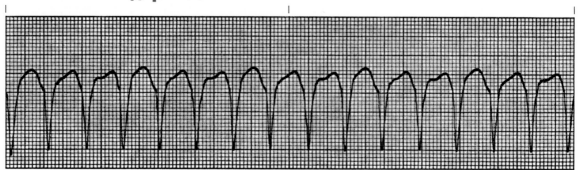

1. Site of origin: one or more ventricular sites
2. P wave: usually not present
3. PR interval: not measurable
4. QRS: usually same size and shape; wide, bizarre, greater than 0.12 second
5. Rhythm: (a) P to P interval: not measurable; (b) R to R interval: usually regular
6. Rate: 101 to 250 or more
7. Occurs: more than three PVCs in a row; sudden onset
8. Duration: usually greater than 30 seconds

TORSADES DE POINTES, p 124

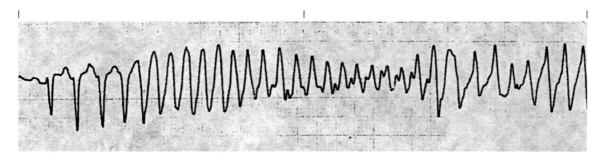

1. Site of origin: one or more ventricular sites
2. P wave: usually not present
3. PR interval: not measurable
4. QRS: usually same shape; varies in size, going from low to high and back to low amplitude
5. Rhythm: (a) P to P interval: not measurable; (b) R to R interval: usually regular
6. Rate: usually greater than 150
7. Occurs: sudden onset; frequently seen in a rhythm with prolonged QT intervals
8. Duration: varies

VENTRICULAR FIBRILLATION, p 125

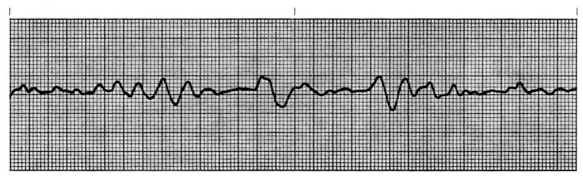

1. Site of origin: many ventricular sites
2. P wave: not present
3. PR interval: not measurable
4. QRS: not present; only a chaotic, wavy line
5. Rhythm: (a) P to P interval: not present; (b) R to R interval: not present
6. Rate: not measurable
7. Wave amplitude: coarse or fine

IDIOVENTRICULAR/AGONAL DYSRHYTHMIAS (DYING HEART), p 127

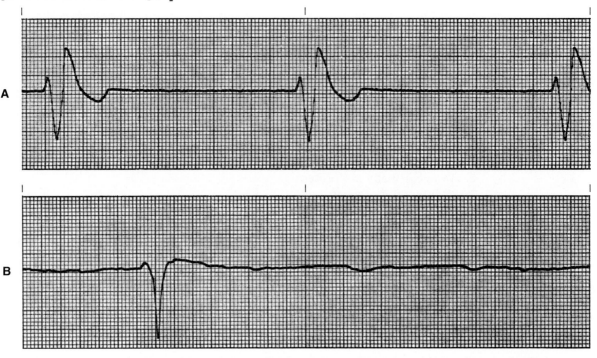

1. Site of origin: usually one ventricular site
2. P wave: not present
3. PR interval: not measurable
4. QRS: gradually *decreases* in amplitude and *increases* in width; wide, bizarre, greater than 0.12 second
5. Rhythm: (a) P to P interval: not present; (b) R to R interval: usually irregular
6. Rate:
   a. Idioventricular: 20 to 40
   b. Agonal: less than 20; becomes slower until it completely stops

NOTE: If the ventricular rate is 41 to 100, it is known as *accelerated idioventricular dysrhythmia* or *slow V Tach.*

VENTRICULAR STANDSTILL, p 128

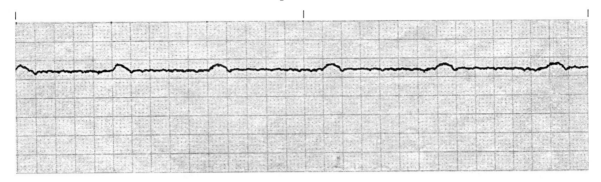

1. Site of origin: atria
2. P wave: seen without QRS; usually same size and shape
3. PR interval: not measurable
4. QRS: not present
5. Rhythm: (a) P to P interval: usually regular; (b) R to R interval: not present
6. Rate:
   a. Atrial: usually 60 to 100
   b. Ventricular: 0

ASYSTOLE, p 128

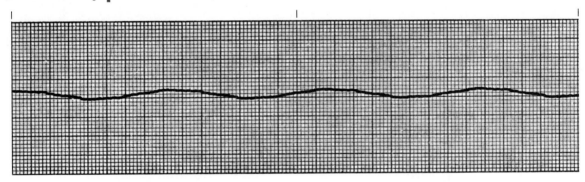

1. Site of origin: no electrical activity in heart muscle
2. P wave: not present
3. PR interval: not present
4. QRS: not present; only a straight or slightly wavy line
5. Rhythm: (a) P to P interval: not present; (b) R to R interval: not present
6. Rate: 0

"FUNNY LOOKING" BEATS (Chapter 7)

ESCAPE BEATS, p 140

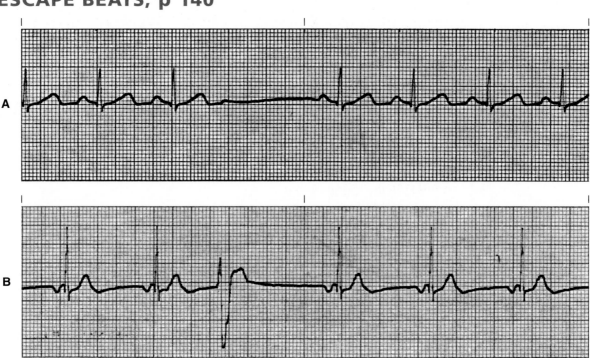

1. Site of origin: single atrial, junctional, or ventricular site; other than the SA node
2. P wave: varies according to site of origin
3. PR interval: varies according to site of origin
4. QRS: varies according to site of origin
5. Rhythm: (a) P to P interval: irregular, if present; (b) R to R interval: irregular
6. Rate: varies according to site of origin and underlying rhythm
7. Occurs:
   a. Complex that ends the pause of a sinus exit block or sinus arrest
   b. Premature complexes that increase the rate of a bradycardic rhythm

ABERRANTLY CONDUCTED COMPLEX, p 140

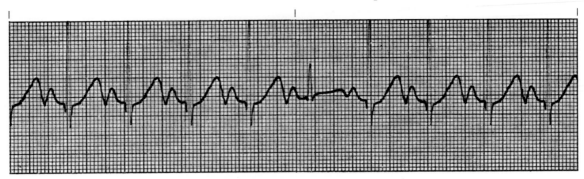

1. Site of origin: varies
2. P wave: varies according to site of origin
3. PR interval: varies according to site of origin
4. QRS: varies according to site of origin
5. Rhythm: (a) P to P interval: varies according to underlying rhythm; (b) R to R interval: varies according to underlying rhythm
6. Rate: varies according to underlying rhythm
7. Occurs:
   a. Single complex that follows different electrical conduction pathway than the underlying rhythm
   b. Complex usually does not occur prematurely

PULSELESS ELECTRICAL ACTIVITY, p 142

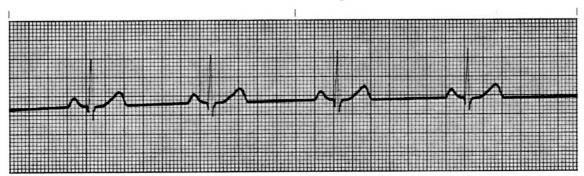

1. Site of origin: **mimics any rhythm**
2. P wave: mimics any rhythm
3. PR interval: mimics any rhythm
4. QRS: mimics any rhythm
5. Rhythm: (a) P to P interval: mimics any rhythm; (b) R to R interval: mimics any rhythm
6. Rate: mimics any rhythm; patient **does not** have a pulse
7. Includes: idioventricular dysrhythmias, bradyasystole dysrhythmias

PACEMAKER RHYTHMS, p 143

A
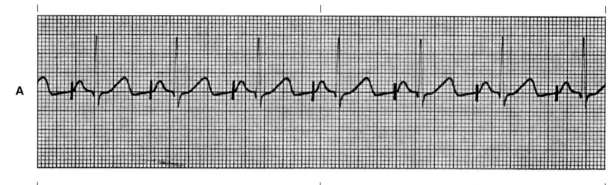

B
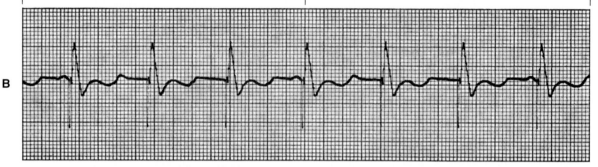

C
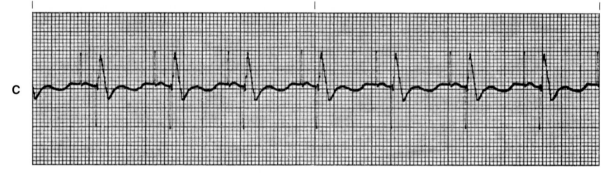

1. Site of origin:
   a. Atrial pacemaker: right atrium (strip **A**)
   b. Ventricular pacemaker: either right atrium or right ventricle (strip **B**)
   c. Sequential pacemaker: either right atrium and right ventricle or only right atrium (strip **C**)
2. P wave: may be replaced by pacer spike
3. PR interval: not measured in paced rhythm
4. QRS: usually greater than 0.12 second; occurs after ventricular pacer spike
5. Rhythm:
   a. P to P interval: varies if present
   b. R to R interval:
      (1) Fixed rate pacemaker: regular
      (2) Demand pacemaker: varies
   c. Pacer spike to pacer spike
      (1) Fixed rate: regular
      (2) Demand rate: varies
6. Rate: varies according to pacemaker; fixed rate or demand rate
7. Pacing: varies
8. Capture: 100%
9. Types:
   a. Temporary
      (1) Transvenous
      (2) Transcutaneous
   b. Permanent

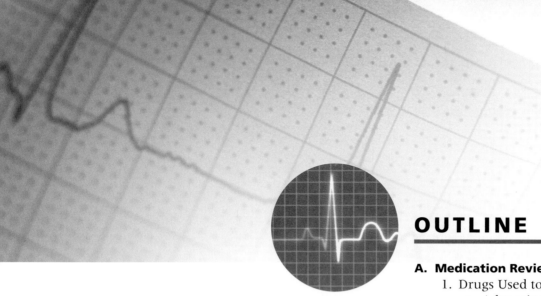

OUTLINE

CHAPTER 9

MEDICATION REVIEW AND ADULT TREATMENT GUIDELINES

This chapter is a brief and simplified summary of the most common drugs used to treat cardiac dysrhythmias in the adult patient. This chapter does **not** include all medications that might be used in the treatment of any dysrhythmia or cardiac disease. This review is not meant to take the place of a pharmacology course. Anyone administering medication should do so only after certification by his or her institution and as governed by the laws of his or her state.

The medication review and treatment guidelines are based on the American Heart Association's advanced cardiac life support (ACLS) protocols of 2000 and include the most recent updates including the *2000 Handbook of Emergency Cardiac Care for Healthcare Providers.*

For the purpose of treatment, it is assumed that all patients are being monitored in Lead II, all patients are adult, and no contraindications exist to any of the treatment protocols. Anyone wishing to learn pediatric treatment protocols is encouraged to attend a pediatric advanced life support (PALS) course offered by the American Heart Association.

The treatments outlined in this chapter are only general guidelines. They should be used in conjunction with, *not instead of,* your institution's policies and procedures. All treatments **must** be performed under the guidance of a physician.

IV medications should be administered at the port closest to the IV site, and followed by elevation of that extremity. These two actions will promote faster circulation of the drug.

As with any dysrhythmia, ongoing assessment of the patient's condition is essential. The patient's tolerance of the dysrhythmia and any subsequent symptoms will determine the appropriate treatment. Patients should be assessed **before** and **after** administering any medication and **before** and **after** each cardioversion attempt.

Patient assessment involves observing the patient's overall condition in addition to monitoring vital signs and interpreting the dysrhythmia on the monitor screen.

Patients who are symptomatic will show signs and symptoms of poor cardiac output. These signs and symptoms include cool, sweaty skin; hypotension (low BP); pallor (pale, grayish skin); cyanosis (bluish tint to lips, nail beds, and skin); dyspnea (difficulty breathing); dizziness; nausea, and vomiting; a decrease in urinary output; and a decrease in the level of consciousness (responsiveness).

Any one of these symptoms, by itself, may not indicate poor cardiac output. However, if these symptoms occur with either tachycardia or bradycardia, it strongly suggests poor cardiac output and treatment should be started immediately.

NOTE: The terms *poor cardiac output* and *medically unstable* are **both** used to describe a patient who is unable to tolerate a dysrhythmia.

MEDICATION REVIEW

DRUGS USED TO TREAT DYSRHYTHMIAS

Adenosine (Adenocard)

Action: Decreases HR by depressing the SA node and AV node activity.

Indications: To treat narrow complex tachycardias such as PAT/PSVT, SVT, or wide complex tachycardias such as VT that started as SVT.

Dosage: 6 mg IV push rapidly over 1 to 3 seconds, followed immediately by a 20-ml IV saline solution flush, followed by elevation of the extremity; if no response in 1 to 2 minutes, repeat adenosine at 12 mg IV push rapidly, followed by 20-ml IV saline solution flush; may repeat once more at 12 mg IV push, if there is no response in 1 to 2 minutes.

Precautions: Side effects usually last only 1 to 2 minutes and include flushing, difficulty breathing, and mild chest pain; may also have short-lasting episodes of bradycardia, asystole, or ventricular ectopy (abnormal beats); PAT/PSVT and SVT may recur because the effects of this medication last only a short time; may interact with theophylline, aminophylline, dipyridamole (Persantine), or carbamazepine (Tegretol). Use with caution in pregnancy and in the elderly. Contraindicated in hypersensitivity to adenosine. May be harmful if used in atrial flutter, A Fib or WPW syndrome.

Amiodarone (Cordarone)

Action: Decreases HR by altering impulses through conduction pathways; slows conduction; and prolongs effective refractory period.

Indications: To treat most narrow complex SVT, VT, V Fib, pulseless VT, and PVCs that do not respond to procainamide.

Dosage: **V Fib/VT:** 300 mg IV push; if no response within 3 to 5 minutes, repeat at 150 mg IV push, for a total dose of 2.2 g IV in 24 hours. **Stable tachycardias:** a rapid infusion of 150 mg IV over 10 minutes can be delivered; if no response, repeat 150 mg IV every 10 minutes, as needed, for a total dose of 2.2 g IV in 24 hours. A slow infusion is 360 mg IV over 6 hours; a maintenance infusion is 540 mg IV over 18 hours.

Precautions: May cause bradycardia, vasodilation, hypotension, and prolonged QT intervals. Use with caution in patients with renal failure, liver disease, and in pregnancy. Contraindicated in hypersensitivity to amiodarone. Amiodarone is incompatible with saline solution and should be administered only in D_5W solution, with the use of an inline filter. Always put in a glass bottle. Has a tendency to foam when shaken.

Atropine Sulfate

Action: Increases HR and sinus node automaticity; improves AV conduction.

Indications: To correct symptomatic bradycardias; asystole; PEA; to increase HR to at least 60 beats/min in a bradycardic rhythm with PVCs.

Dosage: **Symptomatic bradycardia:** 0.5 to 1 mg IV, repeated at 3- to 5-minute intervals to a total of 0.04 mg/kg or a total dose of 3 mg; **asystole:** 1 mg IV, repeated every 5 minutes for a total of 0.04 mg/kg or a total dose of 3 mg; **endotracheal administration:** 2 to 3 mg (total dose), diluted in 10 ml sterile water or sterile saline solution.

Precautions: May cause tachycardia; may increase ischemia due to increased need for oxygen by the myocardium. Use with caution in pregnancy and in the elderly. Contraindicated in hypersensitivity to atropine sulfate.

Beta-Adrenergic Blockers (atenolol [Tenormin, Noten], esmolol hydrochloride [Brevibloc], labetalol [Normodyne], metoprolol

Action: May reduce cardiac ischemia in patients receiving fibrinolytic agents; may reduce occurrence of V Fib after MI.

Indications: Recurrent VT and V Fib; after emergency treatment of MI; severe hypertension, and to decrease ventricular response in patients with SVT, A Fib, or A flutter.

Dosage: **Atenolol:** 5 mg IV over 5 minutes; wait 10 minutes, repeat dose of 5 mg IV over 5 minutes. **Esmolol:** initial dose: 0.5 mg/kg IV over 1 minute, followed by continuous infusion at 0.05 mg/kg per minute. Titrate to a maximum dose of 0.3 mg/kg per minute. **Labetalol:** 10 mg IV push

tartrate [Lopressor], and propranolol hydrochloride [Inderal])		over 1 to 2 minutes. May either repeat or double the dose every 10 minutes to a maximum dose of 150 mg, or follow initial bolus dose with an IV infusion of 2 to 8 mg/min. **Metoprolol:** 5 mg slow IV push over 2 to 5 minutes, repeated at 5-minute intervals to a total dose of 15 mg. **Propranolol:** give total dose of 0.1 mg/kg divided into 3 equal doses IV, given no more than 1 mg/min; give second and third dose at 2- to 3-minute intervals.
	Precautions:	May cause bradycardia, AV conduction delays, and hypotension; should not be used in patients with bradycardias, second- or third-degree heart block, conduction delays, hypotension, left-sided congestive heart failure, or bronchospasm; use with caution in patients with kidney failure and in pregnancy. May be harmful if used in patients with WPW syndrome. Contraindicated in hypersensitivity to these beta-adrenergic blockers. Do not mix with furosemide and sodium bicarbonate.
Calcium Channel Blockers (diltiazem [Dilacor, Tiazac, Cardizem, Cardizem SR]; verapamil [Calan, Covera HS, Verelan, Isoptin])	Action:	Both drugs decrease the HR by slowing conduction of the AV node and by lengthening the refractory periods.
	Indications:	To treat SVT, PAT/PSVT, and rapid ventricular response in atrial flutter and A Fib.
	Dosage:	**Diltiazem:** initial bolus: 0.25 mg/kg (average 15 to 20 mg) IV over 2 minutes; repeat dose: 0.35 mg/kg (average 20 to 25 mg) IV over 2 minutes, 15 minutes after the first dose; maintenance dose: continuous IV infusion of 5 to 15 mg/hr, titrated to HR, not to exceed 15 mg/hr and not to infuse more than 24 hours. **Verapamil:** initial dose: 2.5 to 5 mg IV over 2 minutes; repeat dose: 5 to 10 mg IV over 2 to 4 minutes, 15 to 30 minutes after first dose, if needed; total maximum dosage of 20 mg.
	Precautions:	May cause a short period of hypotension and/or bradycardia. Older patients should be given lower doses (2.5 mg) verapamil at slower rates of infusion (over 3 minutes). Use with caution in pregnancy. Contraindicated in hypersensitivity to these calcium channel blockers. Do not use in the following: patients with WPW syndrome; in wide QRS tachycardias (VT); with beta blockers; in patients with an AV block, unless a temporary pacemaker is available.
Ibutilide (Corvert)	Action:	Decreases the HR by slowing conduction through the AV junction and by lengthening the refractory periods.
	Indications:	To treat SVT, PAT/PSVT, and rapid ventricular response in atrial flutter and A Fib.
	Dosage:	**Adults weighing more than 60 kg:** 1 mg (10 ml) IV over 10 minutes. Repeat the second dose after 10 minutes, at the same rate. **Adults weighing less than 60 kg:** 0.01 mg/kg IV.
	Precautions:	May cause VT, torsades de pointes; should be monitored during use and up to 6 hours after infusion, with a defibrillator readily available; use with caution in liver disease, impaired left ventricular function, in pregnancy, and in the elderly. Contraindicated in hypersensitivity to ibutilide.
Intravenous Fluids (IV Fluids)	Action:	Replaces lost body fluids; provides IV access for administration of medications; used to dilute and deliver medications.
	Indications:	Hypovolemia; IV access for medication administration.
	Dosage:	1000 ml of 0.9 normal saline (NS) solution or lactated Ringer's (LR) solution administered IV. **Hypovolemia:** bolus (rapid infusion) of 300 ml/hr or greater. **IV access:** usually 60 ml/hr or less. IV rate of infusion varies because the rate is titrated (adjusted) to the patient's needs.
	Precautions:	Must be used with caution in elderly patients or patients with chronic lung problems to prevent complications such as congestive heart failure. Must be used with caution in patients with brain injury. Monitor IV site to prevent infiltration (IV catheter slips out of vein and solution infuses into tissue).

Isoproterenol Hydrochloride (Isuprel)	Action:	Increases force and rate of myocardial contractions, improving cardiac output and systolic BP.
	Indications:	Torsades de pointes that does not respond to magnesium sulfate and temporary use for symptomatic bradycardia unresponsive to atropine, until temporary pacing can be established.
	Dosage:	**Continuous infusion:** 2-10 μg/min, titrated to patient's BP and pulse. **Torsades de pointes:** titrate to increase the HR of the underlying rhythm (causing the QT intervals to shorten), until the torsades de pointes is resolved.
	Precautions:	Use with extreme caution. Do not use with other tachycardic dysrhythmias; must be used with infusion pump; incompatible with aminophylline and sodium bicarbonate; use lower doses in the elderly; use with caution in pregnancy and in patients with sulfite allergy (may contain sulfite preservative); do not use with epinephrine—can cause V Fib or VT.
Lidocaine Hydrochloride (Xylocaine, Xylocard, LidoPen)	Action:	Decreases automaticity, helping to decrease ventricular dysrhythmias.
	Indications:	To control ventricular dysrhythmias such as PVCs, VT, or V Fib.
	Dosage:	1 to 1.5 mg/kg IV, repeated at 5- to 10-minute intervals in doses of 0.5 to 0.75 mg/kg IV, until a total of 3 mg/kg has been given; if the ventricular ectopy has been suppressed and the patient has a pulse, begin a continuous infusion at 1 to 4 mg/min. May be given via endotracheal tube at 2 to 4 mg/kg.
	Precautions:	Signs of toxicity include numbness in hands or feet, drowsiness, slurred speech, decreased hearing, confusion, muscle twitching or tremors, or agitation. In severe cases of toxicity, seizures may occur; large doses of lidocaine may cause bradycardia, heart block, or AV conduction dysrhythmias. If underlying rhythm is bradycardic, consider giving atropine first. Use with caution in pregnancy and in the elderly. Contraindicated in hypersensitivity to lidocaine and in patients with WPW syndrome.
Magnesium Sulfate (Slow-Mag)	Action:	Reduces ventricular dysrhythmias that may follow an MI (decreased magnesium levels may cause V Fib and may also prevent VT from responding to treatment).
	Indications:	Treatment of choice in torsades de pointes; may be used in V Fib or pulseless VT; magnesium sulfate should be used whenever magnesium levels are decreased.
	Dosage:	**Cardiac arrest with torsades de pointes or hypomagnesium:** 1 to 2 g diluted in 10 ml D$_5$W IV push. **Torsades de pointes without cardiac arrest:** loading dose of 1 to 2 g in 50 to 100 ml D$_5$W IV, over 5 to 60 minutes. Follow with 0.5 to 1 g/hr IV, titrating dosage to control torsades de pointes.
	Precautions:	May cause flushing, sweating, slight bradycardia, and hypotension. Use with caution in patients with kidney failure and in pregnancy. Contraindicated in hypersensitivity to magnesium sulfate. Should only be diluted in D$_5$W.
Oxygen (O$_2$)	Action:	Increases oxygen available to all tissue cells; helps to reduce shortness of breath; may help to decrease ischemia.
	Indications:	For all patients with respiratory distress, chest pains, dysrhythmias, decreased cardiac output, and in all cardiopulmonary arrests; part of "MONA" protocol for acute MI (acute coronary syndrome [ACS]).
	Dosage:	**For alert patients with mild distress:** 1 to 6 L/min (liters per minute) delivered by nasal cannula. **For patients with moderate respiratory distress:** 4 to 8 L/min by Venturi mask, at 24% to 40%. **For patients with severe respiratory distress:** 6 to 10 L/min of 100% oxygen, delivered by a partial rebreather or non-rebreather mask at 35% to 60%. **During CPR:** give by bag-valve-mask device or endotracheal tube at 15 L/min at 100%. Pulse oximetry may be helpful in oxygen titration.

	Precautions:	Flammable; do not use in presence of flames or sparks. Use with caution in alert patients with chronic lung disease. Should be used at 100% in all resuscitation attempts.
Phenytoin (Dilantin)	Action:	Increases AV conduction; inhibition of sodium channels.
	Indication:	Ventricular dysrhythmias uncontrolled by antidysrhythmics.
	Dosage:	250 mg IV over 5 minutes (not to exceed 50 mg/min) or 100 mg IV every 15 minutes, until either of the following occur: (1) Dysrhythmias subside. (2) A total of 1 g is given.
	Precautions:	May cause nausea, vomiting, hypocalcemia; use with caution in liver or kidney disease, in pregnancy, and in the elderly. Contraindicated in hypersensitivity to phenytoin, bradycardia, SA or AV block, or liver failure.
Procainamide Hydrochloride (Pronestyl)	Action:	Suppresses ventricular ectopy when amiodarone or lidocaine have not been effective.
	Indications:	To control a wide variety of dysrhythmias when amiodarone and lidocaine have not been effective.
	Dosage:	20 mg/min IV until any of the following occur: (1) The dysrhythmia is suppressed. (2) The patient becomes hypotensive. (3) The QRS complex widens by 50% of its original width. (4) A total of 17 mg/kg has been given. If necessary, 50 mg/min IV up to 17 mg/kg IV can be given, until any of the above symptoms occur. A continuous IV infusion of procainamide at a rate of 1 to 4 mg/min should be started if the ventricular dysrhythmia has been suppressed and the patient has a pulse.
	Precautions:	May cause hypotension if administered too quickly; decrease maintenance dose if patient has kidney failure. Use with caution in bradycardia and in pregnancy. Contraindicated in hypersensitivity to procainamide hydrochloride. Avoid using in patients with prolonged QT intervals and in torsades de pointes; monitor BP closely.

DRUGS USED TO TREAT POOR CARDIAC OUTPUT/BLOOD PRESSURE

Acetylsalicylic Acid (Aspirin)	Action:	Prevents platelet formation of clots against the arterial walls.
	Indications:	Part of "MONA" protocol for acute MI (ACS); consider using as a preventive measure for MI, stroke, and angina.
	Dosage:	160 to 325 mg PO immediately in acute MI; recommend chewing over swallowing whole tablet.
	Precautions:	May cause gastrointestinal bleeding, tinnitus (ringing in the ears), dizziness, wheezing, confusion, and convulsions. Giving increased doses (1000 mg) may limit the positive effects that are needed. Use with caution in liver or kidney disease, asthma, Hodgkin's disease, and in pregnancy. Contraindicated in ulcer disease, in the last trimester of pregnancy, in hypersensitivity to salicylates, or in patients taking warfarin (Coumadin).
Amrinone Lactate (Inocor)	Action:	Improves cardiac output by increasing strength of cardiac contractions; decreases BP by relaxing and dilating blood vessel walls.
	Indications:	Consider using in congestive heart failure (CHF) that has not responded to other drug therapy.
	Dosage:	**Initial bolus:** 0.75 mg/kg IV over 10 to 15 minutes. **Maintenance dose:** 5 to 15 µg/kg per minute, titrated to desired BP. Maximum dose is 10 mg/kg in 24 hours.
	Precautions:	May cause stomach upset, fever, liver problems, kidney failure, and reduction of platelets. Increases myocardial demand for oxygen, which can cause cardiac dysrhythmias; may also increase ventricular irritability. Use with caution in pregnancy and in the elderly. Contraindicated in

hypersensitivity to sulfites or patients with an acute MI. Incompatible with furosemide, sodium bicarbonate, and dextrose. Use an infusion pump to administer.

Calcium Chloride (Kalcinate)	Action:	Increases myocardial contractility.
	Indications:	Replace and maintain calcium levels; hyperkalemia (increased potassium level); calcium channel blocker toxicity.
	Dosage:	8 to 16 mg/kg IV; may repeat if necessary; 2 to 4 mg/kg is recommended before giving intravenous calcium channel blockers.
	Precautions:	Give slowly; rapid administration may cause slowing of the HR. May cause spasms of the coronary and cerebral (brain) arteries. Use with caution in patients receiving digitalis, in pregnancy, and in kidney disease. Contraindicated in hypercalcemia and V Fib; incompatible with sodium bicarbonate; not routinely used in cardiac arrest.
Digitalis Glycoside (Digoxin [Lanoxin])	Action:	Increases myocardial contractility, resulting in increased cardiac output; helps control ventricular response to atrial dysrhythmias.
	Indications:	Atrial flutter, A Fib, and is an alternate treatment for atrial tachycardias, including PAT/PSVT and SVT; used in treatment of chronic congestive heart failure.
	Dosage:	10 to 15 µg/kg administered IV.
	Precautions:	Use with caution in patients with acute MI because the drug may cause AV block, sinus bradycardia, or VT; use with caution in pregnancy and in the elderly. Contraindicated for patients with WPW syndrome, digitalis toxicity, torsades de pointes, VT, V Fib, or hypersensitivity to digitalis glycoside. Incompatible with dobutamine; do not administer if HR is less than 60 beats/min; usually not used outside hospital setting because of slow onset of action. Avoid use of cardioversion if patient is taking digoxin, unless condition is life threatening. If necessary, use low settings of 10 to 20 joules.
Digoxin-Specific Antibody Therapy (Digibind)	Action:	Corrects digoxin toxicity.
	Indications:	Used in digoxin toxicity that causes life-threatening dysrhythmias, shock, CHF; hyperkalemia (potassium level greater than 5.0 mEq/L); elevated digitalis blood levels, if patient is symptomatic.
	Dosage:	**Chronic toxicity:** 3 to 5 vials (120 to 200 mg); each vial binds 0.6 mg digoxin. **Acute toxicity:** 10 vials (400 mg), may require up to 20 vials (800 mg). Dosage varies with the amount of digoxin taken.
	Precautions:	Serum digoxin level should not be used to calculate additional dosage of Digibind because serum levels usually rise after treatment. Use with caution in pregnancy and in the elderly. Contraindicated in hypersensitivity to Digibind.
Dobutamine Hydrochloride (Dobutrex)	Action:	Increases force of contraction of heart muscle, increasing cardiac output and increasing coronary artery blood flow.
	Indications:	Short-term treatment of heart failure.
	Dosage:	2 to 20 µg/kg per minute IV. Titrate so HR does not increase by more than 10% of the HR before treatment.
	Precautions:	May cause rapid-rate dysrhythmias, changes in BP, headache, nausea, and vomiting. Monitor vital signs and patient's rhythm continuously; administer with infusion pump; use with caution in patients who have the following:

(1) Atrial fibrillation: increases AV conduction and rapid ventricular response.

(2) MI: high doses may increase myocardium's need for oxygen and increase ischemia.

(3) PVCs: may increase incidence of PVCs.

Use with caution in patients with hypertension and in pregnancy. Contraindicated in hypersensitivity to dobutamine hydrochloride. Do not use in patients with systolic BP less than 100 mm Hg who are in shock, or in shock caused by known poison or drugs. Incompatible with aminophylline, verapamil, digoxin, and heparin. Do not mix with sodium bicarbonate.

Dopamine Hydrochloride (Intropin, Dopastat, Revimine)	Action:	Increases cardiac output by improving myocardial contractility; increases BP by constricting peripheral arteries and veins.
	Indications:	To treat hypotension accompanied by other symptoms, when there is no hypovolemia.
	Dosage:	**To improve urinary output:** 1 to 5 μg/kg per minute continuous IV infusion. **To improve cardiac output:** 5 to 10 μg/kg per minute continuous IV infusion. **To improve BP:** 10 to 20 μg/kg per minute continuous IV infusion; may require higher dose. Not to exceed 50 μg/kg per minute; titrate all doses to patient's response.
	Precautions:	May cause nausea and vomiting. Increased HR may produce supraventricular and ventricular dysrhythmias. May increase need for oxygen by the myocardium, which can lead to ischemia. Use with caution in pregnancy and in the elderly. Contraindicated in V Fib, tachycardic dysrhythmias, and hypersensitivity to dopamine. Use with an infusion pump; monitor vital signs and cardiac rhythm frequently; do not mix with sodium bicarbonate. Discontinue drug administration slowly.
Epinepherine Hydrochloride (Adrenalin)	Action:	Increases rate and force of cardiac contractions; increases coronary and cerebral blood flow; increases automaticity.
	Indications:	During CPR and cardiac resuscitation; V Fib; pulseless VT; asystole; PEA, or anaphylaxis. Use in severe bradycardia or hypotension that has not responded to other therapies.
	Dosage:	**IV bolus:** 1 mg of a 1:10,000 dilution; may be repeated at 3- to 5-minute intervals; follow with a 20-ml IV flush and elevate the arm. **Endotracheal tube:** 2 to 2.5 mg of a 1:1000 dilution in 10 ml NS; may be repeated at 3- to 5-minute intervals. **Continuous IV infusion:** 30 mg (30 cc) of a 1:1000 dilution in 250 ml D_5W or NS, starting at a rate of 2 μg/min at 100 ml/hr and titrated as needed. Up to 0.2 mg/kg may be used.
	Precautions:	May increase ischemia due to increased rate and force of contractions; may cause or increase ventricular ectopy (abnormal beat). Use with caution in patients with hypertension, in pregnancy, and in the elderly. Contraindicated in hypersensitivities to epinephrine. Do not mix with sodium bicarbonate; continuous infusion not used in cardiac arrests until the patient has a pulse.
Fibrinolytic Agents		**("Clot Busters"; Activase, tissue plasminogen activator [t-PA]; Alteplase, tissue plasminogen activator, recombinant; Anistreplase, anisoylated plasminogen-streptokinase activator complex [APSAC]; Eminase, anisoylated plasminogen-streptokinase activator complex [APSAC]; Reteplase, recombinant [Retavase]; Streptokinase [Kabikinase, Streptase]; Tenecteplase [TNKase]; Urokinase [Abbokinase, Ukidan, Win-Kinase])**
	Action:	Dissolves clots in the coronary arteries that cause ischemia and infarction; may reduce number of deaths from MI.
	Indications:	All patients with symptoms and EKG findings of acute MI, within less than 12 hours of onset of symptoms; patients must meet specific criteria determined by the manufacturer and your institution.
	Dosage:	Varies with specific thrombolytic agent; follow manufacturer's instructions or the policy of your institution and specific instructions of the physician.
	Precautions:	May lead to increased bleeding, decreased clot formation, and intracranial bleeding. Use with caution in pregnancy. Should not be used in patients with bleeding disorders, recent surgery, recent CVAs

(hemorrhagic strokes), or with hypersensitivity to these agents. All patients receiving fibrinolytic therapy should receive 160 to 325 mg of aspirin as soon as possible; patients may require heparinization to help keep blood vessels open after fibrinolytic therapy. Streptokinase should not be used in patients with recent streptococcal infections.

NOTE: Urokinase may not be available in the United States.

Furosemide (Lasix, Lasix Special)

Action: Dilates blood vessels; removes excess fluid from tissues; increases formation of urine.

Indications: Acute pulmonary edema; congestive heart failure; cerebral edema after MI; hypertensive emergencies.

Dosage: 0.5 to 1 mg/kg IV, over 1 to 2 minutes; if there is no response, double the dose to 2.0 mg/kg IV over 1 to 2 minutes.

Precautions: May cause severe dehydration, hypotension, hypovolemia, electrolyte imbalances, or high blood glucose levels. Use with caution in pregnancy. Contraindicated in hypersensitivity to sulfonamides.

Heparin (Unfractionated UFH, Heparin Lock Flush, Heparin Leo, Calcilean)

Action: Anticoagulant.

Indications: Acute MI.

Dosage: **Initial bolus:** 60 units/kg, with a maximum dose of 4000 units. **Continuous infusion:** 12 units/kg per hour with maximum dose of 1000 units/hr for patients weighing more than 70 kg. Follow heparin protocol of your institution.

Precautions: May cause active bleeding, severe hypertension, bleeding disorders, and gastrointestinal bleeding. Use with caution in pregnancy and in the elderly. Contraindicated in recent surgery, severe hypertension, liver or kidney disease, known thrombocytopenia (low platelet count), and hypersensitivity to heparin.

Milrinone (Primacor)

Actions: Improves cardiac output by increasing strength of cardiac contractions; decreases BP by relaxing and dilating blood vessel walls.

Indications: Consider using in congestive heart failure that has not responded to other drug therapy.

Dosage: **Initial bolus:** 50 µg/kg IV over 10 minutes. **Maintenance dose:** 0.375 to 0.750 µg/kg per minute for 2 to 3 days.

Precautions: May cause stomach upset, fever, liver problems, kidney failure, or reduction of platelets. Increases myocardial demand for oxygen, which can increase cardiac ischemia; may also increase ventricular irritability. Use with caution in patients with atrial flutter, A Fib, liver or kidney disease; use with caution in pregnancy and in the elderly. Should not be used in acute MI patients or patients who are allergic to sulfites. Incompatible with furosemide, sodium bicarbonate, procainamide, and dextrose. Use an infusion pump to administer.

Morphine Sulfate (Astramorph PF, Duramorph PF)

Action: Narcotic analgesic that provides relief for severe chest pain; reduces need for oxygen in the myocardium.

Indications: Pain relief of choice for MIs. Part of "MONA" protocol for acute MI (ACS); cardiogenic pulmonary edema (with stable BP).

Dosage: 2 to 4 mg IV titrated over 1 to 5 minutes; may repeat in 5 to 30 minutes until pain is relieved; may dilute morphine to a 1 mg/1 ml solution with sterile NS solution for ease in administration.

Precautions: May cause hypotension. Monitor respirations frequently because morphine may depress respiratory function. Use with caution in pregnancy and in the elderly. Contraindicated in hypersensitivity to morphine. Follow your institution's guidelines for use of a narcotic.

**Nitroglycerin
(Nitro-bid, Nitrol,
Nitrostat, Tridil)**

Action: Relieves cardiac chest pain by relaxing smooth muscle in blood vessels and increasing circulation of oxygenated blood to myocardium.

Indications: To treat acute angina, unstable angina, and congestive heart failure associated with MIs; may also be used to reduce pain and hypertension associated with MIs; part of "MONA" protocol for acute MI (ACS).

Dosage: **Sublingual** (under the tongue): One tablet (0.3 or 0.4 mg); repeat at 3- to 5-minute intervals; maximum dose is three tablets. **Spray:** 0.4 mg under or on the tongue by metered-dose canister, for ½ to 1 second (patient should wait 10 seconds before swallowing); maximum dose, three sprays in 15 minutes. **IV:** an initial bolus of 12.5 to 25 μg titrated at 10 to 20 μg/min, until pain and hypertension are relieved.

Precautions: Do not use if systolic BP is less than 90-100 mm Hg. May cause severe hypotension soon after administration of medication (monitor vital signs frequently); headache, nausea, and vomiting may also occur. Use with caution in pregnancy and for IV use in the elderly. Contraindicated in hypersensitivity to nitroglycerin or nitrites. Administer with an infusion pump; incompatible with dobutamine; be aware of other drug incompatibilities. Absorbed by plastic (must be administered in glass bottles with polyethylene tubing). Should also avoid use in patients who have taken Viagra within 24 hours.

**Norepinephrine
Bitartrate
(Levophed)**

Action: Constricts blood vessels, increasing coronary perfusion, BP, and cardiac output; increases force of cardiac contraction and increases HR.

Indications: To treat acute hypotension and severe hypotension after cardiac arrest.

Dosage: 0.5 to 1.0 μg/min IV, titrate infusion to patient's BP; may increase dose to a maximum of 30 μg/min.

Precautions: May cause an increased need for oxygen in myocardium; monitor patient's rhythm continuously for development of dysrhythmias; monitor vital signs frequently, at least every 5 minutes. Use with caution in pregnancy and in the elderly. Contraindicated in patients with V Fib, tachy-dysrhythmias, hypertension, or hypersensitivity to norepinephrine bitartrate. Assess infusion site frequently because infiltration may cause death of tissues around the IV site; incompatible with aminophylline, lidocaine, sodium bicarbonate, and NS solution; use only with D_5W.

**Sodium
Bicarbonate**

Actions: Reverses acidosis by neutralizing some of the excess acid throughout the body.

Indications: Metabolic acidosis; prolonged cardiac arrest; cardiotoxicity with some drug overdoses.

Dosage: 1 mEq/kg IV; repeat every 10 minutes at 0.5 mEq/kg, based on arterial blood gas results, if available.

Precautions: Flush IV with 20 ml NS solution before and after administering medication; monitor electrolytes, arterial blood gases, and renal function. Use with caution in pregnancy, in CHF, and in the elderly. Contraindicated in patients with respiratory acidosis or hypersensitivity to sodium bicarbonate.

Sodium Nitroprusside (Nipride, Nitropress)	Action:	Decreases BP by relaxing smooth muscle of blood vessels; increases cardiac output; reduces myocardium's need for oxygen (may reduce ischemia); relieves chest pain.
	Indications:	Hypertensive emergencies (when high BP will not respond to other drugs), and acute congestive heart failure.
	Dosage:	50 mg diluted in 500 ml D_5W solution for a concentration of 100 µg/ml; **initial IV dose:** 0.1 µg/kg per minute; titrate every 3 to 5 minutes until desired BP or maximum dose of 5 µg/kg per minute. Action occurs within 1 to 2 minutes.
	Precautions:	May cause headache, nausea and vomiting, abdominal cramps, and hypotension. Monitor vital signs frequently because medication may decrease BP rapidly. Use with caution in patients with liver or kidney disease, in pregnancy, and the elderly. Contraindicated in hypersensitivity to sodium nitroprusside. Solution must be protected from light; cover IV bottle with foil or dark plastic; follow your institution's policy regarding covering IV tubing; incompatible with bacteriostatic water and saline solution; use D_5W solution to reconstitute medication; do not add any other drugs or preservatives to nitroprusside solution. Administer with an infusion pump.
Vasopressin (Pitressin)	Action:	Constricts smooth muscle in blood vessels.
	Indications:	Alternative to epinephrine in the treatment of refractory V Fib and pulseless VT.
	Dosage:	40 units IV push, **once only.**
	Precautions:	Potent peripheral vasoconstrictor, which may lead to severe hypertension, increased cardiac ischemia, and chest pain. Use with caution in pregnancy and in the elderly. Not recommended for patients with coronary artery disease, chronic kidney disease, or hypersensitivity to vasopressin.

RESEARCH DRUGS

The medications in this section are currently not approved by the FDA for IV administration in the United States of America, except in research. However, they may be in use in other countries.

Disopyramide (Norpace)

Action: Decreases the HR by slowing conduction through myocardial cells and by lengthening the refractory periods.

Indications: To treat a variety of rapid-rate dysrhythmias.

Dosage: 2 mg/kg IV over 10 minutes, then a continuous IV infusion of 0.4 mg/kg per hour.

Precautions: Infuse slowly; use is limited because of its potent anticholinergic and hypotensive effects, as well as its need to be infused slowly. Use with caution in pregnancy and in the elderly. Contraindicated in hypersensitivity to disopyramide.

Flecainide (Tambocor)

Action: Potent sodium channel blocker with ability to decrease HR.

Indications: To treat dysrhythmias unresponsive to other medications, such as atrial flutter, A Fib, WPW syndrome, ectopic atrial tachycardia, and some ventricular dysrhythmias.

Dosage: 1-2 mg/kg IV at 10 mg/min, infused slowly.

Precautions: Must infuse slowly. May cause bradycardia, other dysrhythmias, hypotension, oral paresthesia (numbness of mouth), and blurred vision. Use with caution in pregnancy and in the elderly. Contraindicated in hypersensitivity to flecainide. Avoid with impaired left ventricular function.

Propafenone (Rhythmol)

Action: Slows speed of conduction; inhibits automaticity.

Indications: To control supraventricular and ventricular dysrhythmias.

Dosage: 1 to 2 mg/kg IV at 10 mg/min.

Precautions: Infuse slowly. May cause bradycardia, hypotension, gastrointestinal upset, and congestive heart failure. Use with caution in pregnancy and in the elderly. Contraindicated in hypersensitivity to propafenone. Avoid with coronary artery disease. Digitalis and warfarin levels may increase when taken with propafenone.

Sotalol (Betapace)

Action: Prolongs absolute refractory period without affecting conduction; suppresses ventricular ectopy when amiodarone, lidocaine, and procainamide have not been effective.

Indications: To control supraventricular and ventricular dysrhythmias.

Dosage: 1 to 1.5 mg/kg IV at 10 mg/min.

Precautions: Must be given slowly. May cause bradycardia, hypotension, and torsades de pointes. Use with caution in pregnancy, in the elderly, and with medications that prolong QT intervals. Contraindicated in hypersensitivity to sotalol.

ADULT TREATMENT GUIDELINES

Please remember that these are only general guidelines. For these guidelines, it is assumed that all patients are being monitored in Lead II, all patients are adults, and no contraindications exist to any of the treatment protocols.

Artifact

1. Artifact is not treated.
2. Correct the cause of the artifact to simplify identification of the rhythm.
3. Initiate treatment, if necessary.

Myocardial Infarction (Acute Coronary Syndrome)

1. Assess the patient; be prepared to initiate morphine, oxygen, nitroglycerin, and aspirin (MONA protocol).
2. Provide oxygen; apply pulse oximetry.
3. Begin IV fluids.
4. Give nitroglycerin sublingual or spray for pain.
5. Obtain a 12-Lead electrocardiograph. Reassess the patient.
6. If no relief from repeated nitroglycerin, administer morphine IV, titrated to pain relief. Consider IV nitroglycerin.
7. Continue to assess and monitor the patient. Treat any dysrhythmias that occur.
8. Once diagnosis of MI has been confirmed, begin fibrinolytic protocol if no contraindications exist and if within 12 hours of onset of symptoms; consider oral aspirin and IV heparin, if included in fibrinolytic protocol.
9. Continued assessment and monitoring of the patient is essential. Transfer patient to care of cardiologist in coronary care unit.

Normal Sinus Rhythm

1. Normal sinus rhythm does not require treatment.
2. **Remember,** the monitor is **not** the patient. The patient must be assessed, and, if symptomatic, treatment must be initiated.
3. Continue to assess and monitor the patient.

Sinus Bradycardia

1. Assess the patient. If the patient is medically unstable, begin treatment.
2. Provide oxygen; apply pulse oximetry.
3. Begin IV fluids.
4. Administer atropine. Reassess the patient; repeat atropine, if necessary.
5. Obtain a 12-Lead electrocardiograph. Reassess the patient.
6. An artificial pacemaker (temporary or permanent) may be necessary. Use a transcutaneous or transvenous pacemaker, if available, until a permanent pacemaker is placed.
7. Dopamine may be administered for a systolic BP less than 80 mm Hg.
8. Epinephrine may be administered to patients who do not respond to atropine.
9. Isoproterenol may be helpful for symptomatic bradycardia, when used at low doses, until a pacemaker is available; use this drug with caution.
10. Continue to assess and monitor the patient.
11. Reassess the patient. If the dysrhythmia has converted to another rhythm and/or rate, reassess the patient; if necessary, treat the new dysrhythmia.

Sinus Tachycardia

1. Assess the patient. If the patient is medically unstable, begin treatment.
2. Determine the cause of the tachycardia:
   a. Fever
      (1) Administer antipyretics, such as aspirin or acetaminophen, to lower fever.
      (2) Provide cool to tepid bath.
   b. Anxiety
      (1) Acknowledge the patient's anxiety.
      (2) Offer reassurance in a calm manner.
   c. Pain
      (1) Administer pain medication as ordered.
      (2) Use relaxation techniques.
   d. Hypovolemia
      (1) Replace fluids or blood.
3. Provide oxygen; apply pulse oximetry.
4. Begin IV fluids.
5. Obtain a 12-Lead electrocardiograph. Reassess the patient.
6. Consider using, beta blockers, diltiazem, or digoxin if the patient's HR is greater than 100 but less than 151 beats/min. If HR is greater than 150 beats/min, treat as SVT.
7. Reassess the patient. If the dysrhythmia has converted to another rhythm and/or rate, reassess the patient; if necessary, treat the new dysrhythmia.

Sinus Arrhythmia

1. Assess the patient. If signs of poor cardiac output are present, begin treatment.
2. Provide oxygen; apply pulse oximetry.
3. Begin IV fluids.
4. If overall HR is bradycardic, administer atropine. Reassess the patient; repeat atropine, if necessary.
5. Obtain a 12-Lead electrocardiograph. Reassess the patient.
6. An artificial pacemaker (temporary or permanent) may be necessary. Use a transcutaneous or transvenous pacemaker, if available, until a permanent pacemaker is placed.
7. Dopamine may be administered for a systolic BP less than 80 mm Hg.
8. Epinephrine may be administered to patients who do not respond to atropine.
9. Isoproterenol may be helpful for symptomatic bradycardia when used at low doses, until a pacemaker is available; use this drug with caution.
10. Consider using digoxin, beta blockers, or diltiazem if the patient's HR is greater than 100 but less than 151 beats/min. If HR is greater than 150 beats/min, treat as SVT.
11. Reassess the patient. If the dysrhythmia has converted to another rhythm and/or rate, reassess the patient; if necessary, treat the new dysrhythmia.

Sinus Exit Block and Sinus Arrest

1. If the sinus exit block or sinus arrest is a new dysrhythmia, observe the patient closely for a change in the cardiac rhythm and/or rate.
2. Provide oxygen; apply pulse oximetry.
3. Begin IV fluids.
4. If overall HR is bradycardic, administer atropine. Reassess the patient; repeat atropine, if necessary.
5. Obtain a 12-Lead electrocardiograph. Reassess the patient.

6. Sinus exit block and sinus arrest are both indications of damage or injury to the SA node. If the pauses are frequent or long, the patient may become medically unstable and require an artificial pacemaker.
7. Dopamine may be administered for a systolic BP less than 80 mm Hg.
8. Epinephrine may be administered to patients who do not respond to atropine.
9. Isoproterenol may be helpful for symptomatic bradycardia when used at low doses, until a pacemaker is available; use this drug with caution.
10. Reassess the patient. If the dysrhythmia has converted to another rhythm and/or rate, reassess the patient; if necessary, treat the new dysrhythmia.

Premature Atrial Contraction

1. Assess the patient. A PAC by itself does not require treatment. If the patient is medically unstable or shows signs of poor cardiac output, treat the underlying rhythm and/or rate.
2. If the cause of the PAC is caffeine or nicotine, decrease or eliminate the stimulant in the patient's daily intake.
3. If the PAC is a new occurrence, observe the patient closely for a change in the cardiac rhythm and/or rate.
4. Continue to reassess and monitor the patient.

Paroxysmal Atrial Tachycardia/Paroxysmal Supraventricular Tachycardia

1. Assess the patient. If the patient is medically stable, continue to observe the patient; if the patient is medically unstable, begin treatment.
2. Provide oxygen; apply pulse oximetry.
3. Begin IV fluids.
4. The physician may perform vagal stimulation, such as Valsalva's maneuver (have the patient bear down) or carotid massage. Reassess the patient.
5. Obtain a 12-Lead electrocardiograph. Reassess the patient.
6. Administer adenosine.
7. If PAT/PSVT continues, repeat adenosine at higher dose; may repeat this dose once after 1 to 2 minutes.
8. If PAT/PSVT continues, monitor BP. If systolic pressure is normal or high, administer verapamil. Reassess the patient.
9. Wait 15 to 30 minutes; if PAT/PSVT continues, repeat verapamil. If the patient is medically **stable,** consider using these drugs in the following order: calcium channel blockers, beta blockers, and amiodarone, to convert the PAT/PSVT to a normal or more stable rhythm.
10. Reassess the patient.
11. If the patient is medically **unstable,** consider using amiodarone or diltiazem.
12. Reassess the patient. If the dysrhythmia has converted to another rhythm and/or rate, reassess the patient; if necessary, treat the new dysrhythmia.

Supraventricular Tachycardia

1. Assess the patient. If the patient is medically stable, continue to observe the patient. If the patient is medically unstable, begin treatment, following the guidelines for the treatment of PAT/PSVT.
2. Provide oxygen; apply pulse oximetry.
3. Begin IV fluids.
4. The physician may perform vagal stimulation, such as Valsalva's maneuver (have the patient bear down) or carotid massage. Reassess the patient.
5. Obtain a 12-Lead electrocardiograph. Reassess the patient.

6. Administer adenosine; must be pushed rapidly to be effective.
7. If SVT continues, administer adenosine again at a higher dose; may repeat the higher dose once after 1 to 2 minutes.
8. If SVT continues, reassess the patient and monitor BP. If the systolic pressure is normal or high, administer verapamil.
9. Wait 15 to 30 minutes; if SVT continues, repeat verapamil.
10. If the patient is medically **stable,** consider using these drugs and treatment in the following order: calcium channel blockers, beta blockers, digoxin, synchronized cardioversion, procainamide, and amiodarone, to convert the SVT to a normal or more stable rhythm.
11. Reassess the patient.
12. If the patient is medically **unstable,** consider using digoxin, amiodarone, or diltiazem.
13. Reassess the patient. If the dysrhythmia has converted to another rhythm and/or rate, reassess the patient; if necessary, treat the new dysrhythmia.

Atrial Flutter/Atrial Fibrillation/Wolff-Parkinson-White Syndrome

1. Assess the patient. If the patient is medically stable, continue to observe the patient. If the patient is medically unstable, begin treatment.
2. Provide oxygen; apply pulse oximetry.
3. Begin IV fluids.
4. If overall HR is bradycardic, administer atropine. Reassess the patient; repeat atropine, if necessary.
5. An artificial pacemaker (temporary or permanent) may be necessary. Use a transcutaneous or transvenous pacemaker, if available, until a permanent pacemaker is placed.
6. Obtain a 12-Lead electrocardiograph. Reassess the patient.
7. Dopamine may be administered for a systolic BP less than 80 mm Hg.
8. Epinephrine may be administered to patients who do not respond to atropine.
9. Isoproterenol may be helpful for symptomatic bradycardia when used at low doses, until a pacemaker is available; use this drug with caution.
10. Consider using vagal stimulation, digoxin, beta blockers, verapamil, amiodarone, ibutilide, procainamide, or diltiazem if the patient's HR is greater than 100 but less than 151 beats/min. If HR is greater than 150 beats/min, treat as SVT. (Do **not** use adenosine, beta blockers, calcium channel blockers, or digoxin in WPW syndrome.)
11. Synchronized cardioversion may be indicated.
12. Reassess the patient. If the dysrhythmia has converted to another rhythm and/or rate, reassess the patient; if necessary, treat the new dysrhythmia.

NOTE: In Wolff-Parkinson-White syndrome, if standard drug treatment is not successful, radio frequency catheter ablation (if available) may be the next line of therapy.

Junctional Dysrhythmia

1. Assess the patient. If the patient is medically stable, continue observing him or her.
2. If the patient is medically unstable, begin treatment, following appropriate junctional guidelines.

Junctional Bradycardia

1. Assess the patient. If the patient is medically stable, continue to observe the patient. If the patient is medically unstable, begin treatment.
2. Provide oxygen; apply pulse oximetry.
3. Begin IV infusion.
4. Administer atropine. Reassess the patient; repeat atropine, if necessary.
5. Obtain a 12-Lead electrocardiograph. Reassess the patient.
6. An artificial pacemaker (temporary or permanent) may be necessary. Use a transcutaneous or transvenous pacemaker, if available, until a permanent pacemaker is placed.
7. Dopamine may be administered for a systolic BP less than 80 mm Hg.
8. Epinephrine may be administered to patients who do not respond to atropine.
9. Isoproterenol may be helpful for symptomatic bradycardia when used at low doses, until a pacemaker is available; use this drug with caution.
10. Reassess the patient. If the dysrhythmia has converted to another rhythm and/or rate, reassess the patient; if necessary, treat the new dysrhythmia.

Accelerated Junctional Dysrhythmia/Junctional Tachycardia

1. Assess the patient. If the patient is medically unstable, begin treatment.
2. Determine the cause of the tachycardia:
   a. Fever
      (1) Administer antipyretics, such as aspirin or acetaminophen, to lower fever.
      (2) Provide cool to tepid bath.
   b. Anxiety
      (1) Acknowledge the patient's anxiety.
      (2) Offer reassurance in a calm manner.
   c. Pain
      (1) Administer pain medication as ordered.
      (2) Use relaxation techniques.
   d. Hypovolemia
      (1) Replace fluids or blood.
   e. Consider digoxin toxicity
3. Provide oxygen; apply pulse oximetry.
4. Begin IV fluids.
5. Obtain a 12-Lead electrocardiograph. Reassess the patient.
6. Consider using vagal stimulation, beta blockers, or diltiazem if the HR is greater than 100 but less than 151 beats/min. If HR is greater than 150 beats/min, treat as SVT.
7. Reassess the patient. If the dysrhythmia has converted to another rhythm and/or rate, reassess the patient; if necessary, treat the new dysrhythmia.

Premature Junctional Contraction

1. Assess the patient. PJCs are not treated unless the patient becomes medically unstable.
2. If the cause of the PJC is caffeine or nicotine, decrease or eliminate the stimulant in the patient's daily intake.
3. If the PJCs are a new occurrence, observe the patient closely for a change in the cardiac rhythm and/or rate.
4. If necessary, treat the underlying rhythm and/or HR according to the patient's symptoms.
5. Reassess the patient. If the dysrhythmia has converted to another rhythm and/or rate, reassess the patient; if necessary, treat the new dysrhythmia.

Wandering Junctional Pacemaker

1. Assess the patient. If the patient is medically stable, continue to observe the patient; if the patient shows signs of poor cardiac output, begin treatment.
2. Provide oxygen; apply pulse oximetry.
3. Begin IV fluids. Reassess the patient.
4. If overall HR is bradycardic, administer atropine. Reassess the patient; repeat atropine, if necessary.
5. Obtain a 12-Lead electrocardiograph. Reassess the patient.
6. An artificial pacemaker (temporary or permanent) may be necessary. Use a transcutaneous or transvenous pacemaker, if available, until a permanent pacemaker is placed.
7. Dopamine may be administered for a systolic BP less than 80 mm Hg.
8. Epinephrine may be administered to patients who do not respond to atropine.
9. Isoproterenol may be helpful for symptomatic bradycardia when used at low doses, until a pacemaker is available; use this drug with caution.
10. Consider using vagal stimulation, beta blockers, or diltiazem if the patient's HR is greater than 100 but less than 151 beats/min. If HR is greater than 150 beats/min, treat as SVT.
11. Reassess the patient. If the dysrhythmia has converted to another rhythm and/or rate, reassess the patient; if necessary, treat the new dysrhythmia.

Wandering Atrial Pacemaker

1. Assess the patient. If patient is medically stable, continue to observe the patient; if patient shows signs of poor cardiac output, begin treatment.
2. Provide oxygen; apply pulse oximetry.
3. Begin IV fluids.
4. If overall HR is bradycardic, administer atropine. Reassess the patient; repeat atropine, if necessary.
5. An artificial pacemaker (temporary or permanent) may be necessary. Use a transcutaneous or transvenous pacemaker, if available, until a permanent pacemaker is placed.
6. Obtain a 12-Lead electrocardiograph. Reassess the patient.
7. Dopamine may be administered for a systolic BP less than 80 mm Hg. Reassess the patient.
8. Epinephrine may be administered to patients who do not respond to atropine.
9. Isoproterenol may be helpful for symptomatic bradycardia when used at low doses, until a pacemaker is available; use this drug with caution.
10. Consider using vagal stimulation, digoxin, beta blockers, or diltiazem if the patient's HR is greater than 100 but less than 151 beats/min. If HR is greater than 150 beats/min, treat as SVT.
11. Reassess the patient. If the dysrhythmia has converted to another rhythm and/or rate, reassess the patient; if necessary, treat the new dysrhythmia.

First-Degree Heart Block

1. Assess the patient. A first-degree block by itself does not require treatment.
2. If the first-degree block is a new occurrence, observe the patient closely for a change in the cardiac rhythm and/or rate.
3. If the patient is medically unstable or is showing signs of poor cardiac output, treat the underlying rhythm and/or rate.
4. Continue to reassess and monitor the patient.
5. Reassess the patient. If the dysrhythmia has converted to another rhythm and/or rate, reassess the patient; if necessary, treat the new dysrhythmia.

Second-Degree Heart Block, Type I (Wenckebach, Mobitz I)

1. Assess the patient. A second-degree heart block, Type I, by itself does not usually require treatment.
2. If the Wenckebach is a new occurrence, observe the patient closely for a change in the cardiac rhythm and/or rate.
3. If the patient is showing signs of poor cardiac output, treat the underlying rhythm and/or rate.
4. Continue to reassess and monitor the patient.
5. Reassess the patient. If the dysrhythmia has converted to another rhythm and/or rate, reassess the patient; if necessary, treat the new dysrhythmia.

Second-Degree Heart Block, Type II (Mobitz II)

1. Assess the patient. Remember, this may become a lethal dysrhythmia. If the patient is medically unstable or is showing signs of poor cardiac output, treatment should be started immediately.
2. Provide oxygen; apply pulse oximetry.
3. Begin IV fluids. Reassess the patient.
4. If overall HR is bradycardic, administer atropine. (Atropine should be used with caution in a second-degree heart block, Type II, because it may only increase the atrial rate, which may increase the block.) Reassess the patient.
5. Obtain a 12-Lead electrocardiograph. Reassess the patient.
6. An artificial pacemaker (temporary or permanent) may be necessary. Use a transcutaneous or transvenous pacemaker, if available, until a permanent pacemaker is placed.
7. Dopamine may be administered for a systolic BP less than 80 mm Hg.
8. Epinephrine may be administered to patients who do not respond to atropine. Reassess the patient.
9. Reassess the patient. If the dysrhythmia has converted to another rhythm and/or rate, reassess the patient; if necessary, treat the new dysrhythmia.

Third-Degree Heart Block (Complete Heart Block, Complete AV Dissociation)

1. Assess the patient. Remember, this is a lethal dysrhythmia. If the patient is medically stable, continue to observe the patient while setting up a pacemaker. If the patient shows signs of poor cardiac output, begin treatment immediately.
2. Provide oxygen; apply pulse oximetry.
3. Begin IV fluids.
4. If overall HR is bradycardic, administer atropine. (Atropine may be contraindicated if the QRS is wider than 0.12 seconds; atropine may worsen the block by increasing only the atrial rate.) Reassess the patient.
5. Obtain a 12-Lead electrocardiograph. Reassess the patient.
6. An artificial pacemaker (temporary or permanent) may be necessary. Use a transcutaneous or transvenous pacemaker, if available, until a permanent pacemaker is placed.
7. Dopamine may be administered for a systolic BP less than 80 mm Hg.
8. Epinephrine IV may be administered to patients who do not respond to atropine. Reassess the patient.
9. Reassess the patient. If the dysrhythmia has converted to another rhythm and/or rate, reassess the patient; if necessary, treat the new dysrhythmia.

Bundle Branch Block

1. Assess the patient. A bundle branch block by itself does not require treatment.
2. If the bundle branch block is a new occurrence, observe the patient closely for a change in the cardiac rhythm and/or rate.
3. If the patient is medically unstable and is showing signs of poor cardiac output, treat the underlying rhythm and/or rate.
4. Continue to monitor and reassess the patient.

Premature Ventricular Contraction

1. Assess the patient. Begin treatment if the patient is showing signs of poor cardiac output or if any of the following "danger signals" are present:
   a. More than six PVCs in 1 minute
   b. Bigeminy
   c. Multifocal PVCs
   d. R on T phenomenon
   e. Run of V Tach
2. Provide oxygen; apply pulse oximetry.
3. Begin IV fluids.
4. If the rate is bradycardic, administer atropine. Reassess the patient; repeat atropine, if necessary.
5. Obtain a 12-Lead electrocardiograph. Reassess the patient.
6. If the HR is not bradycardic, administer procainamide. Remember, the patient's HR must be at least 60 beats/min, without counting PVCs, before starting procainamide.
7. Administer procainamide until any one of the following occurs:
   a. Total of 17 mg/kg has been given
   b. The PVCs stop
   c. The patient becomes hypotensive
   d. The QRS becomes 50% wider than before administration of procainamide
8. If the PVCs have been controlled and the patient has a pulse, start an IV infusion of procainamide.
9. Reassess the patient.
10. If procainamide is not successful, start an amiodarone IV infusion.
11. If neither procainamide nor amiodarone control the PVCs, administer lidocaine.
12. If lidocaine has controlled the PVCs and the patient has a pulse, start a continuous lidocaine infusion.
13. Reassess the patient. If the dysrhythmia has converted to another rhythm and/or rate, reassess the patient; if necessary, treat the new dysrhythmia.

Ventricular Tachycardia

1. Assess the patient. Remember, this may be a lethal dysrhythmia. If the patient has a pulse and is in stable condition, begin treatment. (If the patient is medically unstable, see #7 below; if the patient has no pulse, see #8 below.)
2. Provide oxygen; apply pulse oximetry.
3. Start IV fluids. Reassess the patient.
4. Administer procainamide until any one of the following occurs:
   a. Total of 17 mg/kg has been given.
   b. The PVCs stop or the dysrhythmia has converted.
   c. The patient becomes hypotensive.
   d. The QRS becomes 50% wider than before administration of procainamide.

5. Start a procainamide infusion, if the procainamide has controlled the VT and the patient has a pulse.
6. Reassess the patient. If procainamide did not control the VT, administer amiodarone or lidocaine.
7. Continue to assess and monitor the patient. If the patient has a pulse but shows signs of poor cardiac output, begin the following treatment:
   a. Perform synchronized cardioversion if the HR is greater than 150 beats/min.
   b. If cardioversion is unsuccessful, administer amiodarone if maximum dose has not been given.
   c. Continue cardioversion attempts.
   d. If amiodarone is not successful, lidocaine may be used, as administered in the treatment of PVCs.
8. If the patient does not have a pulse **or** loses the pulse at any time during treatment, begin CPR and follow the treatment guidelines for V Fib, which is also the treatment for *pulseless ventricular tachycardia.*
9. Reassess the patient. If the dysrhythmia has converted to another rhythm and/or rate, reassess the patient; if necessary, treat the new dysrhythmia.

Torsades de Pointes

Torsades de pointes may result from a prolonged QT interval. Amiodarone, lidocaine, procainamide, and quinidine may **all** prolong QT intervals.
1. Assess the patient. If the patient has a pulse and is medically stable, continue to observe the patient. If the patient shows any signs of poor cardiac output, begin treatment.
2. Provide oxygen; apply pulse oximetry.
3. Begin IV fluids. Reassess the patient.
4. Obtain electrolyte panel and treat abnormal levels.
5. Consider overdrive pacing with a transcutaneous or transvenous pacemaker. Initiate a permanent pacemaker as soon as possible, if the patient is medically unstable.
6. Magnesium sulfate may be used. Reassess the patient.
7. Isoproterenol, phenytoin (Dilantin), and lidocaine may be used. Reassess the patient.
8. If the patient does not have a pulse **or** loses the pulse at any time during treatment, begin CPR and follow the treatment guidelines for V Fib, which is also the treatment for pulseless ventricular tachycardia.
9. Reassess the patient. If the dysrhythmia has converted to another rhythm and/or rate, reassess the patient; if necessary, treat the new dysrhythmia.

Ventricular Fibrillation

1. Assess the patient. Remember to check lead placement as some types of artifact can mimic ventricular fibrillation. If the dysrhythmia **is** V Fib or pulseless V Tach, remember, these are lethal dysrhythmias. Treatment must be started immediately.
2. Begin CPR. Continue CPR **except** during defibrillation.
3. Defibrillate. Initially, three consecutive defibrillation attempts of 200, 200 to 300, and 360 joules should be used; defibrillate at 360 joules during the remaining treatment. Reassess the patient **before** and **after** each defibrillation attempt.
4. Administer 100% oxygen by bag-valve-mask device. Intubate the patient as soon as possible.
5. Begin IV fluids. Reassess the patient.
6. Administer epinephrine. Repeat every 3 to 5 minutes, or give one single dose of vasopressin. Reassess the patient after **any** medication has been administered.
7. Defibrillate at 360 joules within 60 seconds of administering epinephrine.

8. Administer amiodarone or lidocaine IV.
9. Defibrillate at 360 joules after the administration of every medication.
10. Use magnesium sulfate in severe V Fib that does not respond to defibrillation and usual medication administration; the rhythm may be torsades de pointes.
11. Administer procainamide if amiodarone and/or lidocaine has not been effective.
12. Once the patient has a pulse, start an infusion drip of the medication that was successful in ending the V Fib.
13. Assess the patient for a change in rhythm and/or rate after each dose of medication and before and after each defibrillation attempt. When the rhythm and/or rate changes, reassess the patient; treat the new dysrhythmia, if necessary.

Idioventricular/Agonal Dysrhythmias

1. Assess the patient. Remember, these are lethal dysrhythmias, and treatment **must** be started immediately.
2. If pulseless, treat as pulseless electrical activity (PEA).
3. If patient has a pulse, treat as unstable bradycardia.
4. Reassess the patient. If the dysrhythmia has converted to another rhythm and/or rate, reassess the patient; if necessary, treat the new dysrhythmia.

Ventricular Standstill

1. Assess the patient. Remember, this is a lethal dysrhythmia, and treatment **must** be started immediately.
2. Treat as asystole.

Asystole

1. Assess the patient. Remember, this is a lethal dysrhythmia, and treatment **must** be started immediately.
2. Check lead placement. Confirm asystole in two different monitor leads (for example, Lead II and MCL I).
3. Begin CPR.
4. If unable to distinguish between fine V Fib and asystole, treat as V Fib. If the dysrhythmia is identified as asystole, continue with the following guidelines:
   a. Reassess the patient.
   b. Administer 100% oxygen by bag-valve-mask device; the patient should be intubated as soon as possible.
   c. Begin IV fluids; reassess the patient.
   d. An artificial pacemaker (temporary or permanent) may be necessary. Use a transcutaneous or transvenous pacemaker, if available, until a permanent pacemaker is placed.
   e. Administer epinephrine; may repeat every 3 to 5 minutes.
   f. Atropine may be administered IV; may repeat every 3 to 5 minutes.
5. Reassess the patient after each medication. If the cardiac dysrhythmia and/or rate changes, treat the new dysrhythmia, if necessary.

Escape Beats

1. Assess the patient. Escape beats by themselves do not require treatment.
2. If the escape beat is a new occurrence, observe the patient closely for a change in the cardiac rhythm and/or rate.
3. If the patient is medically unstable or is showing signs of poor cardiac output, treat the underlying rhythm and/or rate.
4. Continue to reassess and monitor the patient.

Aberrantly Conducted Beats

1. Assess the patient. Aberrantly conducted beats (complexes) by themselves do not require treatment.
2. If the aberrantly conducted complex is a new occurrence, observe the patient closely for a change in the cardiac rhythm and/or rate.
3. If the patient is medically unstable or is showing signs of poor cardiac output, treat the underlying rhythm and/or rate.
4. Continue to assess and monitor the patient.

Pulseless Electrical Activity

PEA, formerly known as *electromechanical dissociation*, includes idioventricular dysrhythmias and bradyasystole dysrhythmias.

1. Assess the patient. Remember, this is a lethal dysrhythmia, and treatment **must** be started immediately, **regardless** of what the monitor shows.
2. Begin CPR.
3. Provide 100% oxygen by bag-valve-mask device. Intubate the patient as soon as possible.
4. Start IV fluids. Reassess the patient.
5. Consider possible causes:
   a. Hypovolemia—give fluid replacement; reassess the patient.
   b. Hypoxia—increase ventilations and oxygen; reassess the patient.
   c. Cardiac tamponade—physician performs pericardiocentesis; reassess the patient.
   d. Tension pneumothorax—perform needle decompression; reassess the patient.
   e. Acidosis—obtain arterial blood gas values (ABGs); evaluate and treat appropriately.
   f. Hypokalemia or hyperkalemia—obtain electrolyte panel and treat accordingly.
   g. Hypothermia—assess patient for low body temperature and treat accordingly.
   h. Assess patient for any of the following additional causes:
      (1) Drug overdose
      (2) Coronary thrombosis (ACS)
      (3) Pulmonary thrombosis (embolism)
6. Administer epinephrine; may repeat every 3 to 5 minutes.
7. Reassess the patient.
8. If dysrhythmia is bradycardic, administer atropine; may repeat every 3 to 5 minutes until the maximum dose is given; reassess patient after each dose.
9. Reassess the patient. If the dysrhythmia has converted to another rhythm and/or rate, reassess the patient; if necessary, treat the new dysrhythmia.

Pacemaker Rhythms

1. Assess the patient. If the patient is medically unstable, treat the underlying rhythm and/or rate.
2. If the pacemaker is malfunctioning (not pacing), the pacemaker must be repaired or replaced. A transcutaneous or transvenous pacemaker may be used temporarily until the permanent pacemaker is repaired or replaced.
3. Provide oxygen; apply pulse oximetry.
4. Start IV fluids.
5. Reassure the patient by giving frequent explanations of the procedures being performed and by acting in a calm manner.
6. Continue to reassess and monitor the patient.

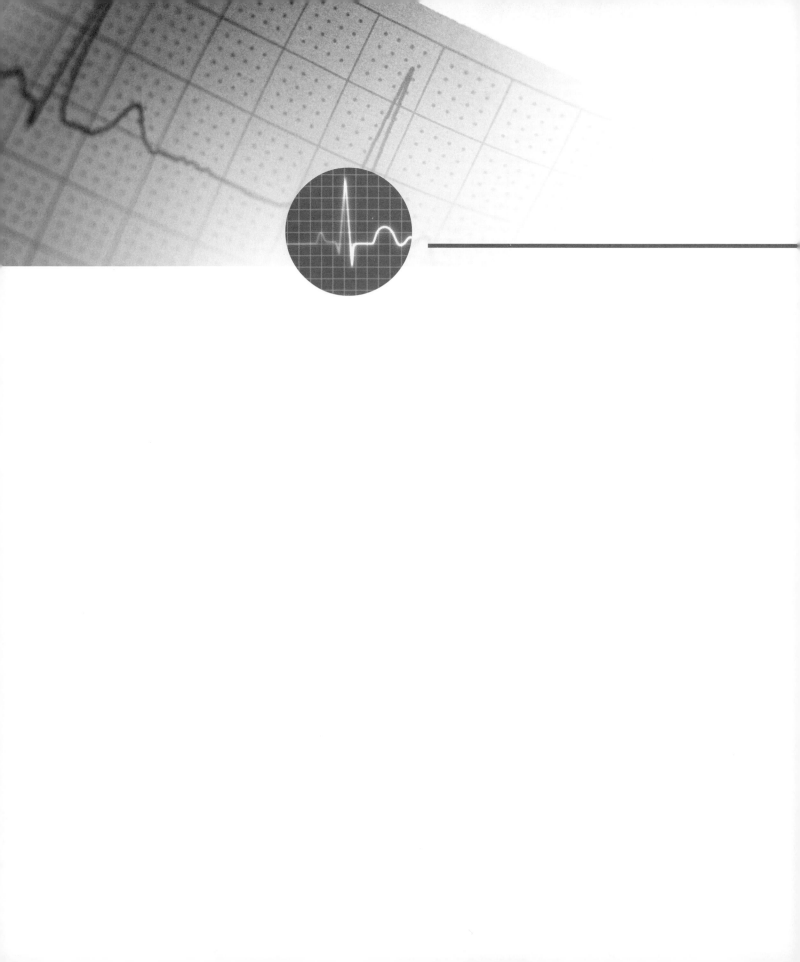

CHAPTER 10

DYSRHYTHMIA INTERPRETATION PRACTICE

As with most skills, interpreting cardiac rhythm strips takes practice, practice, and more practice. Use any rhythm strips that are available to you, since the more strips you look at and interpret, the easier it will become.

This chapter is designed for you to practice all that you have learned, in order to interpret cardiac dysrhythmia strips. The practice strips range from simple to complicated, but all have been discussed in the previous chapters. Take your time and remember to look at each strip using the steps you learned in chapter two. Just as a reminder, to accurately interpret a cardiac rhythm strip, you must:

1. Evaluate the P waves, including the ratio of P waves to QRS complexes.
2. Measure the PR intervals.
3. Evaluate the QRS complexes, including shape and size.
4. Identify any abnormalities in the ST segments, T waves, and QT intervals.
5. Count both the atrial and ventricular rates.
6. Look for any unusual markings on the strip, such as pacer spikes or aberrantly conducted complexes.

Because this is a practice chapter, take as much time as you need. When you are finished, compare your answers to the answer section in the back of the book. If you have a problem with any particular group of dysrhythmias, review that chapter again.

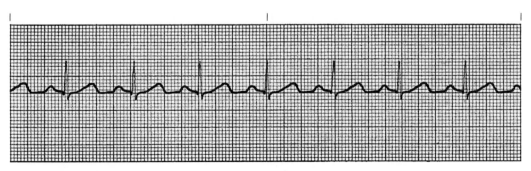

1. MEASURE: PR interval _____ Rhythm _____
               QRS complex _____ Heart rate _____
   INTERPRETATION: _____

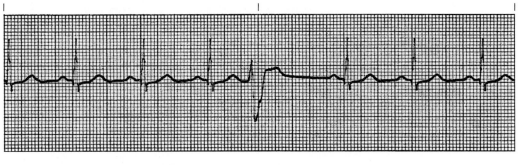

2. MEASURE: PR interval _____ Rhythm _____
                 QRS complex _____ Heart rate _____
INTERPRETATION: _____

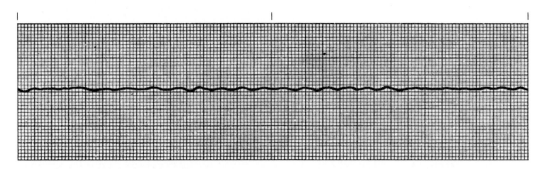

3. MEASURE: PR interval _____ Rhythm _____
                 QRS complex _____ Heart rate _____
INTERPRETATION: _____

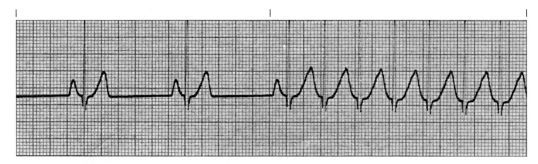

4. MEASURE: PR interval _____ Rhythm _____
                 QRS complex _____ Heart rate _____
INTERPRETATION: _____

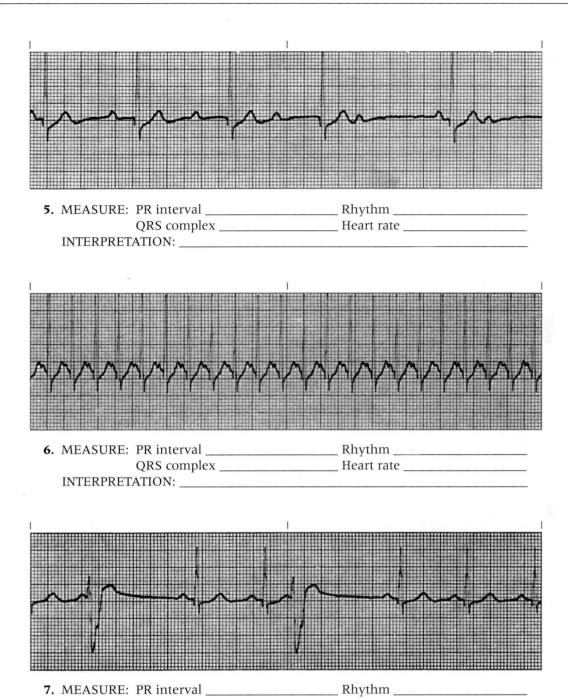

5. MEASURE: PR interval _____ Rhythm _____
                    QRS complex _____ Heart rate _____
        INTERPRETATION: _____

6. MEASURE: PR interval _____ Rhythm _____
                    QRS complex _____ Heart rate _____
        INTERPRETATION: _____

7. MEASURE: PR interval _____ Rhythm _____
                    QRS complex _____ Heart rate _____
        INTERPRETATION: _____

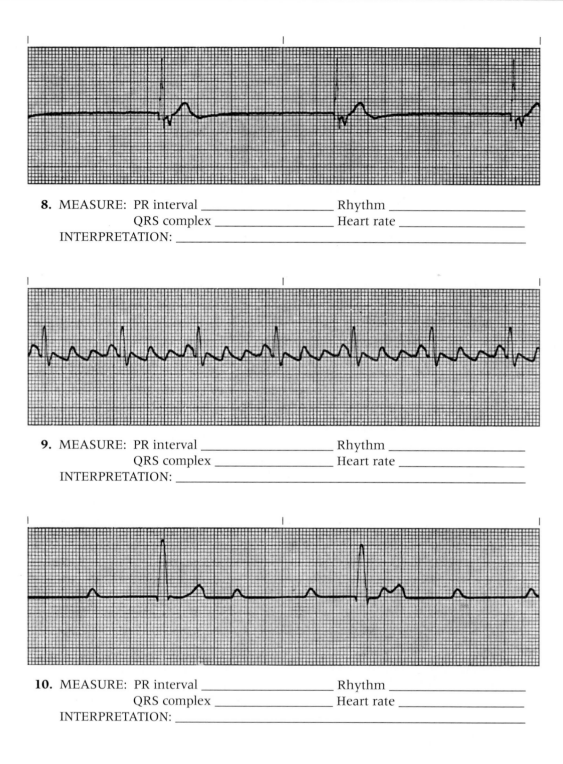

8. MEASURE: PR interval _____ Rhythm _____

QRS complex _____ Heart rate _____

INTERPRETATION: _____

9. MEASURE: PR interval _____ Rhythm _____

QRS complex _____ Heart rate _____

INTERPRETATION: _____

10. MEASURE: PR interval _____ Rhythm _____

QRS complex _____ Heart rate _____

INTERPRETATION: _____

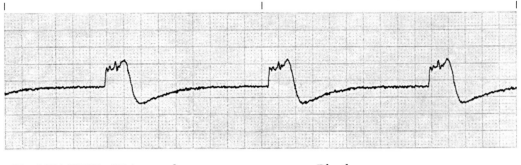

11. MEASURE: PR interval _____ Rhythm _____

QRS complex _____ Heart rate _____

INTERPRETATION: _____

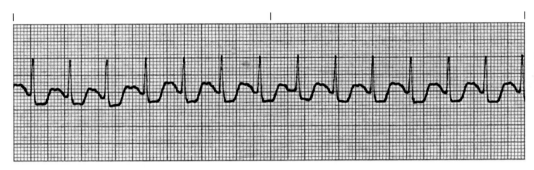

12. MEASURE: PR interval _____ Rhythm _____

QRS complex _____ Heart rate _____

INTERPRETATION: _____

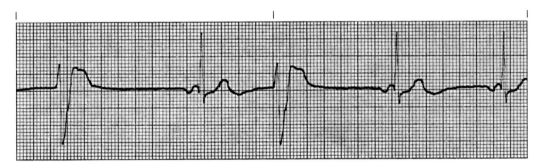

13. MEASURE: PR interval _____ Rhythm _____

QRS complex _____ Heart rate _____

INTERPRETATION: _____

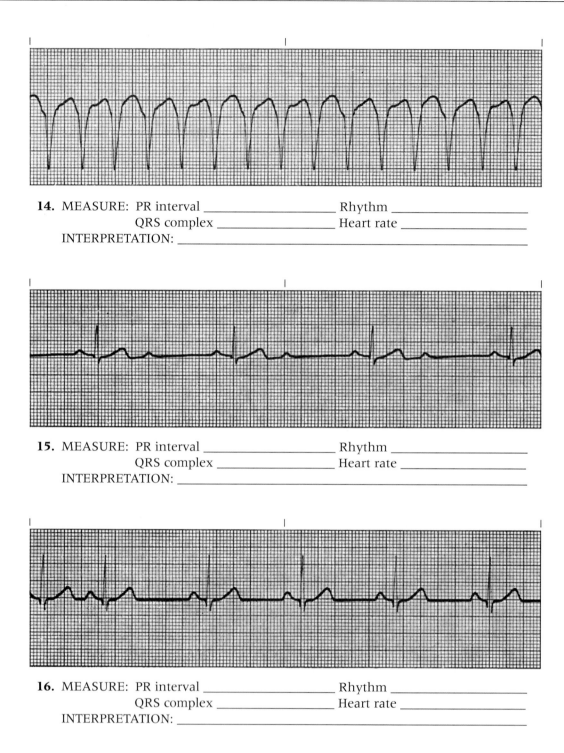

14. MEASURE: PR interval _____ Rhythm _____
    QRS complex _____ Heart rate _____
    INTERPRETATION: _____

15. MEASURE: PR interval _____ Rhythm _____
    QRS complex _____ Heart rate _____
    INTERPRETATION: _____

16. MEASURE: PR interval _____ Rhythm _____
    QRS complex _____ Heart rate _____
    INTERPRETATION: _____

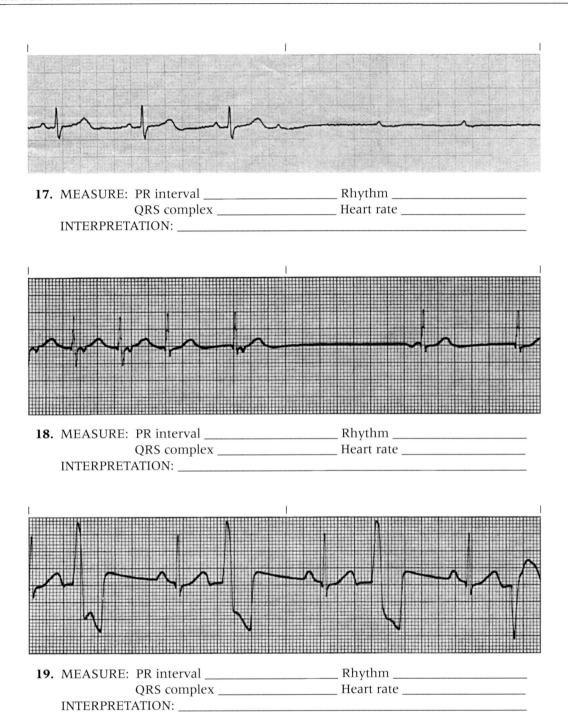

17. MEASURE: PR interval _____ Rhythm _____

QRS complex _____ Heart rate _____

INTERPRETATION: _____

18. MEASURE: PR interval _____ Rhythm _____

QRS complex _____ Heart rate _____

INTERPRETATION: _____

19. MEASURE: PR interval _____ Rhythm _____

QRS complex _____ Heart rate _____

INTERPRETATION: _____

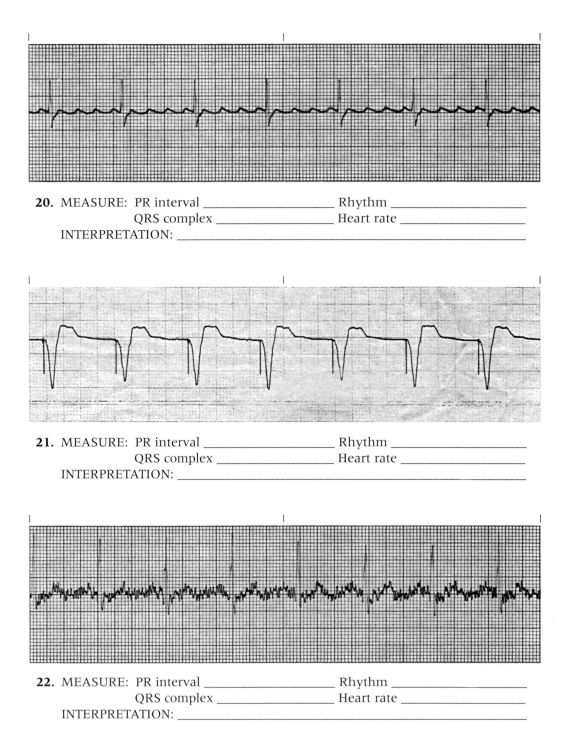

20. MEASURE: PR interval _____ Rhythm _____

QRS complex _____ Heart rate _____

INTERPRETATION: _____

21. MEASURE: PR interval _____ Rhythm _____

QRS complex _____ Heart rate _____

INTERPRETATION: _____

22. MEASURE: PR interval _____ Rhythm _____

QRS complex _____ Heart rate _____

INTERPRETATION: _____

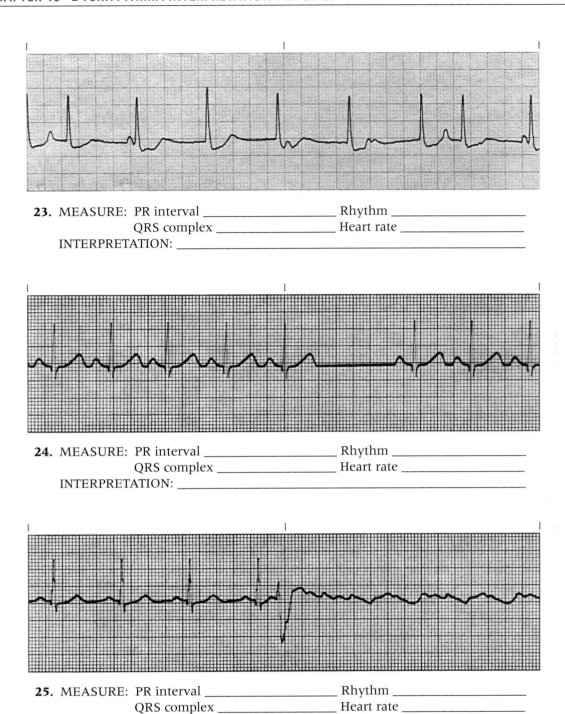

23. MEASURE: PR interval _____ Rhythm _____
         QRS complex _____ Heart rate _____
INTERPRETATION: _____

24. MEASURE: PR interval _____ Rhythm _____
         QRS complex _____ Heart rate _____
INTERPRETATION: _____

25. MEASURE: PR interval _____ Rhythm _____
         QRS complex _____ Heart rate _____
INTERPRETATION: _____

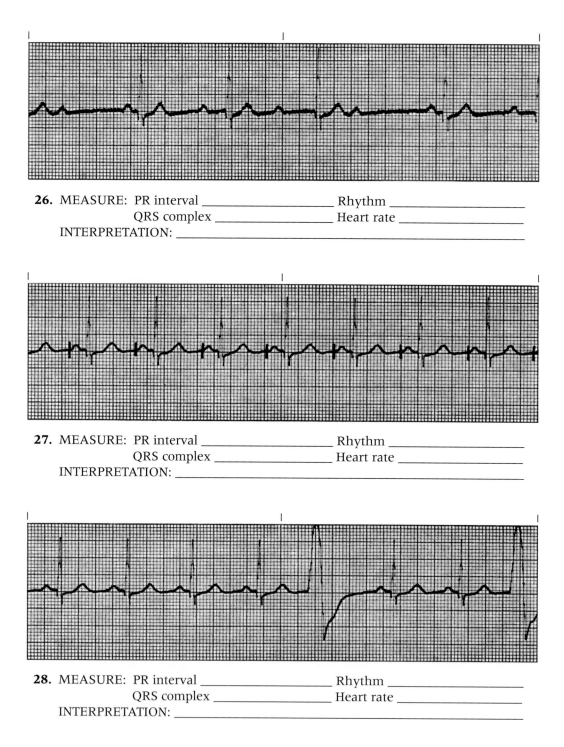

26. MEASURE: PR interval _____ Rhythm _____
QRS complex _____ Heart rate _____
INTERPRETATION: _____

27. MEASURE: PR interval _____ Rhythm _____
QRS complex _____ Heart rate _____
INTERPRETATION: _____

28. MEASURE: PR interval _____ Rhythm _____
QRS complex _____ Heart rate _____
INTERPRETATION: _____

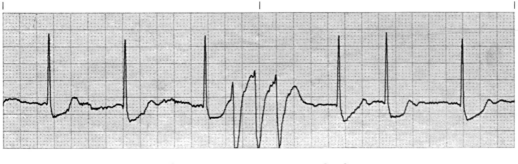

29. MEASURE: PR interval _____ Rhythm _____
                 QRS complex _____ Heart rate _____
    INTERPRETATION: _____

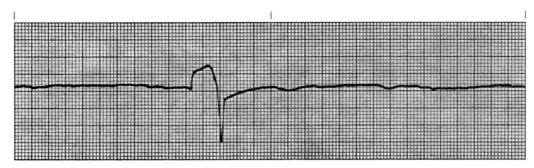

30. MEASURE: PR interval _____ Rhythm _____
                 QRS complex _____ Heart rate _____
    INTERPRETATION: _____

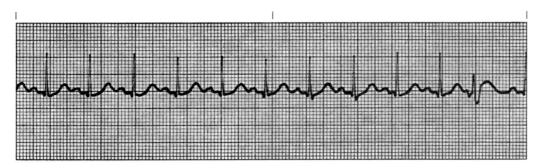

31. MEASURE: PR interval _____ Rhythm _____
                 QRS complex _____ Heart rate _____
    INTERPRETATION: _____

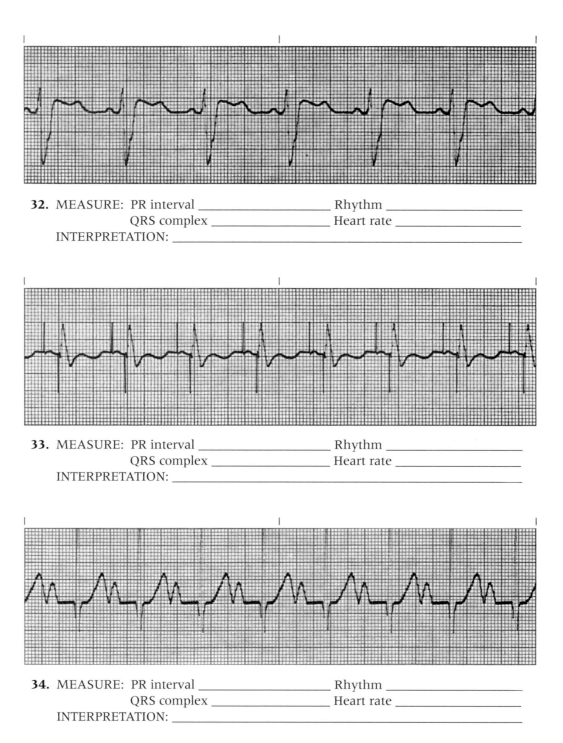

32. MEASURE: PR interval _____   Rhythm _____

QRS complex _____   Heart rate _____

INTERPRETATION: _____

33. MEASURE: PR interval _____   Rhythm _____

QRS complex _____   Heart rate _____

INTERPRETATION: _____

34. MEASURE: PR interval _____   Rhythm _____

QRS complex _____   Heart rate _____

INTERPRETATION: _____

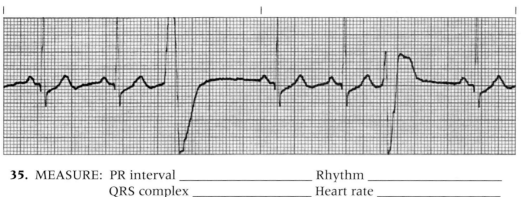

35. MEASURE: PR interval _____ Rhythm _____
QRS complex _____ Heart rate _____
INTERPRETATION: _____

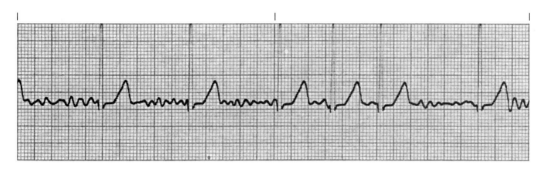

36. MEASURE: PR interval _____ Rhythm _____
QRS complex _____ Heart rate _____
INTERPRETATION: _____

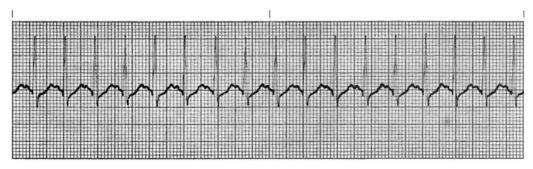

37. MEASURE: PR interval _____ Rhythm _____
QRS complex _____ Heart rate _____
INTERPRETATION: _____

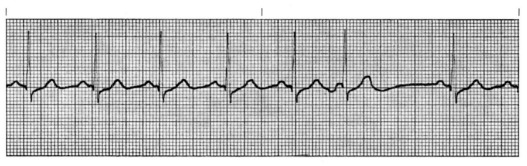

38. MEASURE: PR interval _____ Rhythm _____
QRS complex _____ Heart rate _____
INTERPRETATION: _____

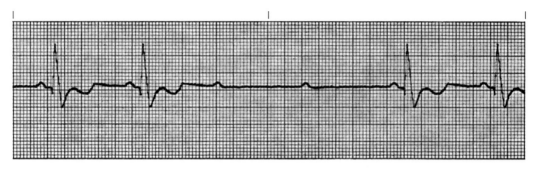

39. MEASURE: PR interval _____ Rhythm _____
QRS complex _____ Heart rate _____
INTERPRETATION: _____

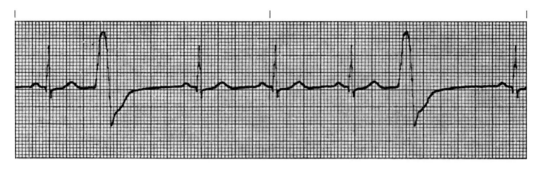

40. MEASURE: PR interval _____ Rhythm _____
QRS complex _____ Heart rate _____
INTERPRETATION: _____

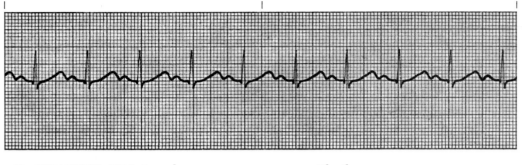

41. MEASURE: PR interval _____ Rhythm _____

QRS complex _____ Heart rate _____

INTERPRETATION: _____

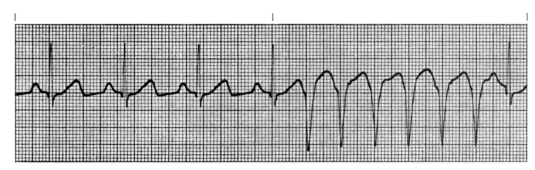

42. MEASURE: PR interval _____ Rhythm _____

QRS complex _____ Heart rate _____

INTERPRETATION: _____

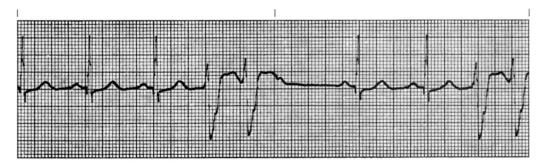

43. MEASURE: PR interval _____ Rhythm _____

QRS complex _____ Heart rate _____

INTERPRETATION: _____

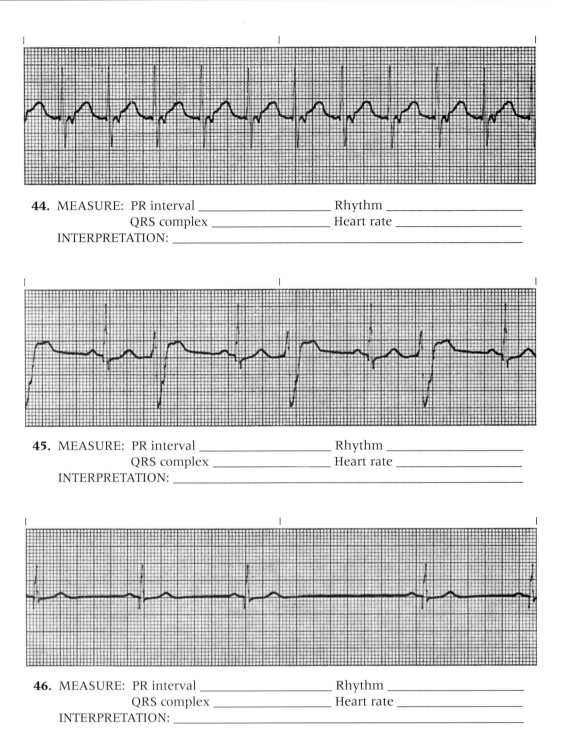

44. MEASURE: PR interval _____ Rhythm _____

                QRS complex _____ Heart rate _____

INTERPRETATION: _____

45. MEASURE: PR interval _____ Rhythm _____

                QRS complex _____ Heart rate _____

INTERPRETATION: _____

46. MEASURE: PR interval _____ Rhythm _____

                QRS complex _____ Heart rate _____

INTERPRETATION: _____

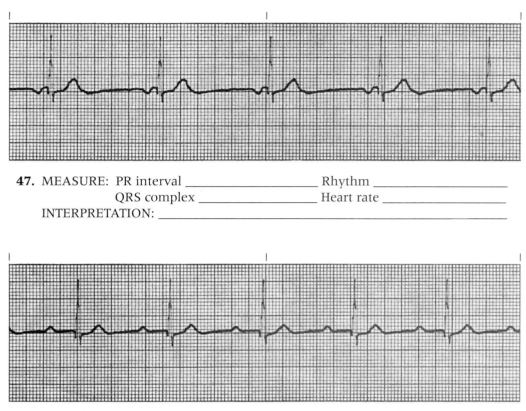

47. MEASURE: PR interval _____ Rhythm _____

QRS complex _____ Heart rate _____

INTERPRETATION: _____

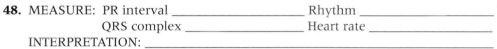

48. MEASURE: PR interval _____ Rhythm _____

QRS complex _____ Heart rate _____

INTERPRETATION: _____

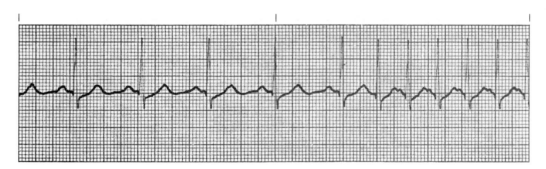

49. MEASURE: PR interval _____ Rhythm _____

QRS complex _____ Heart rate _____

INTERPRETATION: _____

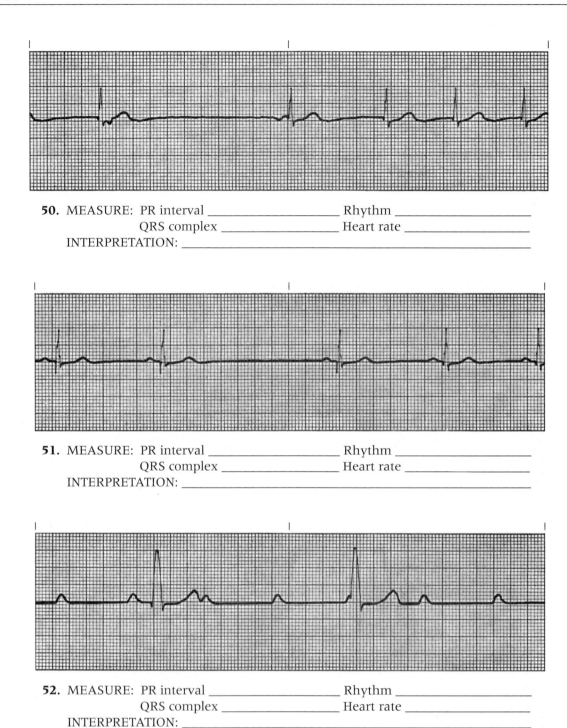

50. MEASURE: PR interval _____ Rhythm _____

QRS complex _____ Heart rate _____

INTERPRETATION: _____

51. MEASURE: PR interval _____ Rhythm _____

QRS complex _____ Heart rate _____

INTERPRETATION: _____

52. MEASURE: PR interval _____ Rhythm _____

QRS complex _____ Heart rate _____

INTERPRETATION: _____

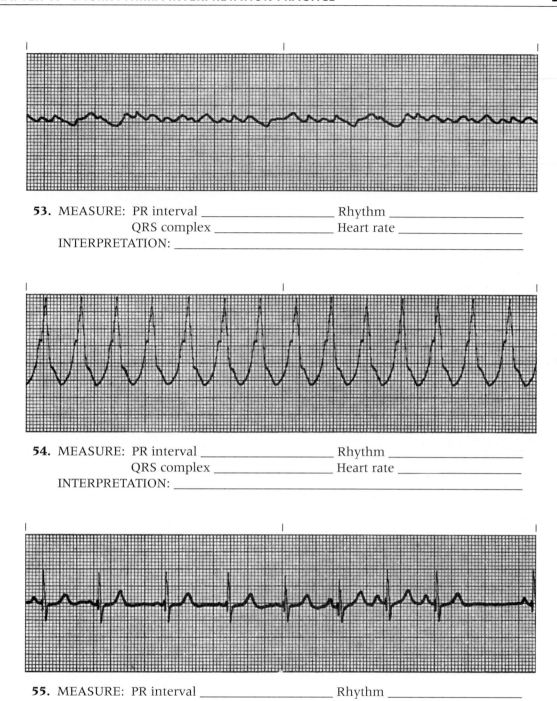

53. MEASURE: PR interval _____ Rhythm _____

QRS complex _____ Heart rate _____

INTERPRETATION: _____

54. MEASURE: PR interval _____ Rhythm _____

QRS complex _____ Heart rate _____

INTERPRETATION: _____

55. MEASURE: PR interval _____ Rhythm _____

QRS complex _____ Heart rate _____

INTERPRETATION: _____

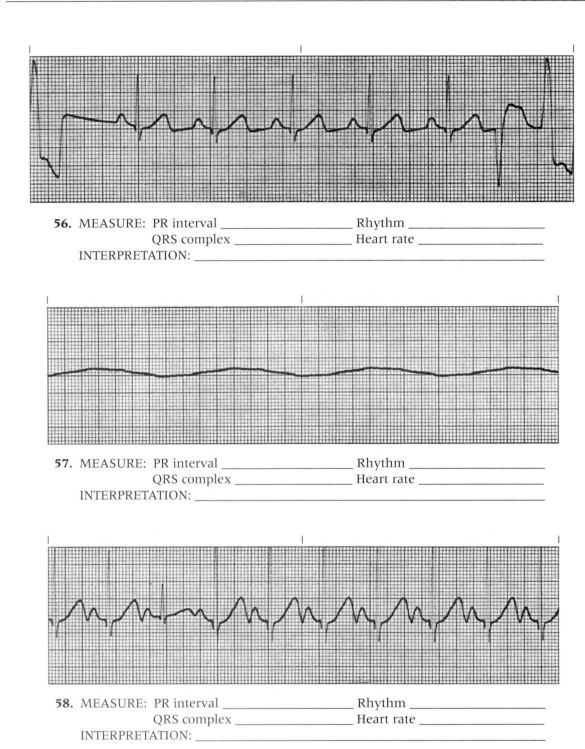

56. MEASURE: PR interval _____ Rhythm _____
                   QRS complex _____ Heart rate _____
     INTERPRETATION: _____

57. MEASURE: PR interval _____ Rhythm _____
                   QRS complex _____ Heart rate _____
     INTERPRETATION: _____

58. MEASURE: PR interval _____ Rhythm _____
                   QRS complex _____ Heart rate _____
     INTERPRETATION: _____

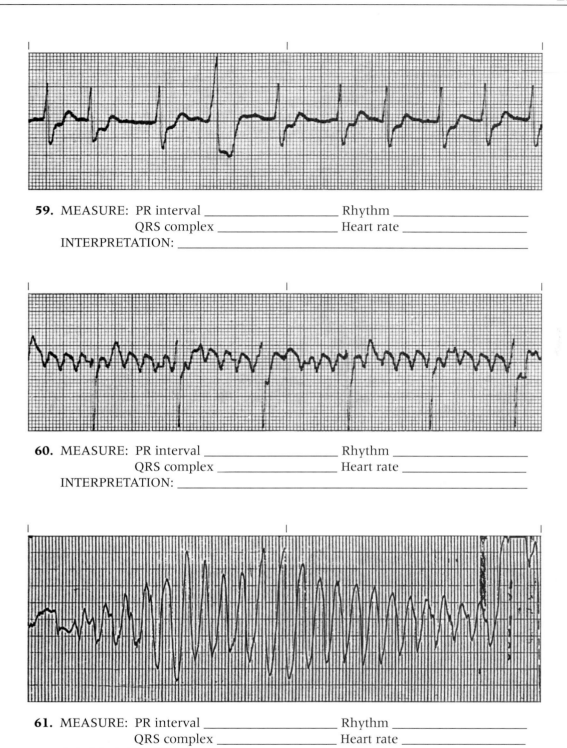

59. MEASURE: PR interval _____ Rhythm _____

QRS complex _____ Heart rate _____

INTERPRETATION: _____

60. MEASURE: PR interval _____ Rhythm _____

QRS complex _____ Heart rate _____

INTERPRETATION: _____

61. MEASURE: PR interval _____ Rhythm _____

QRS complex _____ Heart rate _____

INTERPRETATION: _____

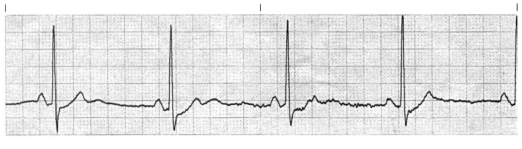

62. MEASURE: PR interval _____ Rhythm _____

QRS complex _____ Heart rate _____

INTERPRETATION: _____

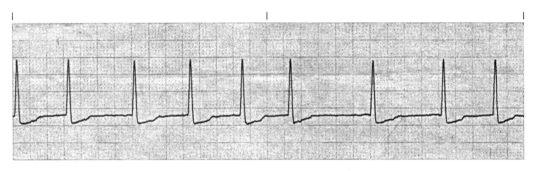

63. MEASURE: PR interval _____ Rhythm _____

QRS complex _____ Heart rate _____

INTERPRETATION: _____

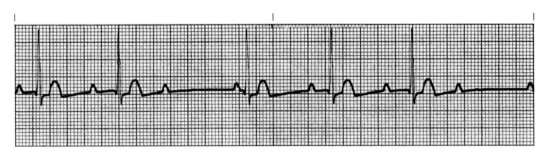

64. MEASURE: PR interval _____ Rhythm _____

QRS complex _____ Heart rate _____

INTERPRETATION: _____

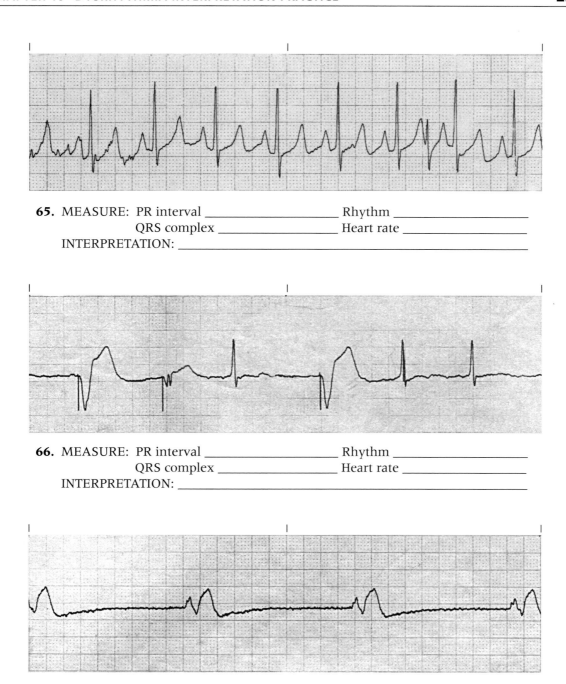

65. MEASURE: PR interval _____ Rhythm _____
                 QRS complex _____ Heart rate _____
        INTERPRETATION: _____

66. MEASURE: PR interval _____ Rhythm _____
                 QRS complex _____ Heart rate _____
        INTERPRETATION: _____

67. MEASURE: PR interval _____ Rhythm _____
                 QRS complex _____ Heart rate _____
        INTERPRETATION: _____

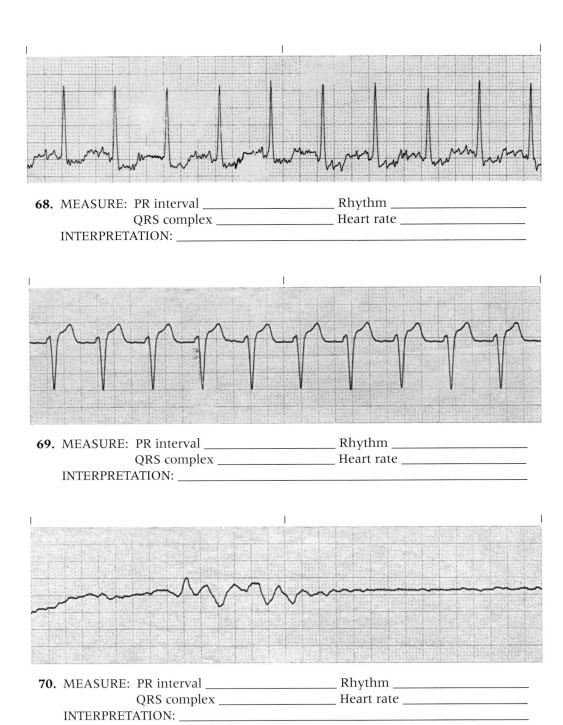

68. MEASURE: PR interval _____ Rhythm _____
QRS complex _____ Heart rate _____
INTERPRETATION: _____

69. MEASURE: PR interval _____ Rhythm _____
QRS complex _____ Heart rate _____
INTERPRETATION: _____

70. MEASURE: PR interval _____ Rhythm _____
QRS complex _____ Heart rate _____
INTERPRETATION: _____

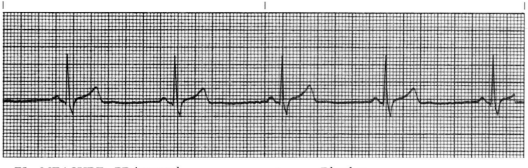

71. MEASURE: PR interval _____ Rhythm _____

QRS complex _____ Heart rate _____

INTERPRETATION: _____

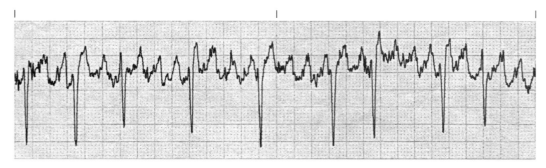

72. MEASURE: PR interval _____ Rhythm _____

QRS complex _____ Heart rate _____

INTERPRETATION: _____

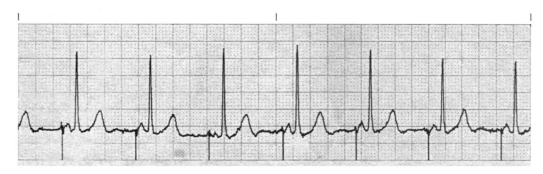

73. MEASURE: PR interval _____ Rhythm _____

QRS complex _____ Heart rate _____

INTERPRETATION: _____

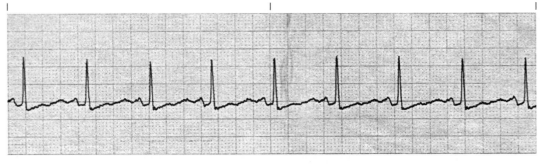

74. MEASURE: PR interval _____ Rhythm _____
                   QRS complex _____ Heart rate _____
INTERPRETATION: _____

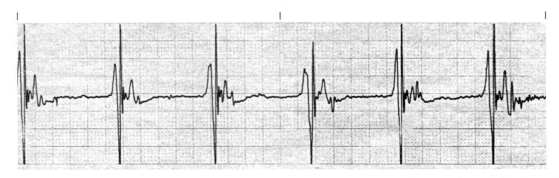

75. MEASURE: PR interval _____ Rhythm _____
                   QRS complex _____ Heart rate _____
INTERPRETATION: _____

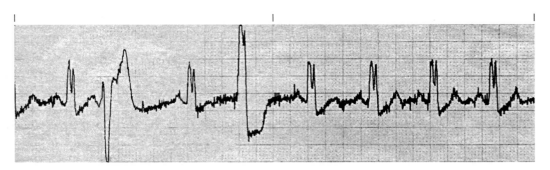

76. MEASURE: PR interval _____ Rhythm _____
                   QRS complex _____ Heart rate _____
INTERPRETATION: _____

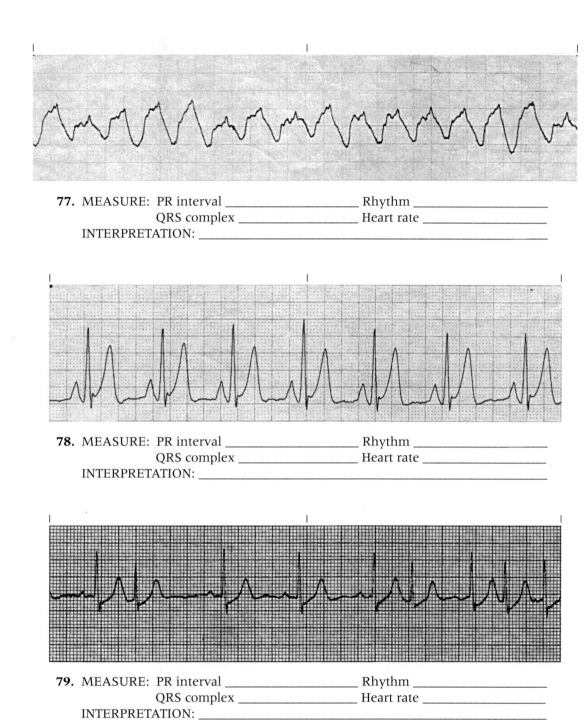

77. MEASURE: PR interval _____ Rhythm _____

QRS complex _____ Heart rate _____

INTERPRETATION: _____

78. MEASURE: PR interval _____ Rhythm _____

QRS complex _____ Heart rate _____

INTERPRETATION: _____

79. MEASURE: PR interval _____ Rhythm _____

QRS complex _____ Heart rate _____

INTERPRETATION: _____

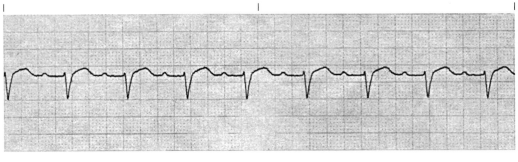

80. MEASURE: PR interval _____ Rhythm _____
QRS complex _____ Heart rate _____
INTERPRETATION: _____

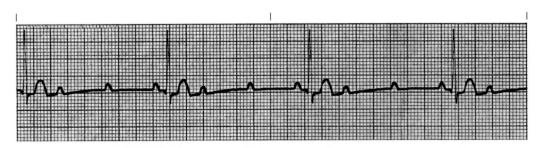

81. MEASURE: PR interval _____ Rhythm _____
QRS complex _____ Heart rate _____
INTERPRETATION: _____

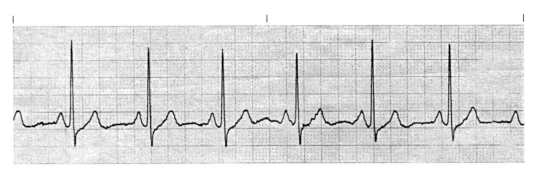

82. MEASURE: PR interval _____ Rhythm _____
QRS complex _____ Heart rate _____
INTERPRETATION: _____

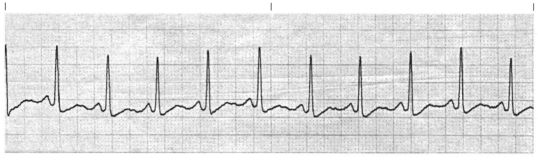

83. MEASURE: PR interval _____ Rhythm _____
              QRS complex _____ Heart rate _____
    INTERPRETATION: _____

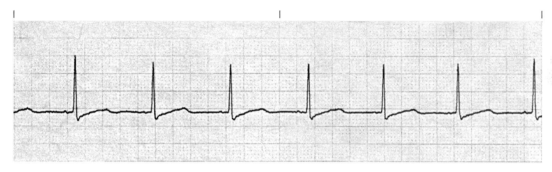

84. MEASURE: PR interval _____ Rhythm _____
              QRS complex _____ Heart rate _____
    INTERPRETATION: _____

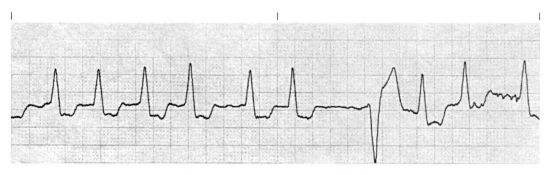

85. MEASURE: PR interval _____ Rhythm _____
              QRS complex _____ Heart rate _____
    INTERPRETATION: _____

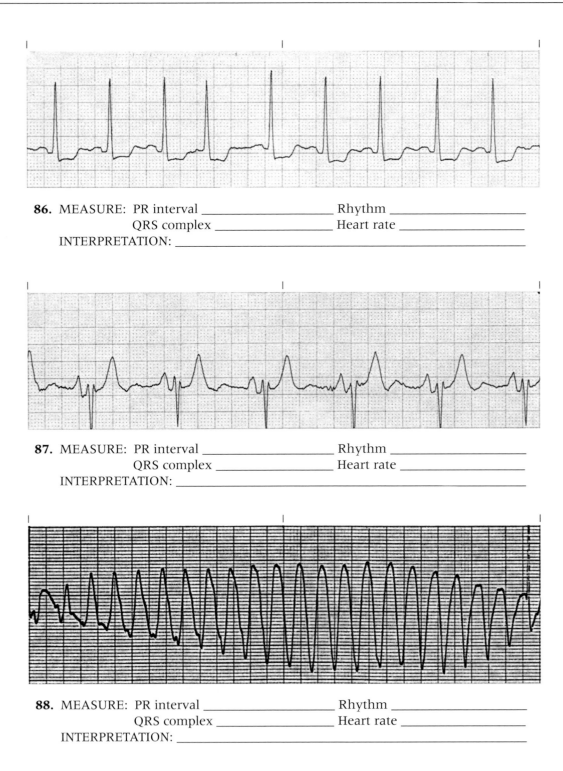

86. MEASURE: PR interval _____ Rhythm _____
QRS complex _____ Heart rate _____
INTERPRETATION: _____

87. MEASURE: PR interval _____ Rhythm _____
QRS complex _____ Heart rate _____
INTERPRETATION: _____

88. MEASURE: PR interval _____ Rhythm _____
QRS complex _____ Heart rate _____
INTERPRETATION: _____

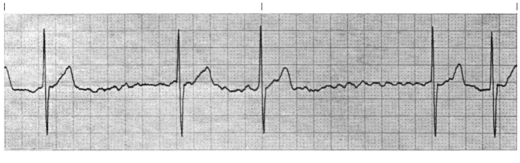

89. MEASURE: PR interval _____ Rhythm _____
QRS complex _____ Heart rate _____
INTERPRETATION: _____

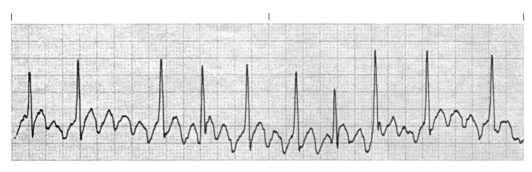

90. MEASURE: PR interval _____ Rhythm _____
QRS complex _____ Heart rate _____
INTERPRETATION: _____

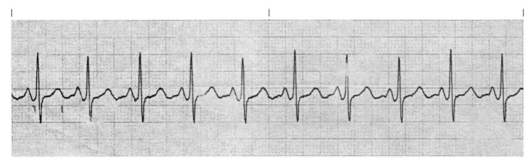

91. MEASURE: PR interval _____ Rhythm _____
QRS complex _____ Heart rate _____
INTERPRETATION: _____

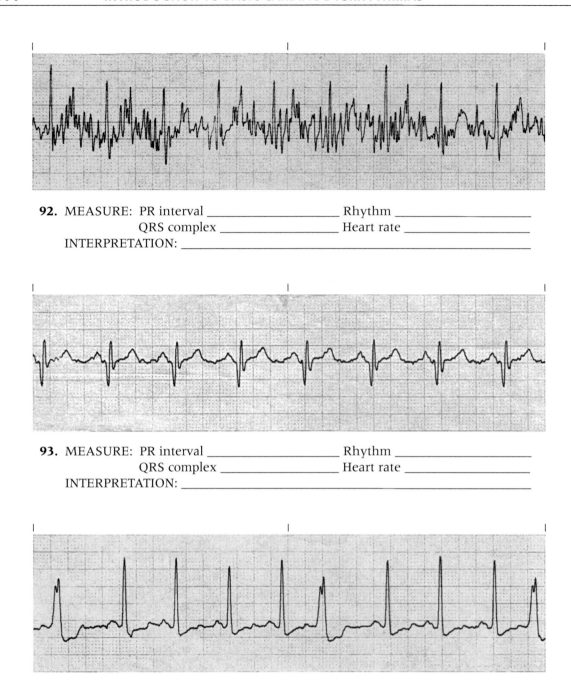

92. MEASURE: PR interval _____ Rhythm _____

QRS complex _____ Heart rate _____

INTERPRETATION: _____

93. MEASURE: PR interval _____ Rhythm _____

QRS complex _____ Heart rate _____

INTERPRETATION: _____

94. MEASURE: PR interval _____ Rhythm _____

QRS complex _____ Heart rate _____

INTERPRETATION: _____

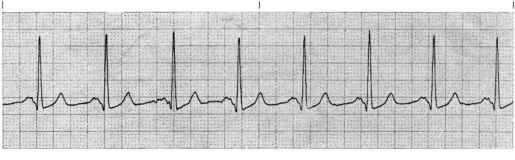

95. MEASURE: PR interval _____ Rhythm _____
                  QRS complex _____ Heart rate _____
INTERPRETATION: _____

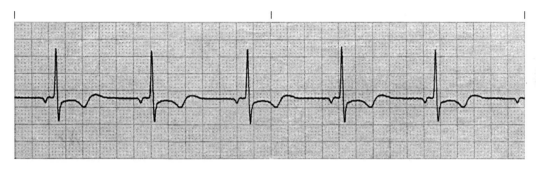

96. MEASURE: PR interval _____ Rhythm _____
                  QRS complex _____ Heart rate _____
INTERPRETATION: _____

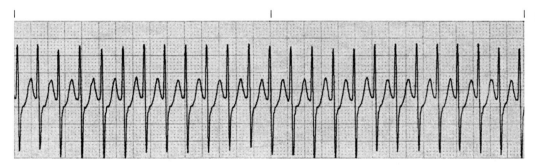

97. MEASURE: PR interval _____ Rhythm _____
                  QRS complex _____ Heart rate _____
INTERPRETATION: _____

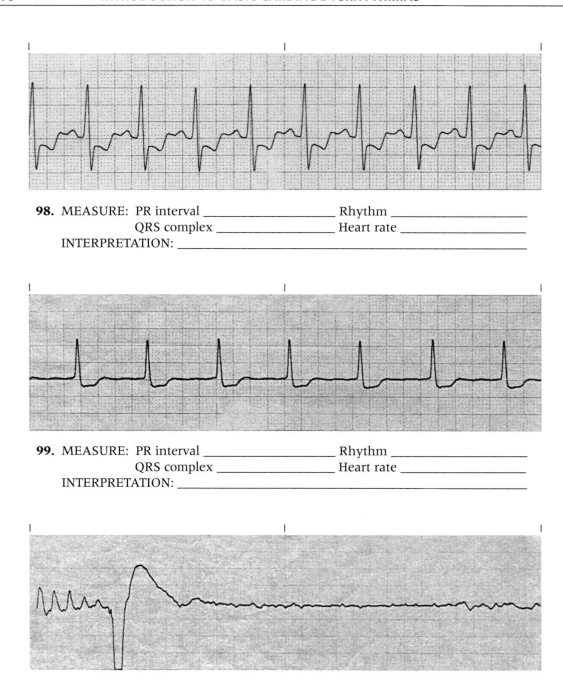

98. MEASURE: PR interval _____ Rhythm _____

QRS complex _____ Heart rate _____

INTERPRETATION: _____

99. MEASURE: PR interval _____ Rhythm _____

QRS complex _____ Heart rate _____

INTERPRETATION: _____

100. MEASURE: PR interval _____ Rhythm _____

QRS complex _____ Heart rate _____

INTERPRETATION: _____

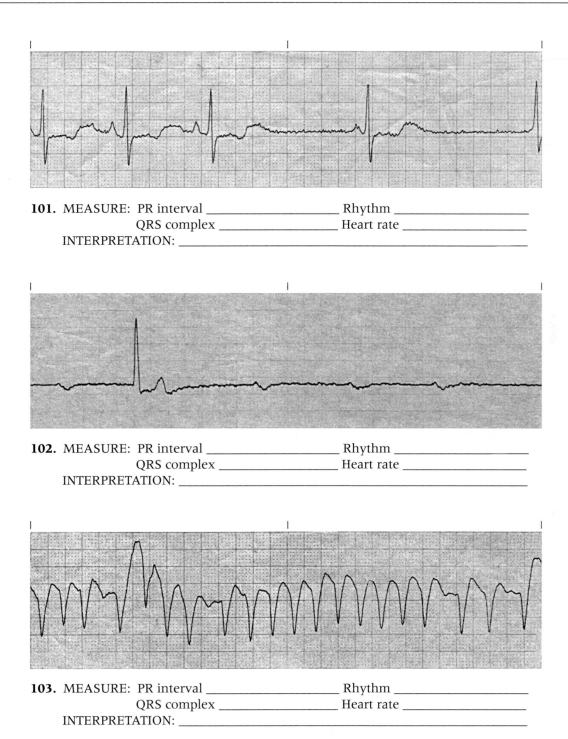

101. MEASURE: PR interval _____ Rhythm _____
QRS complex _____ Heart rate _____
INTERPRETATION: _____

102. MEASURE: PR interval _____ Rhythm _____
QRS complex _____ Heart rate _____
INTERPRETATION: _____

103. MEASURE: PR interval _____ Rhythm _____
QRS complex _____ Heart rate _____
INTERPRETATION: _____

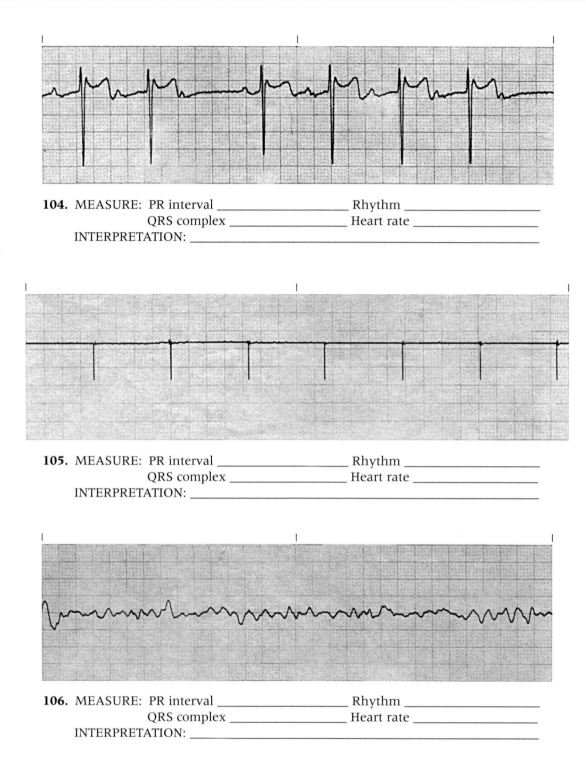

104. MEASURE: PR interval _____ Rhythm _____

QRS complex _____ Heart rate _____

INTERPRETATION: _____

105. MEASURE: PR interval _____ Rhythm _____

QRS complex _____ Heart rate _____

INTERPRETATION: _____

106. MEASURE: PR interval _____ Rhythm _____

QRS complex _____ Heart rate _____

INTERPRETATION: _____

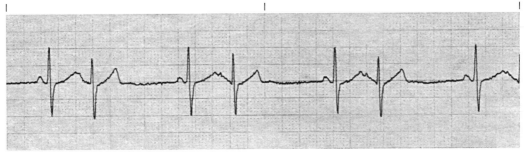

107. MEASURE: PR interval _____ Rhythm _____

QRS complex _____ Heart rate _____

INTERPRETATION: _____

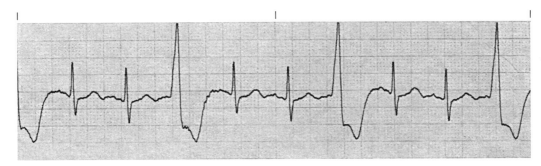

108. MEASURE: PR interval _____ Rhythm _____

QRS complex _____ Heart rate _____

INTERPRETATION: _____

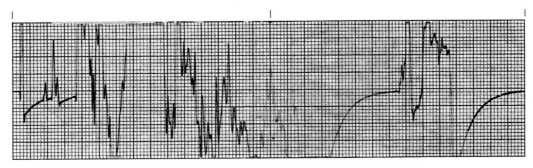

109. MEASURE: PR interval _____ Rhythm _____

QRS complex _____ Heart rate _____

INTERPRETATION: _____

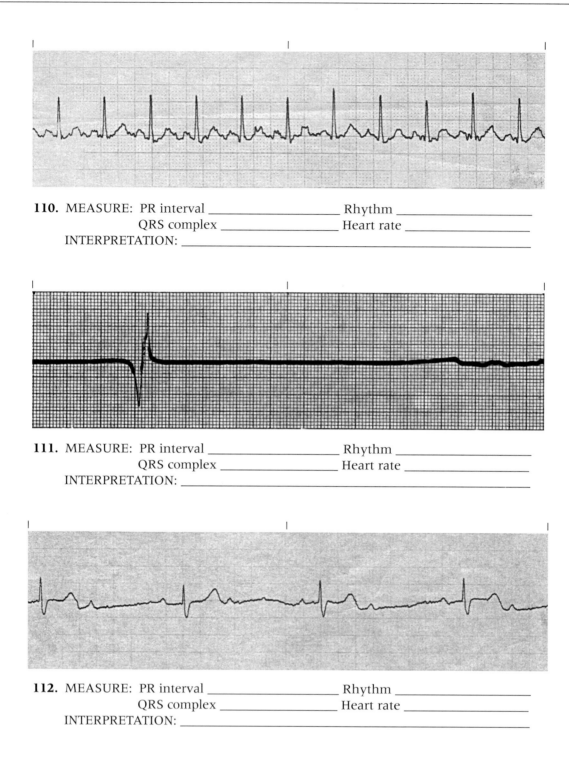

110. MEASURE: PR interval _____ Rhythm _____
                QRS complex _____ Heart rate _____
INTERPRETATION: _____

111. MEASURE: PR interval _____ Rhythm _____
                QRS complex _____ Heart rate _____
INTERPRETATION: _____

112. MEASURE: PR interval _____ Rhythm _____
                QRS complex _____ Heart rate _____
INTERPRETATION: _____

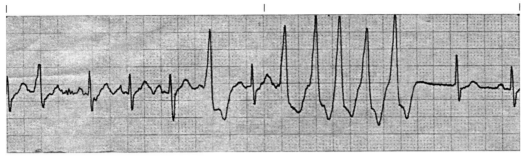

113. MEASURE: PR interval _____ Rhythm _____

QRS complex _____ Heart rate _____

INTERPRETATION: _____

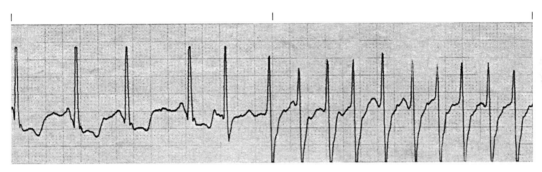

114. MEASURE: PR interval _____ Rhythm _____

QRS complex _____ Heart rate _____

INTERPRETATION: _____

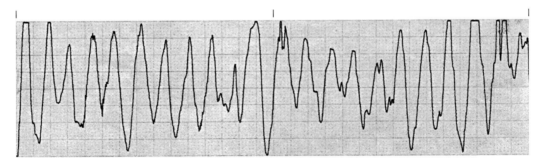

115. MEASURE: PR interval _____ Rhythm _____

QRS complex _____ Heart rate _____

INTERPRETATION: _____

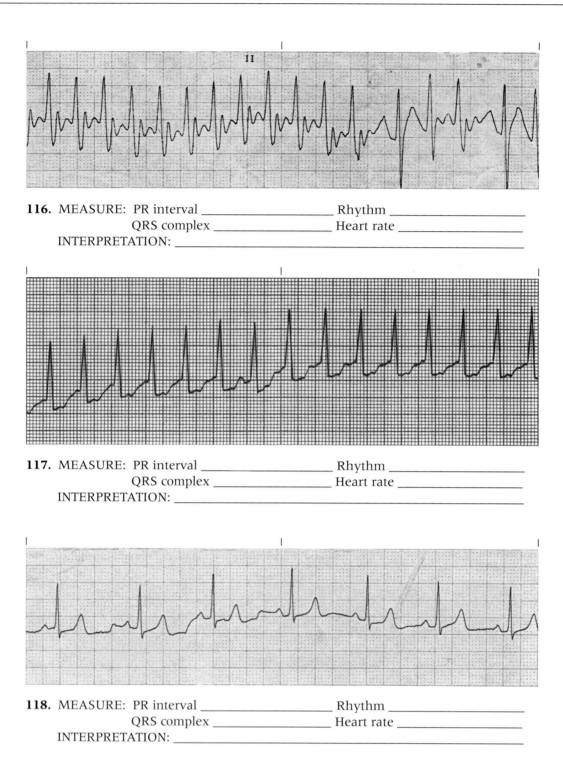

116. MEASURE: PR interval _____ Rhythm _____
　　　　　　　　QRS complex _____ Heart rate _____
　　　　INTERPRETATION: _____

117. MEASURE: PR interval _____ Rhythm _____
　　　　　　　　QRS complex _____ Heart rate _____
　　　　INTERPRETATION: _____

118. MEASURE: PR interval _____ Rhythm _____
　　　　　　　　QRS complex _____ Heart rate _____
　　　　INTERPRETATION: _____

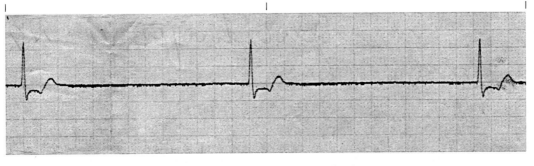

119. MEASURE: PR interval _____ Rhythm _____

QRS complex _____ Heart rate _____

INTERPRETATION: _____

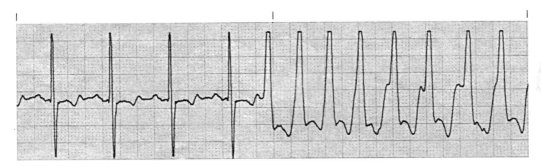

120. MEASURE: PR interval _____ Rhythm _____

QRS complex _____ Heart rate _____

INTERPRETATION: _____

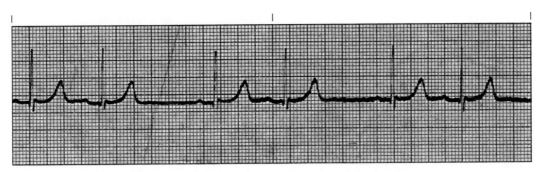

121. MEASURE: PR interval _____ Rhythm _____

QRS complex _____ Heart rate _____

INTERPRETATION: _____

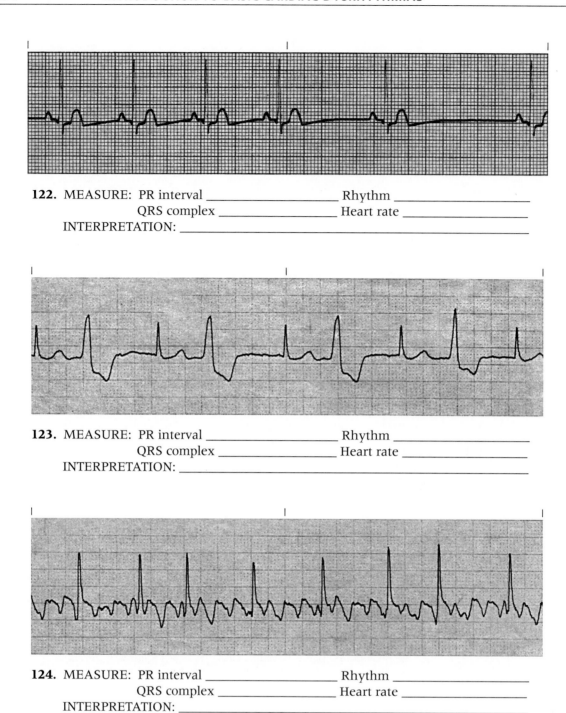

122. MEASURE: PR interval _____ Rhythm _____
QRS complex _____ Heart rate _____
INTERPRETATION: _____

123. MEASURE: PR interval _____ Rhythm _____
QRS complex _____ Heart rate _____
INTERPRETATION: _____

124. MEASURE: PR interval _____ Rhythm _____
QRS complex _____ Heart rate _____
INTERPRETATION: _____

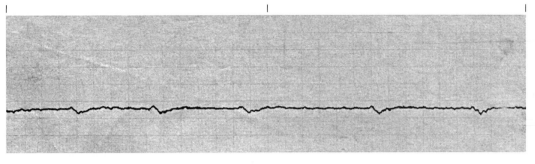

125. MEASURE: PR interval _____ Rhythm _____

  QRS complex _____ Heart rate _____

INTERPRETATION: _____

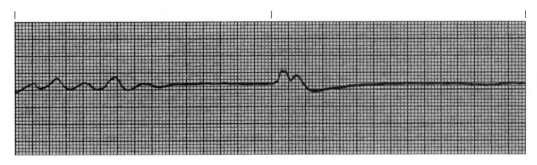

126. MEASURE: PR interval _____ Rhythm _____

  QRS complex _____ Heart rate _____

INTERPRETATION: _____

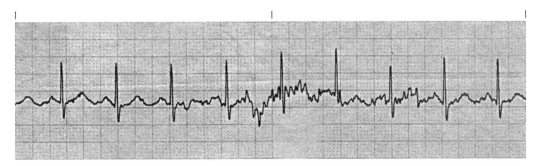

127. MEASURE: PR interval _____ Rhythm _____

  QRS complex _____ Heart rate _____

INTERPRETATION: _____

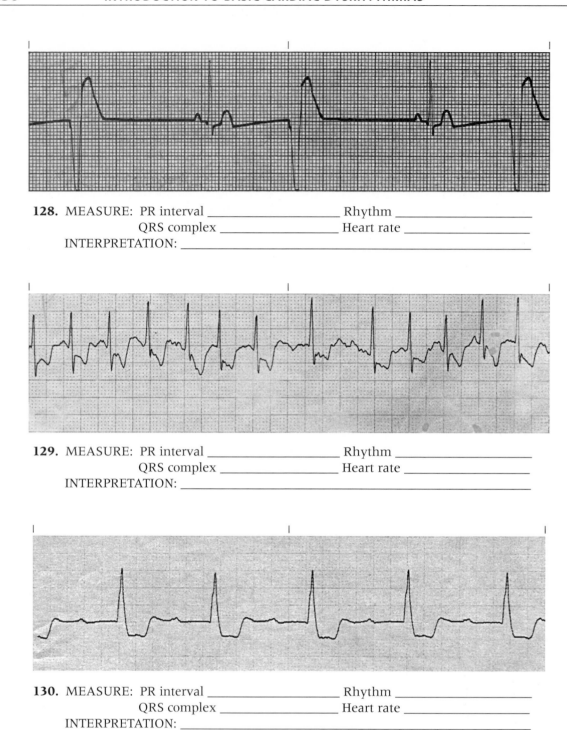

128. MEASURE: PR interval _____ Rhythm _____

QRS complex _____ Heart rate _____

INTERPRETATION: _____

129. MEASURE: PR interval _____ Rhythm _____

QRS complex _____ Heart rate _____

INTERPRETATION: _____

130. MEASURE: PR interval _____ Rhythm _____

QRS complex _____ Heart rate _____

INTERPRETATION: _____

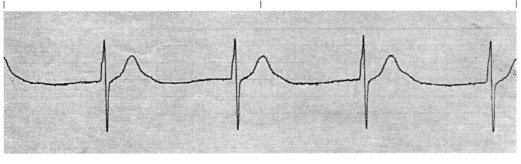

131. MEASURE: PR interval _____ Rhythm _____

QRS complex _____ Heart rate _____

INTERPRETATION: _____

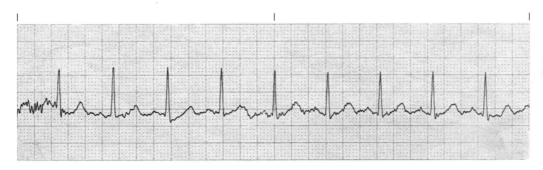

132. MEASURE: PR interval _____ Rhythm _____

QRS complex _____ Heart rate _____

INTERPRETATION: _____

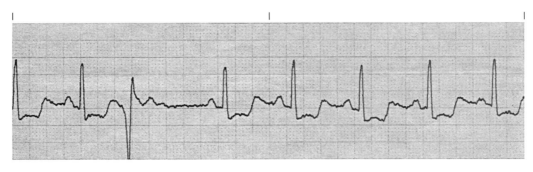

133. MEASURE: PR interval _____ Rhythm _____

QRS complex _____ Heart rate _____

INTERPRETATION: _____

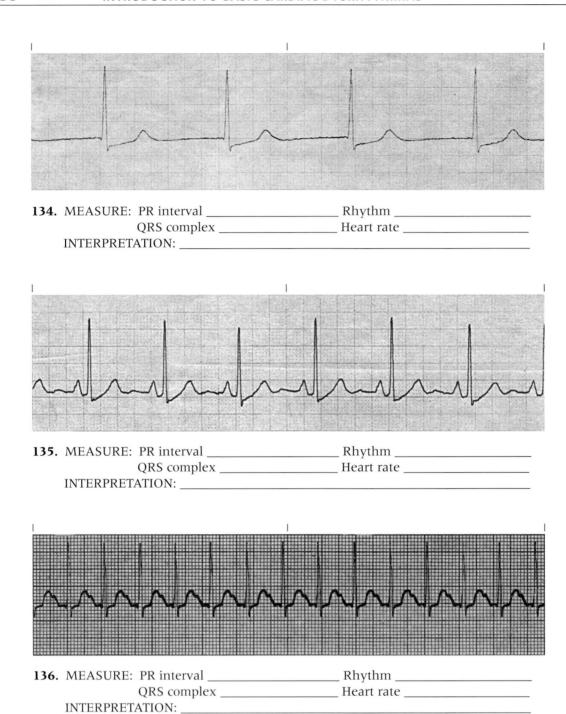

134. MEASURE: PR interval _____   Rhythm _____

QRS complex _____   Heart rate _____

INTERPRETATION: _____

135. MEASURE: PR interval _____   Rhythm _____

QRS complex _____   Heart rate _____

INTERPRETATION: _____

136. MEASURE: PR interval _____   Rhythm _____

QRS complex _____   Heart rate _____

INTERPRETATION: _____

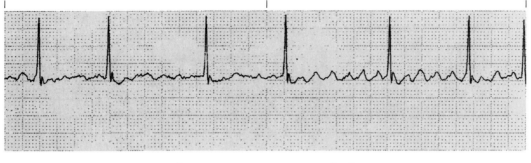

137. MEASURE: PR interval _____   Rhythm _____
                 QRS complex _____   Heart rate _____
INTERPRETATION: _____

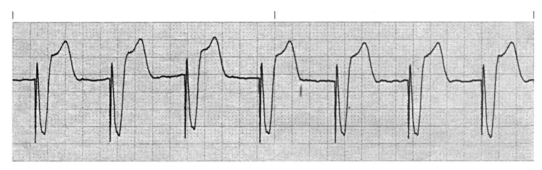

138. MEASURE: PR interval _____   Rhythm _____
                 QRS complex _____   Heart rate _____
INTERPRETATION: _____

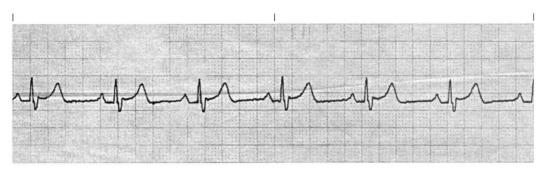

139. MEASURE: PR interval _____   Rhythm _____
                 QRS complex _____   Heart rate _____
INTERPRETATION: _____

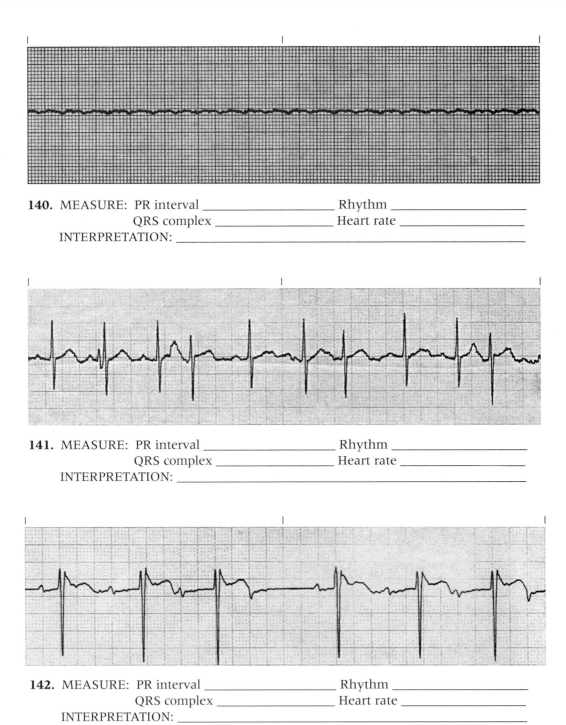

140. MEASURE: PR interval _____ Rhythm _____
QRS complex _____ Heart rate _____
INTERPRETATION: _____

141. MEASURE: PR interval _____ Rhythm _____
QRS complex _____ Heart rate _____
INTERPRETATION: _____

142. MEASURE: PR interval _____ Rhythm _____
QRS complex _____ Heart rate _____
INTERPRETATION: _____

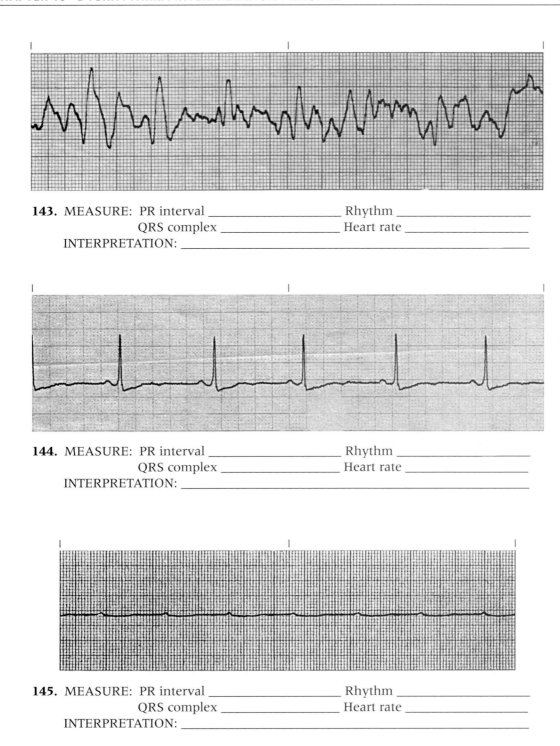

143. MEASURE: PR interval _____ Rhythm _____

QRS complex _____ Heart rate _____

INTERPRETATION: _____

144. MEASURE: PR interval _____ Rhythm _____

QRS complex _____ Heart rate _____

INTERPRETATION: _____

145. MEASURE: PR interval _____ Rhythm _____

QRS complex _____ Heart rate _____

INTERPRETATION: _____

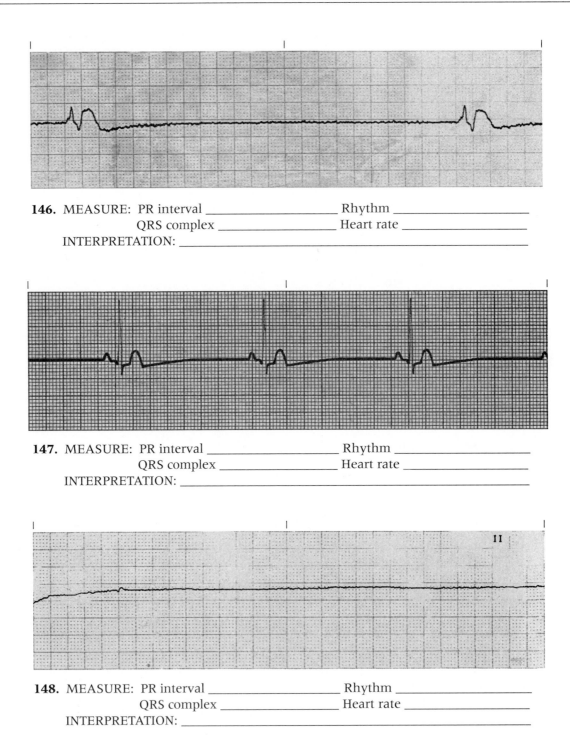

146. MEASURE: PR interval _____ Rhythm _____
QRS complex _____ Heart rate _____
INTERPRETATION: _____

147. MEASURE: PR interval _____ Rhythm _____
QRS complex _____ Heart rate _____
INTERPRETATION: _____

148. MEASURE: PR interval _____ Rhythm _____
QRS complex _____ Heart rate _____
INTERPRETATION: _____

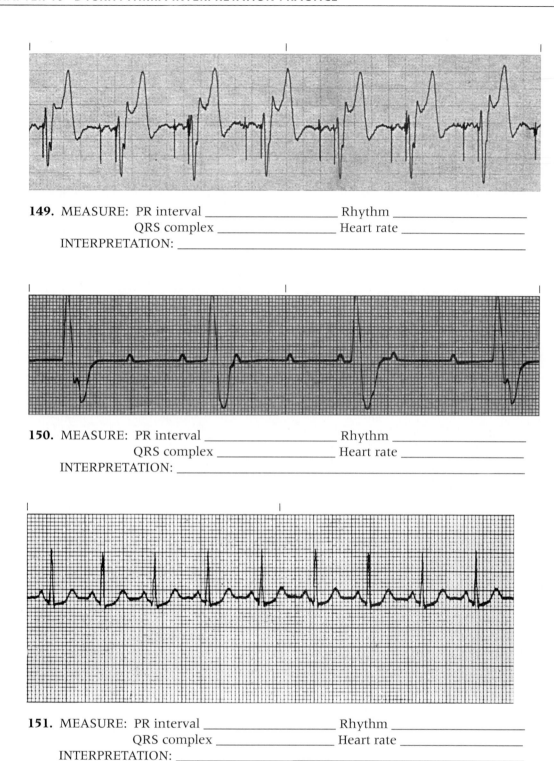

149. MEASURE: PR interval _____ Rhythm _____
            QRS complex _____ Heart rate _____
INTERPRETATION: _____

150. MEASURE: PR interval _____ Rhythm _____
            QRS complex _____ Heart rate _____
INTERPRETATION: _____

151. MEASURE: PR interval _____ Rhythm _____
            QRS complex _____ Heart rate _____
INTERPRETATION: _____

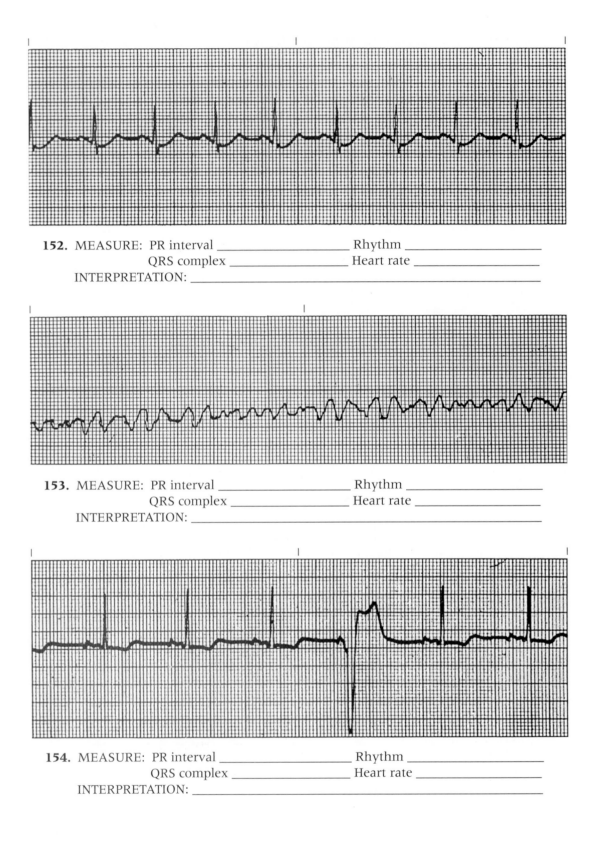

152. MEASURE: PR interval _____ Rhythm _____

QRS complex _____ Heart rate _____

INTERPRETATION: _____

153. MEASURE: PR interval _____ Rhythm _____

QRS complex _____ Heart rate _____

INTERPRETATION: _____

154. MEASURE: PR interval _____ Rhythm _____

QRS complex _____ Heart rate _____

INTERPRETATION: _____

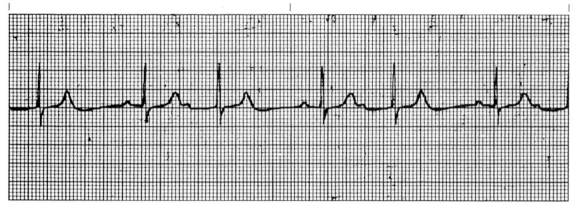

155. MEASURE: PR interval _____ Rhythm _____

QRS complex _____ Heart rate _____

INTERPRETATION: _____

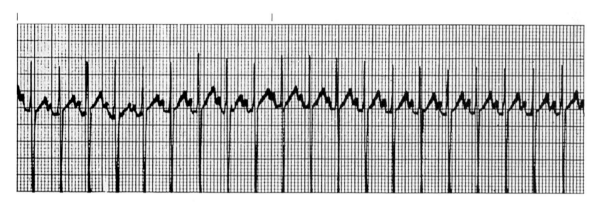

156. MEASURE: PR interval _____ Rhythm _____

QRS complex _____ Heart rate _____

INTERPRETATION: _____

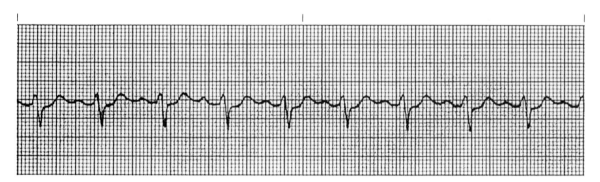

157. MEASURE: PR interval _____ Rhythm _____

QRS complex _____ Heart rate _____

INTERPRETATION: _____

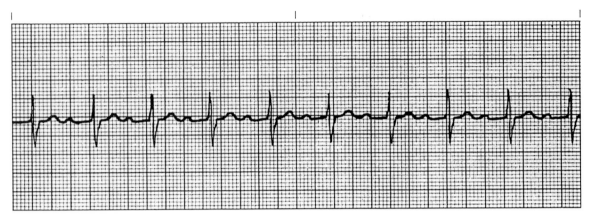

158. MEASURE: PR interval _____   Rhythm _____
                  QRS complex _____   Heart rate _____
         INTERPRETATION: _____

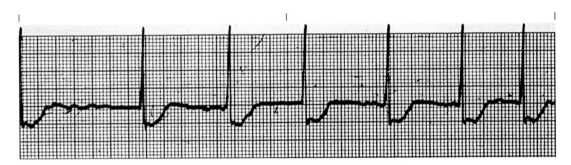

159. MEASURE: PR interval _____   Rhythm _____
                  QRS complex _____   Heart rate _____
         INTERPRETATION: _____

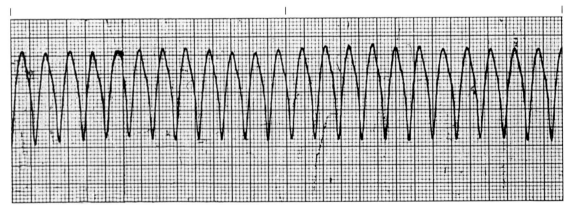

160. MEASURE: PR interval _____   Rhythm _____
                  QRS complex _____   Heart rate _____
         INTERPRETATION: _____

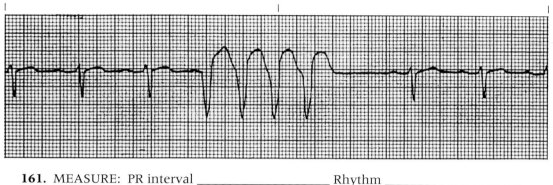

161. MEASURE: PR interval _____ Rhythm _____

QRS complex _____ Heart rate _____

INTERPRETATION: _____

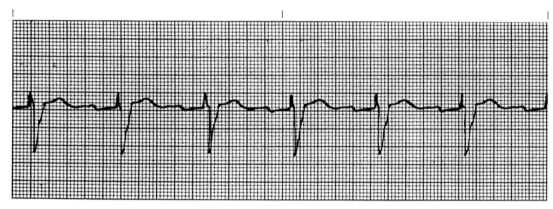

162. MEASURE: PR interval _____ Rhythm _____

QRS complex _____ Heart rate _____

INTERPRETATION: _____

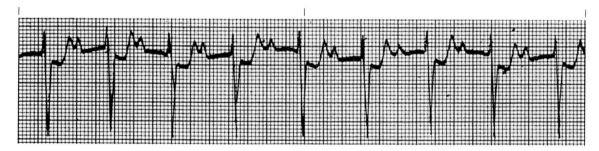

163. MEASURE: PR interval _____ Rhythm _____

QRS complex _____ Heart rate _____

INTERPRETATION: _____

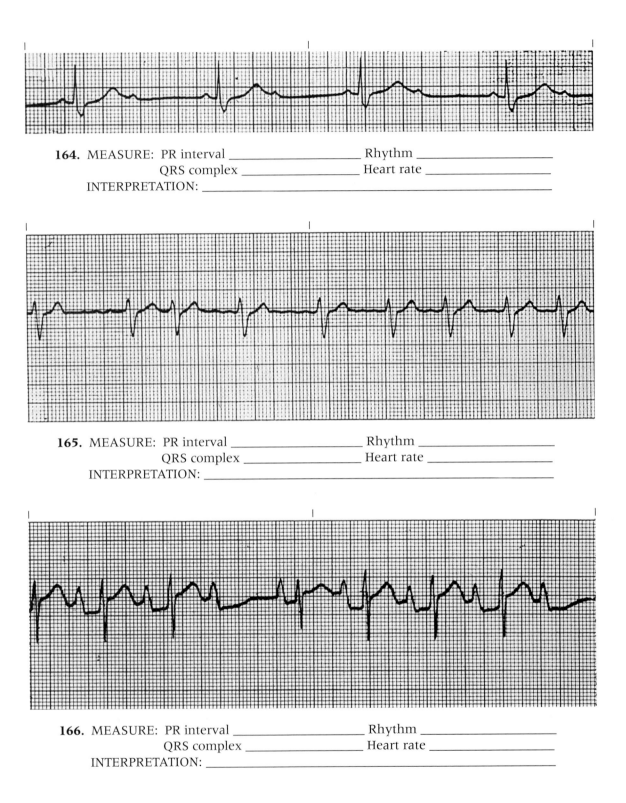

164. MEASURE: PR interval _____ Rhythm _____
QRS complex _____ Heart rate _____
INTERPRETATION: _____

165. MEASURE: PR interval _____ Rhythm _____
QRS complex _____ Heart rate _____
INTERPRETATION: _____

166. MEASURE: PR interval _____ Rhythm _____
QRS complex _____ Heart rate _____
INTERPRETATION: _____

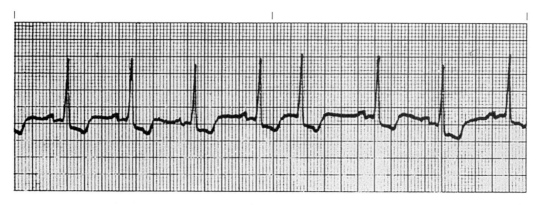

167. MEASURE: PR interval _____ Rhythm _____

QRS complex _____ Heart rate _____

INTERPRETATION: _____

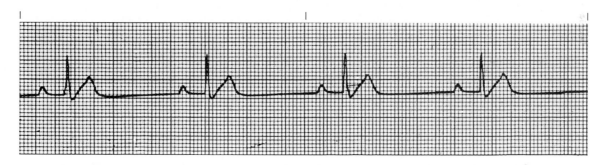

168. MEASURE: PR interval _____ Rhythm _____

QRS complex _____ Heart rate _____

INTERPRETATION: _____

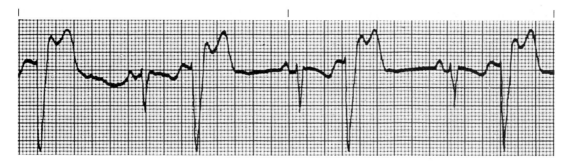

169. MEASURE: PR interval _____ Rhythm _____

QRS complex _____ Heart rate _____

INTERPRETATION: _____

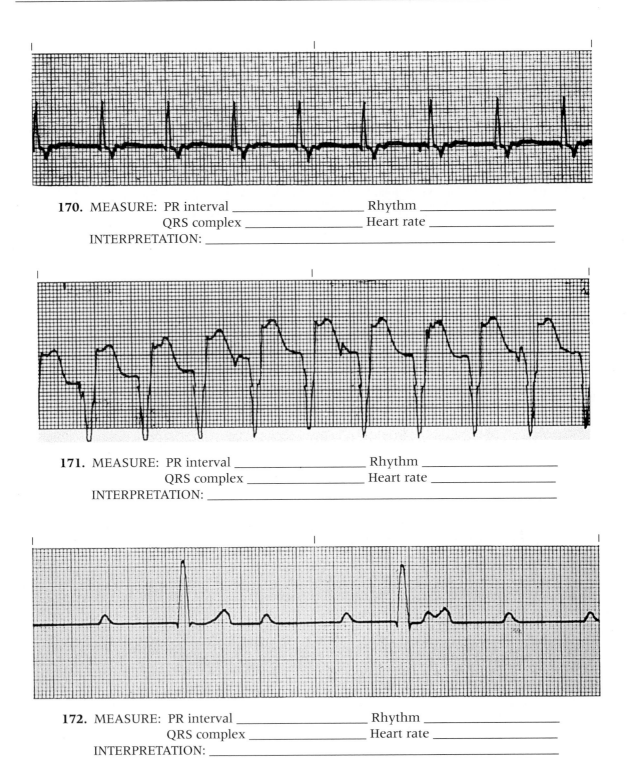

170. MEASURE: PR interval _____ Rhythm _____
                  QRS complex _____ Heart rate _____
          INTERPRETATION: _____

171. MEASURE: PR interval _____ Rhythm _____
                  QRS complex _____ Heart rate _____
          INTERPRETATION: _____

172. MEASURE: PR interval _____ Rhythm _____
                  QRS complex _____ Heart rate _____
          INTERPRETATION: _____

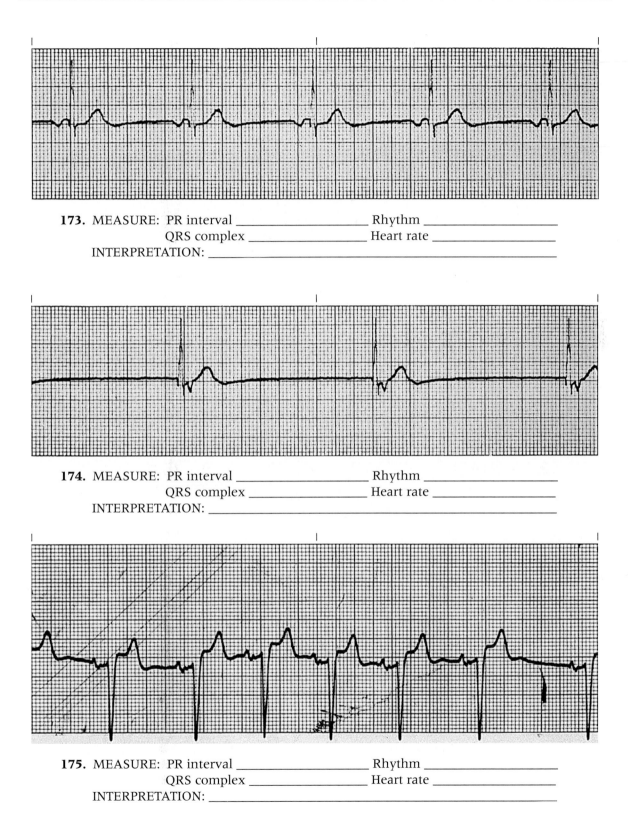

173. MEASURE: PR interval _____ Rhythm _____

QRS complex _____ Heart rate _____

INTERPRETATION: _____

174. MEASURE: PR interval _____ Rhythm _____

QRS complex _____ Heart rate _____

INTERPRETATION: _____

175. MEASURE: PR interval _____ Rhythm _____

QRS complex _____ Heart rate _____

INTERPRETATION: _____

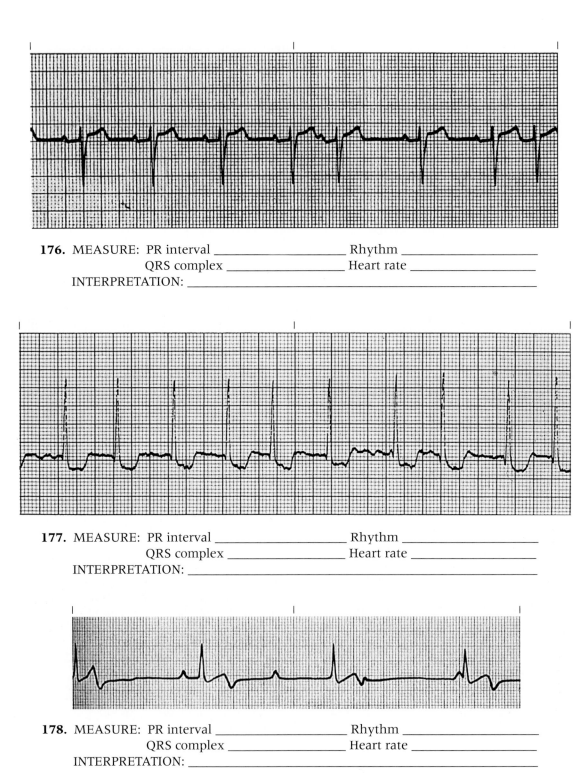

176. MEASURE: PR interval _____ Rhythm _____

QRS complex _____ Heart rate _____

INTERPRETATION: _____

177. MEASURE: PR interval _____ Rhythm _____

QRS complex _____ Heart rate _____

INTERPRETATION: _____

178. MEASURE: PR interval _____ Rhythm _____

QRS complex _____ Heart rate _____

INTERPRETATION: _____

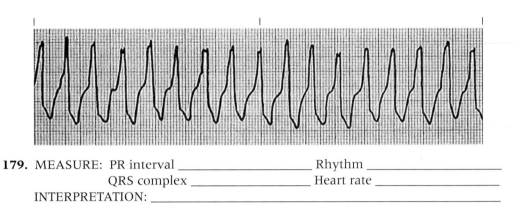

179. MEASURE: PR interval _____ Rhythm _____

QRS complex _____ Heart rate _____

INTERPRETATION: _____

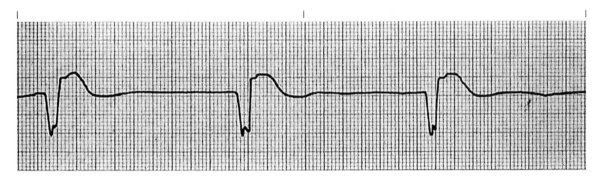

180. MEASURE: PR interval _____ Rhythm _____

QRS complex _____ Heart rate _____

INTERPRETATION: _____

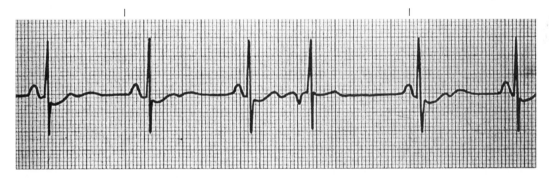

181. MEASURE: PR interval _____ Rhythm _____

QRS complex _____ Heart rate _____

INTERPRETATION: _____

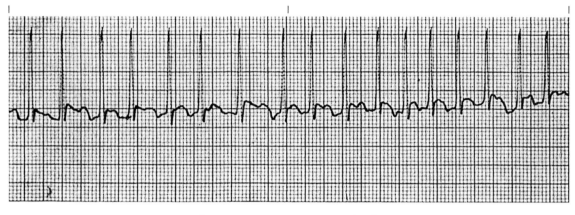

182. MEASURE: PR interval _____ Rhythm _____
                 QRS complex _____ Heart rate _____
INTERPRETATION: _____

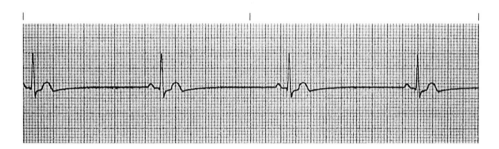

183. MEASURE: PR interval _____ Rhythm _____
                 QRS complex _____ Heart rate _____
INTERPRETATION: _____

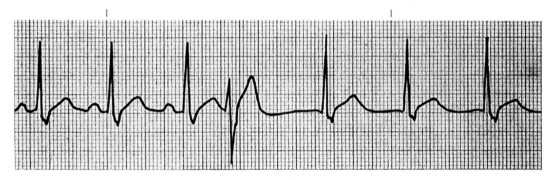

184. MEASURE: PR interval _____ Rhythm _____
                 QRS complex _____ Heart rate _____
INTERPRETATION: _____

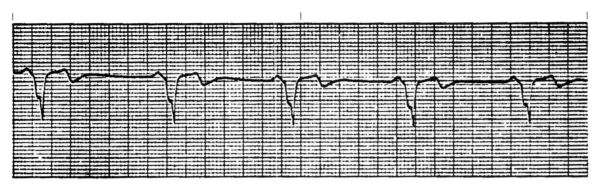

185. MEASURE: PR interval _____ Rhythm _____
        QRS complex _____ Heart rate _____
        INTERPRETATION: _____

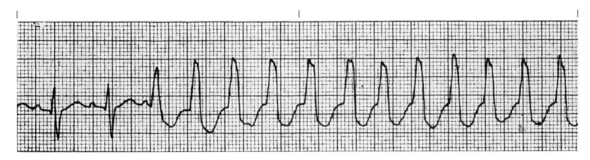

186. MEASURE: PR interval _____ Rhythm _____
        QRS complex _____ Heart rate _____
        INTERPRETATION: _____

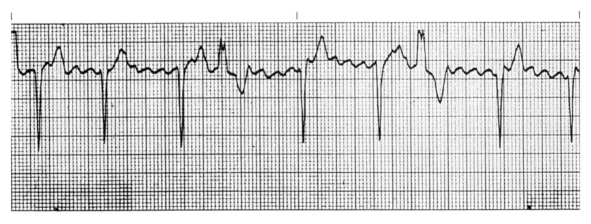

187. MEASURE: PR interval _____ Rhythm _____
        QRS complex _____ Heart rate _____
        INTERPRETATION: _____

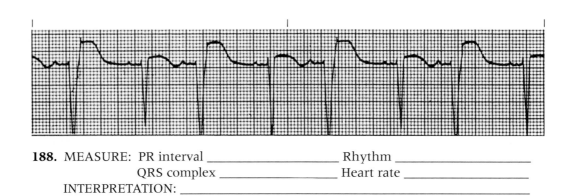

188. MEASURE: PR interval _____   Rhythm _____

                 QRS complex _____   Heart rate _____

INTERPRETATION: _____

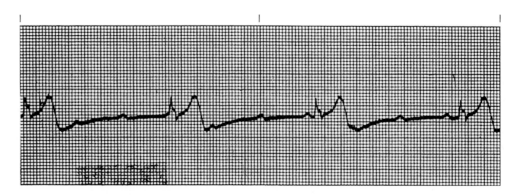

189. MEASURE: PR interval _____   Rhythm _____

                 QRS complex _____   Heart rate _____

INTERPRETATION: _____

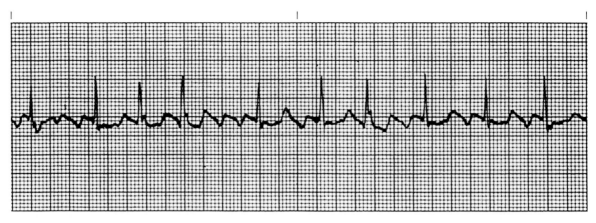

190. MEASURE: PR interval _____   Rhythm _____

                 QRS complex _____   Heart rate _____

INTERPRETATION: _____

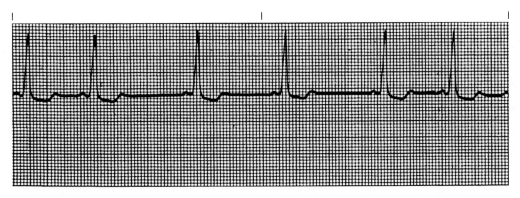

191. MEASURE: PR interval _____ Rhythm _____
                    QRS complex _____ Heart rate _____
      INTERPRETATION: _____

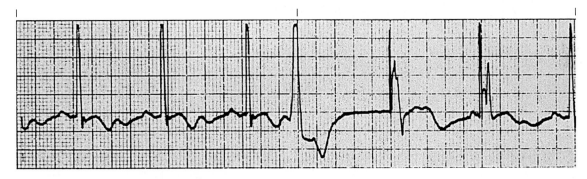

192. MEASURE: PR interval _____ Rhythm _____
                    QRS complex _____ Heart rate _____
      INTERPRETATION: _____

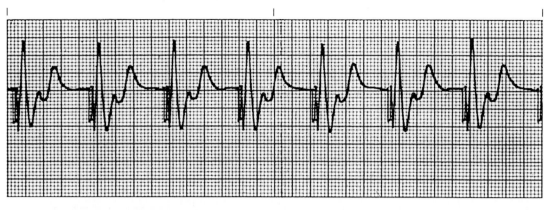

193. MEASURE: PR interval _____ Rhythm _____

QRS complex _____ Heart rate _____

INTERPRETATION: _____

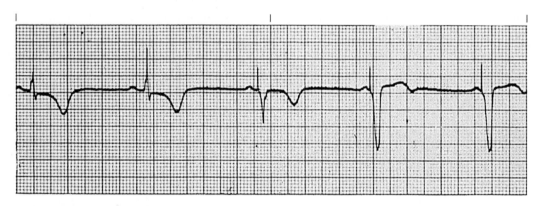

194. MEASURE: PR interval _____ Rhythm _____

QRS complex _____ Heart rate _____

INTERPRETATION: _____

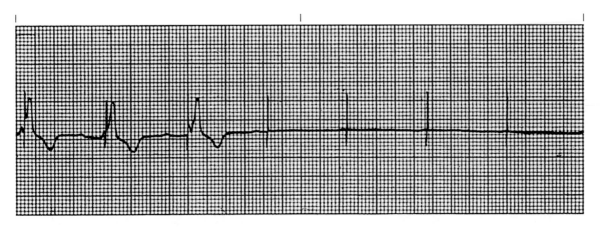

195. MEASURE: PR interval _____ Rhythm _____

QRS complex _____ Heart rate _____

INTERPRETATION: _____

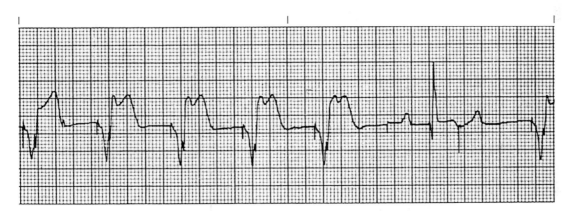

196. MEASURE: PR interval _____ Rhythm _____

QRS complex _____ Heart rate _____

INTERPRETATION: _____

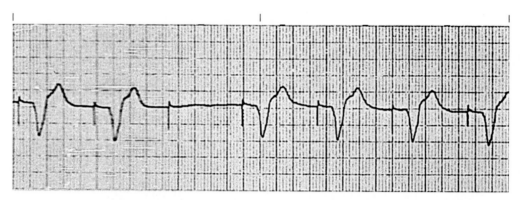

197. MEASURE: PR interval _____ Rhythm _____
QRS complex _____ Heart rate _____
INTERPRETATION: _____

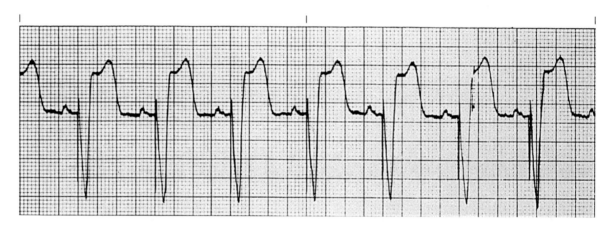

198. MEASURE: PR interval _____ Rhythm _____
QRS complex _____ Heart rate _____
INTERPRETATION: _____

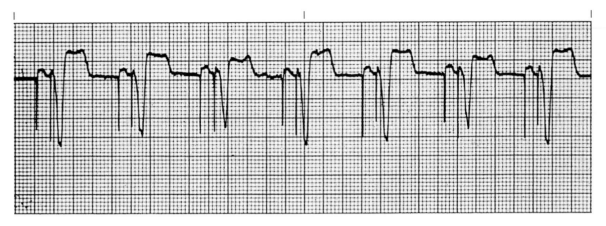

199. MEASURE: PR interval _____ Rhythm _____
          QRS complex _____ Heart rate _____
          INTERPRETATION: _____

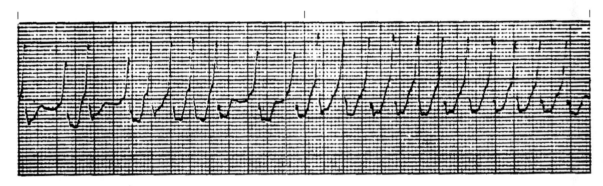

200. MEASURE: PR interval _____ Rhythm _____
          QRS complex _____ Heart rate _____
          INTERPRETATION: _____

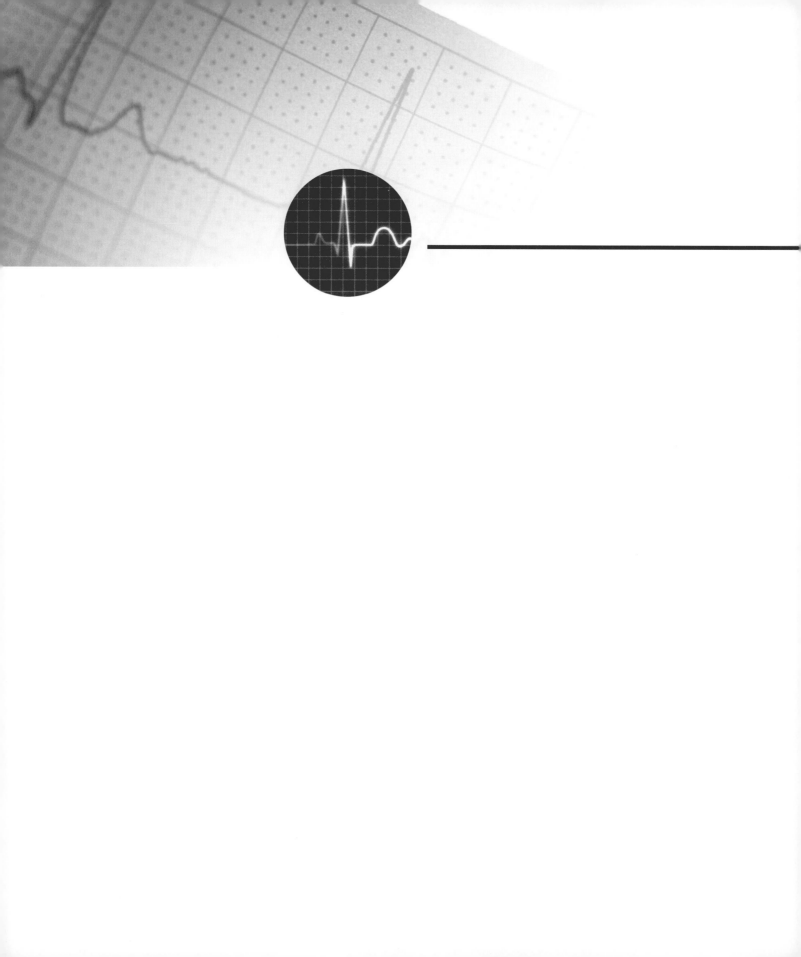

CHAPTER 11

CASE STUDIES

This chapter uses case studies to help you "put it all together." They are an excellent way to learn and remember new material. They also increase your ability to relate signs and symptoms to patient care, and to recognize potential patient problems.

The case studies involve you in medical situations, giving examples of how patient assessment, dysrhythmia identification, medications, and procedures all contribute to treatment of the patient.

The treatments used in these case studies are based on the guidelines of the American Heart Association, as listed in Chapter 9. Remember that these are only general guidelines and should be used in conjunction with, not instead of, the policies and procedures of your institution. All treatment **must** be performed under the guidance of a physician. Only properly trained individuals should administer medications or treatments.

To use these case studies, first assess the patient, next identify the dysrhythmia, and then determine the appropriate treatment, based on your findings. Keep in mind that all patients must be assessed initially, as well as before and after each medication or treatment. This will help you evaluate the patient's tolerance of the dysrhythmia and their response to the medications or treatments.

Assessing the patient for poor cardiac output involves more than taking the blood pressure, heart rate, and looking at the monitor screen. It also includes evaluating the patient's respirations, skin temperature, and level of consciousness. This can be done by talking to, looking at, listening to, and touching the patient. To learn the proper way to evaluate patients, consider attending a physical assessment course.

For the purpose of this chapter, it is assumed that all patients are adult, being monitored on Lead II, have no contraindications for any treatments, are being assessed before and after each medication or treatment, and that all appropriate laboratory tests have been ordered, when available.

We encourage you to use these case studies and to also make up additional situations. Just as interpreting rhythm strips becomes easier with practice, so will patient assessments and treatments.

CASE STUDY 1

You are caring for a 26-year-old patient on the telemetry unit who complains that her heart is "racing" and "pounding" in her chest. The monitor shows the rhythm seen in Fig. 11-1.

FIG. 11-1

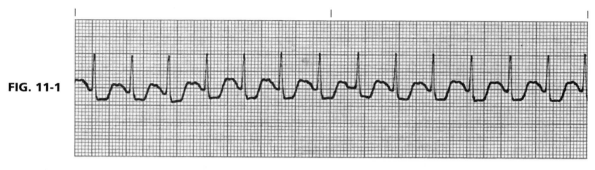

1-A. You identify the dysrhythmia as _____.

As you enter her room to assess the patient, you notice several empty coffee cups and soda cans scattered around the room. The patient is pacing back and forth, and is unable to sit still for long. The patient's vital signs are BP 136/84, HR 140, and respiratory rate (RR) of 26.

As you talk with the patient, she admits to being very anxious about waiting for the results of tests that had been done that morning.

1-B. Your next actions include:

       a. _____

       b. _____

       c. _____

You see that the patient appears less anxious and is now able to relax in bed. The monitor now displays the rhythm shown in Fig. 11-2.

FIG. 11-2

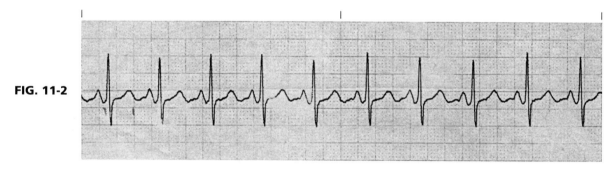

1-C. You identify the rhythm as _____.

You reassess the patient and find BP 128/72, HR 100, and RR 20. You continue to monitor the patient for any further changes.

CASE STUDY 2

A 70-kg patient is brought to the emergency department by his co-worker. The patient states that he has been having occasional dizzy spells for a few days and today he fainted. The monitor shows the dysrhythmia seen in Fig. 11-3. You assess the patient and find signs of poor cardiac output, including: pale, cool, clammy, skin; mild chest pain; light-headedness; mild nausea; slight shortness of breath. Vital signs are BP 92/46, HR 40, and RR 22.

FIG. 11-3

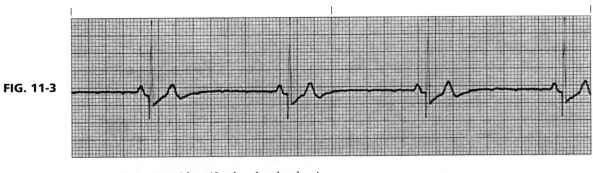

2-A. You identify the dysrhythmia as _____.

2-B. Acting on the pre-printed physician orders of the department, your next actions are:

    a. _____

    b. _____

    c. _____

    d. _____

    e. _____

The doctor is evaluating the patient's response to the above actions. You reassess the patient and find a slight improvement. The chest pain, shortness of breath, and nausea are decreased. Vital signs are BP 96/52, HR 46, and RR 20. There is no change in the dysrhythmia.

2-C. The physician orders you to repeat _____.

2-D. Because there is no change in the dysrhythmia or the patient's condition, the physician has you initiate the use of a _____.

The patient shows immediate signs of improvement. His skin is now pink, warm, and dry. He denies any nausea, chest pain, or shortness of breath. Vital signs are BP 106/68, HR 70, and RR 18.

The monitor shows the rhythm seen in Fig. 11-4.

FIG. 11-4

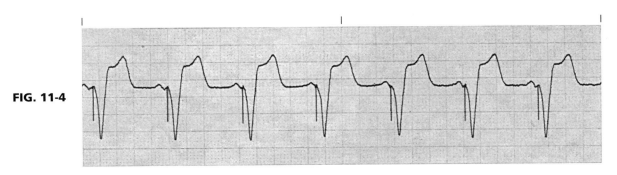

2-E. You identify this rhythm as a _____.

2-F. This rhythm should have (a) _____ capture, even if it is not 100 % (b) _____.

CASE STUDY 3

A new 70-kg patient is admitted to the telemetry unit. During the assessment of the patient, you find vital signs of BP 120/78, HR 70, and RR 22. You attach the patient to a heart monitor, which displays the rhythm seen in Fig. 11-5.

FIG. 11-5
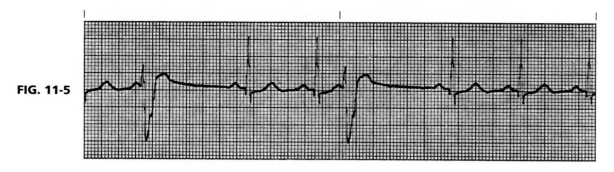

3-A. You identify the rhythm as _____.

You place a call to the physician. Before she can return your call, you see that the rhythm on the monitor has changed to the one seen in Fig. 11-6.

FIG. 11-6
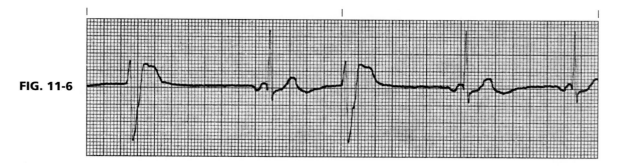

3-B. You identify the dysrhythmia as _____.

3-C. Following the unit's pre-printed physician orders, you initiate the following:

    a. _____

    b. _____

    c. _____

You reassess the patient and find her vital signs to be BP 104/60, HR 50, and RR 26. The patient is pale, cool, clammy, and anxious.

3-D. You immediately _____.

The patient's skin is warm and dry and she appears less anxious. The BP is now 110/70, HR 70, and RR 22. The monitor displays the rhythm seen in Fig. 11-7.

FIG. 11-7

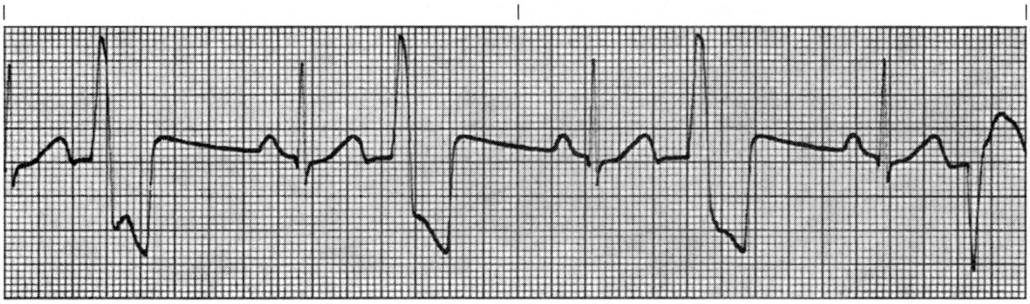

3-E. You interpret the dysrhythmia as _____.

3-F. The physician arrives and orders (a) _____
to be followed by a continuous infusion of (b) _____
when the dysrhythmia has been controlled.

You continue to monitor the patient for any signs of poor cardiac output or change in the rhythm, especially for any of the "danger signs" for PVCs.

3-G. These danger signs include:

    a. _____

    b. _____

    c. _____

    d. _____

    e. _____

CASE STUDY 4

A patient is admitted to the emergency department. You assess the patient and find he is pale, diaphoretic, and complaining of chest pain. His vital signs include a BP of 100/50, HR of 170, and RR of 26. The monitor shows the rhythm as seen in Fig. 11-8.

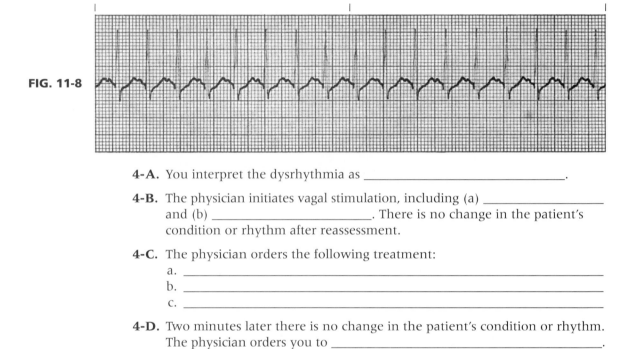

FIG. 11-8

4-A. You interpret the dysrhythmia as _____.

4-B. The physician initiates vagal stimulation, including (a) _____ and (b) _____. There is no change in the patient's condition or rhythm after reassessment.

4-C. The physician orders the following treatment:
a. _____
b. _____
c. _____

4-D. Two minutes later there is no change in the patient's condition or rhythm. The physician orders you to _____.

4-E. Because there is still no change in the patient's condition, the physician orders _____.

After 20 minutes there is no improvement, so the physician decides to cardiovert the patient. You prepare for the cardioversion by administering a sedative to the patient.

4-F. You make sure the defibrillator is set for _____ cardioversion.

You assess the patient after the cardioversion and find no signs of poor cardiac output. The BP is 110/64, HR 70, and RR 20. The monitor now shows the rhythm as seen in Fig. 11-9.

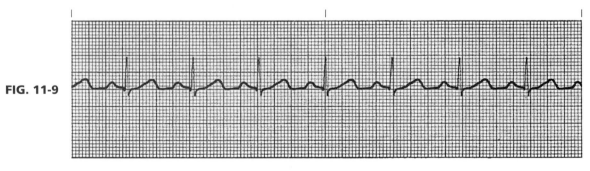

FIG. 11-9

4-G. You identify the rhythm as _____. You continue to monitor the patient and transfer the patient to the coronary care unit.

CASE STUDY 5

During a 5K run, a 27-year-old man is brought to the first-aid station, complaining of weakness and dizziness. You find he is warm, pale, and sweaty with BP 138/82, HR 100-110, and RR 30 on the initial assessment. He denies any pain. You attach him to a heart monitor, which displays the rhythm seen in Fig. 11-10.

FIG. 11-10

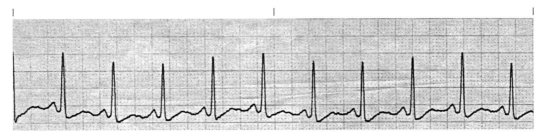

5-A. You identify the rhythm as _____.

5-B. Your initial treatment of this patient includes:

a. _____

b. _____

c. _____

d. _____

You reassess the patient after 20 minutes of rest. Vital signs are BP 110/64, HR 100, and RR 16. The monitor now shows the rhythm in Fig. 11-11.

FIG. 11-11

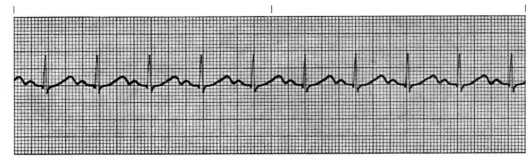

5-C. You identify the rhythm as _____.

Because of the new prolonged QT interval, you notify the patient's physician, who recommends transportation to the emergency department for evaluation.

CASE STUDY 6

A patient is waiting for admission to the hospital after being treated in the emergency department for a drug overdose. The monitor shows a new rhythm as seen in Fig. 11-12.

FIG. 11-12

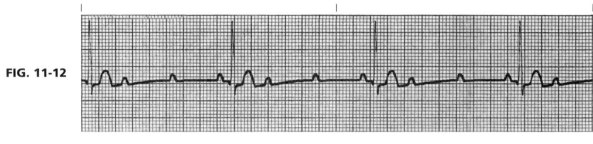

6-A. You identify the dysrhythmia as _____.

You notify the physician and begin the following pre-printed physician orders as the physician re-evaluates the patient:

6-B. a. _____

b. _____

c. _____

The patient has a BP 100/48, HR 40, and RR 22 and is pale, clammy, and lethargic. The monitor suddenly shows the dysrhythmia seen in Fig. 11-13.

FIG. 11-13

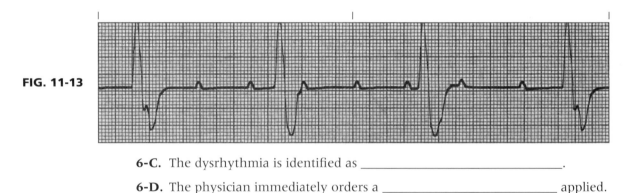

6-C. The dysrhythmia is identified as _____.

6-D. The physician immediately orders a _____ applied.

The patient's cardiac output improves as his heart rate increases as a result of the pacemaker. The patient is admitted to the cardiac care unit.

CASE STUDY 7

You are watching the monitors in the unit and notice that one patient has an episode of R on T phenomenon. The monitor now shows the rhythm seen in Fig. 11-14.

FIG. 11-14

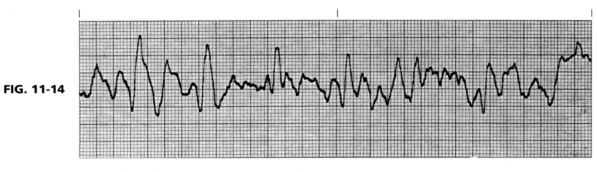

7-A. You identify the dysrhythmia as _____.

7-B. You immediately rush to the patient's room and your first action is to _____.

You find the patient awake, alert, and talking on the telephone.

7-C. Your next actions include:
  a. _____
  b. _____
  c. _____

CASE STUDY 8

You are a member of the ambulance crew responding to a 911 call for an unresponsive male. When you arrive at the scene, you assess the patient, as another crewmember attaches the patient to a heart monitor. You see the rhythm shown in Fig. 11-15.

FIG. 11-15

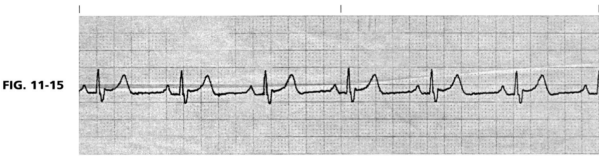

8-A. You identify the rhythm on the monitor as _____.
However, you found no vital signs during your assessment.

8-B. You correctly identify the dysrhythmia as _____.

8-C. You and your crew immediately begin the following treatments:

a. _____

b. _____

c. _____

d. _____

e. _____

f. _____

g. _____

After transporting the patient to the nearest hospital, the emergency physician reassesses the patient.

8-D. The physician decides to perform a pericardiocentesis to relieve a

_____.

8-E. List three causes of PEA; include the treatment:

a. _____; _____

b. _____; _____

c. _____; _____

After the procedure, the patient's dysrhythmia converts to that seen in Fig. 11-16.

FIG. 11-16

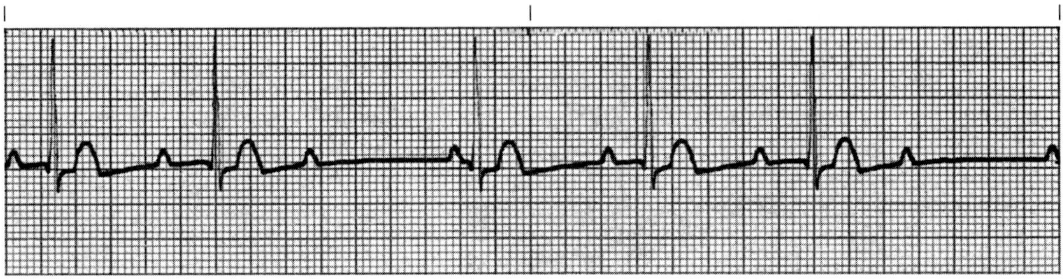

8-F. The new rhythm is identified as _____. The patient's vital signs are BP 100/48, HR 50, with respirations of 16 provided by a bag-valve-mask device at 100% oxygen. The patient's cardiac output has improved.

8-G. You continue to _____.

CASE STUDY 9

A patient's cardiac monitor on your unit suddenly shows the dysrhythmia seen in Fig. 11-17.

FIG. 11-17

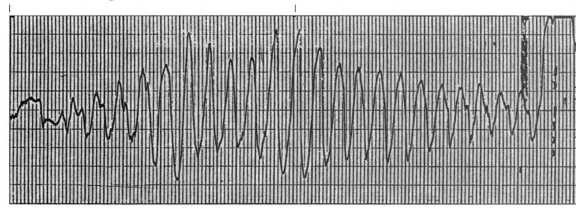

9-A. You identify the dysrhythmia as _____,

Careful assessment of the patient indicates signs and symptoms of poor cardiac output.

9-B. List five signs or symptoms of poor cardiac output:

a. _____
b. _____
c. _____
d. _____
e. _____

9-C. Your initial treatment includes:

a. _____
b. _____
c. _____
d. _____
e. _____
f. _____

9-D. The patient has converted to the rhythm shown in Fig. 11-18. You identify the rhythm as _____.

FIG. 11-18

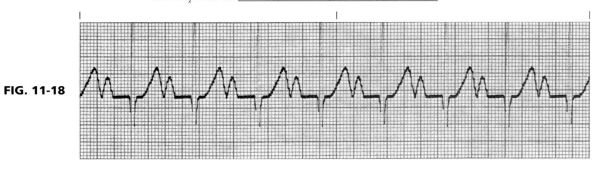

The patient no longer has signs of poor cardiac output. You continue to monitor the patient and his cardiac rhythm.

CASE STUDY 10

A patient returns to the cardiac care unit after a minor procedure. He has an IV infusing and is receiving oxygen at 2 L/min by nasal cannula. On assessment, the patient is awake, oriented, and talking about how well he feels. Vital signs are BP 118/88, HR 50, and RR 20. There is a new dysrhythmia on the monitor screen; see Fig.11-19.

FIG. 11-19

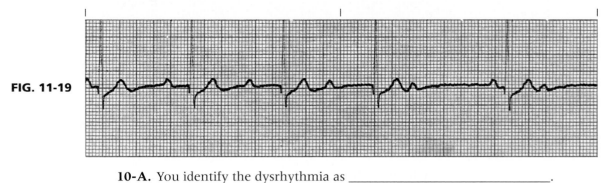

10-A. You identify the dysrhythmia as _____.

Since the patient is tolerating the dysrhythmia, your next actions are to:

10-B. a. _____
  b. _____

After continued observation of the patient, you see the rhythm on the monitor screen change to that seen in Fig. 11-20.

FIG. 11-20

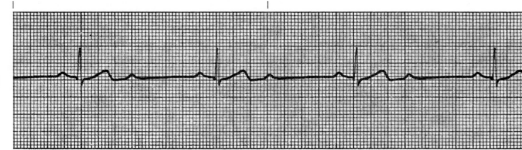

10-C. You identify the dysrhythmia as _____.

The patient's BP is 98/60, HR 40, and the patient is now pale, cool, sweaty, and short of breath.

10-D. You have pre-printed physician orders and you initiate the following:
  a. _____
  b. _____
  c. _____
  d. _____
  e. _____
  f. _____

10-E. The cardiac dysrhythmia has converted to _____;
see Fig. 11-21.

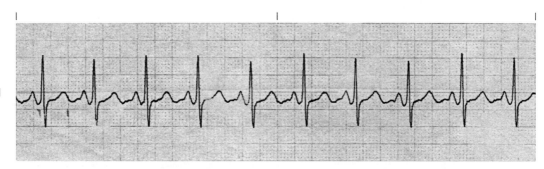

FIG. 11-21

The patient's symptoms have improved, indicating improved cardiac output
with BP 108/72, HR 100, and RR 22. You continue to monitor and observe the
patient.

CASE STUDY 11

A 52-year-old man, weighing 100 kg, is brought to the emergency department,
complaining of pressure in the middle of his chest, difficulty breathing, and nausea. You find his vital signs are BP 110/60, HR 80, and RR 22. The patient is pale,
cool, and diaphoretic.

11-A. These are indications of poor _____.

11-B. The patient is connected to a heart monitor. You identify the dysrhythmia
in Fig. 11-22 as _____.

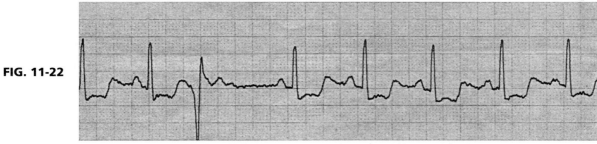

FIG. 11-22

11-C. The physician evaluates the patient and orders the following:
   a. _____
   b. _____
   c. _____

As you are completing these orders, the patient suddenly slumps over. You quickly assess the patient and find no vital signs. The monitor now shows the rhythm seen in Fig. 11-23.

FIG. 11-23

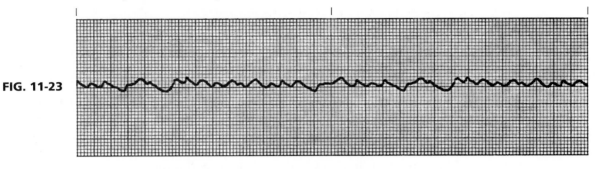

11-D. You identify the dysrhythmia as _____.

11-E. You begin the following treatments:

a. _____
b. _____
c. _____
d. _____
e. _____
f. _____
g. _____
h. _____
i. _____
j. _____
k. _____

11-F. The dysrhythmia has converted to the one shown in Fig. 11-24. The physician identifies it as _____.

FIG. 11-24

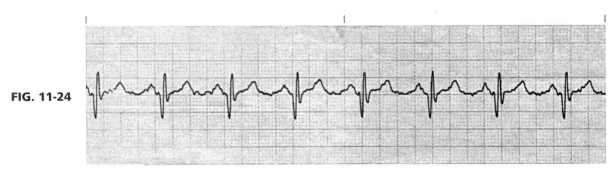

The patient is showing signs of improving cardiac output and has a BP of 96/56, HR of 80, and continues to have respirations of 16, assisted by the use of a bag-valve-mask device. The patient is transferred to the cardiac care unit while you continue to reassess him.

CASE STUDY 12

You come on duty and study the monitors. You observe the dysrhythmia shown in Fig. 11-25 on one of the monitors.

FIG. 11-25

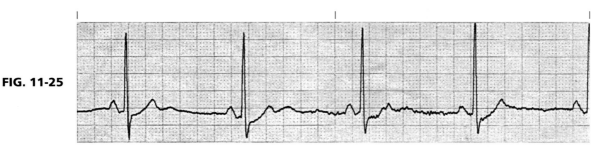

12-A. You identify the dysrhythmia as _____.

You go to the room to assess the patient; He is in his early twenties and appears to be asleep. His BP is 102/58, HR is 50, and his respirations are deep and even with a rate of 14. He has no indications of poor cardiac output.

12-B. Your next actions are to:

a. _____

b. _____

CASE STUDY 13

A 56-year-old woman is brought to the emergency department complaining of episodes of a "racing heart." Her vital signs are stable, and she shows no signs of poor cardiac output. When connected to a heart monitor, she has the rhythm shown in Fig. 11-26.

FIG. 11-26

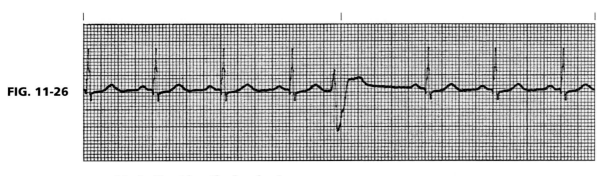

13-A. You identify the rhythm as _____.

As you continue your assessment, the patient suddenly complains of dizziness, shortness of breath, and mild chest pain. She is now pale, clammy, and her vital signs are BP 94/50, HR 220, and RR 28.

The monitor shows the change in rhythm seen in Fig. 11-27.

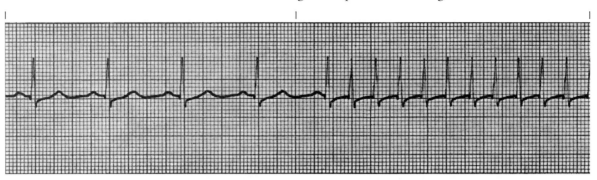

FIG. 11-27

13-B. You identify this rhythm as _____.

13-C. You notify the physician who orders the following treatment:

a. _____

b. _____

c. _____

d. _____

e. _____

f. _____

g. _____

h. _____

13-D. The dysrhythmia has converted to _____; as shown in Fig. 11-28.

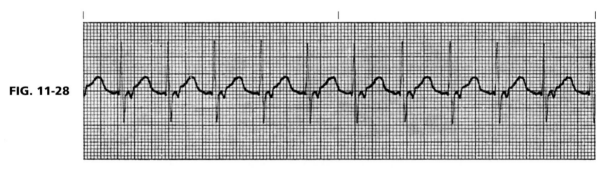

FIG. 11-28

Her vital signs are BP 106/54, HR 110, and RR 22, and she has no further signs of poor cardiac output. The patient continues to be monitored while being transferred to the cardiac care unit.

CASE STUDY 14

You respond with the ambulance crew to a man complaining of chest pains. When you arrive, you find the patient lying on the bed. He is pale, cool, and clammy, is short of breath, and has mild chest pains with BP 92/48, HR 50 and irregular, and RR 26.

14-A. These are signs of _____.

14-B. You attach the monitor and identify the rhythm shown in Fig. 11-29 as

_____.

FIG. 11-29

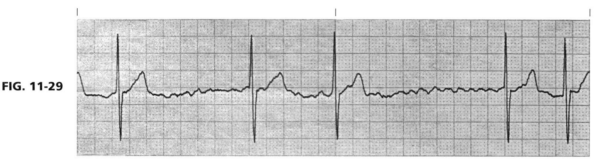

14-C. You call a report to the hospital and start your pre-printed physician orders that include:

a. _____

b. _____

c. _____

d. _____

e. _____

You continue to assess the patient while transporting him to the emergency department. His symptoms of poor cardiac output improve, BP 105/60, HR 76, and RR 20, and his skin is pink, warm, and dry. After arriving at the hospital, the patient is transferred to the emergency department's monitor. The patient complains that "it felt like his heart stopped for a just a second then started up again." The monitor is now showing the rhythm seen in Fig. 11-30.

FIG. 11-30

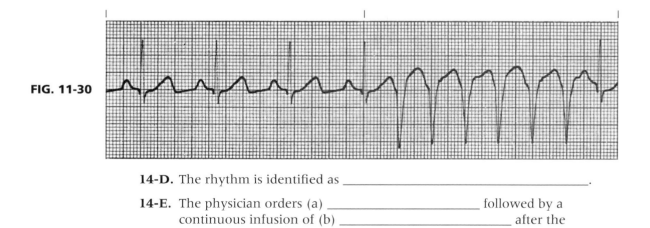

14-D. The rhythm is identified as _____.

14-E. The physician orders (a) _____ followed by a continuous infusion of (b) _____ after the dysrhythmia is controlled.

Vital signs are BP 110/70, HR 76, and RR 22. The patient is transferred to the cardiac care unit.

CASE STUDY 15

A 45-year-old man is brought to the emergency department by his wife. The patient complains of indigestion, lasting 2 to 3 hours, which was not relieved by antacids. He also complains that his shoulders feel heavy and his jaw is beginning to ache. His wife states that earlier, he had been sweating a lot and vomited twice.

On your assessment, the patient is clammy, pale, nauseated, slightly short of breath, and is now complaining of chest pain. Vital signs are BP 122/75, HR 70, and RR 24.

15-A. You identify the rhythm on the monitor (Fig. 11-31) as _____.

FIG. 11-31

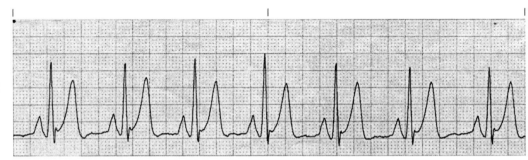

15-B. Because your department has pre-printed physician orders, you begin the following treatments:
a. _____
b. _____
c. _____
d. _____

The physician enters the treatment room and examines the patient. You reassess the patient and find no change in the patient's condition, vital signs, or in his cardiac rhythm. The physician orders you to continue following the pre-printed physician orders.

15-C. You repeat the (a) _____ tablets two times without success. You administer a titrated dose of (b)_____ to control the pain.

You reassess the patient. He continues to complain of pain and shortness of breath. Vital signs are now BP 152/94, HR 72, and RR of 22. You increase the oxygen to 4 L/min.

15-D. While the ECG is being completed, you prepare to administer an infusion of nitroglycerine using an _____, as ordered by the physician.

You reassess the patient after the infusion is started and find that the pain has decreased and the vital signs are now BP 110/78, HR 82, and RR 20.

15-E. The physician has determined that the patient is having an acute myocardial infarction. After determining that there are no contraindications, the doctor decides to begin _____.

Following hospital policy, you begin treatment by starting a continuous heparin infusion, administering a bolus of heparin and giving aspirin, unless already administered, while another nurse prepares the ordered fibrinolytic medication.

15-F. You continue to _____ the patient and his cardiac rhythm.

The patient is transferred to the care of a cardiologist and is moved to the cardiac care unit.

CASE STUDY 16

Your ambulance is called to the scene of a 70-kg man who complains of dizziness and difficulty breathing. His vital signs are BP 92/46, HR 40, and RR 26.

16-A. The monitor shows _____; see Fig. 11-32.

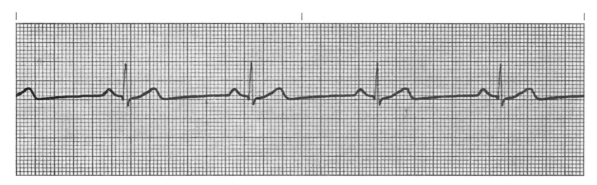

FIG. 11-32

16-B. You follow the pre-printed physician orders of your institution, and begin the following treatments:

a. _____

b. _____

c. _____

After 5 minutes, you reassess the patient and find BP 102/60, HR 50, and RR 20. The patient states it is easier to breathe now and that he is less dizzy.

16-C. You identify the dysrhythmia now seen on the monitor as _____; see Fig. 11-33.

FIG. 11-33

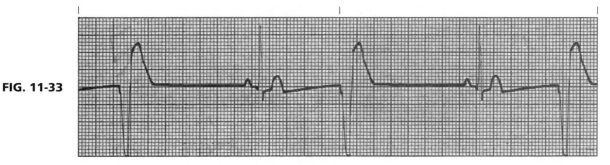

16-D. Your next action is to _____.

16-E. On the next assessment, the monitor shows _____
as seen in Fig 11-34. Vital signs are BP 110/60, HR 80, and RR 20, with
no signs of poor cardiac output. You transport the patient to the hospital.

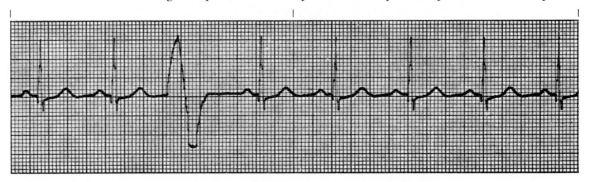

FIG. 11-34   **16-F.** En route to the hospital, the monitor changes to _____
as seen in Fig. 11-35.

FIG. 11-35

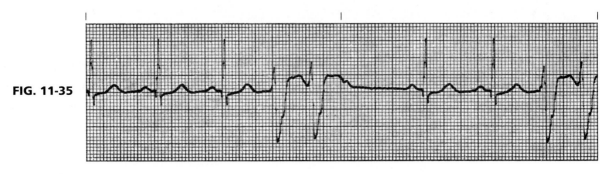

16-G. The patient's condition is stable. You begin an infusion of

_____.

16-H. The monitor now shows _____ as seen in
Fig. 11-36.

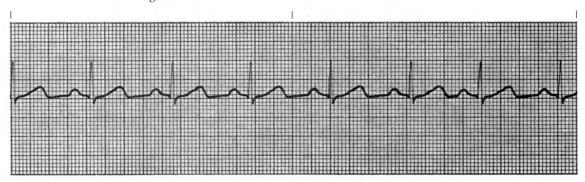

FIG. 11-36   **16-I.** The patient is stable with BP 112/70, HR 70-80, and RR 20. You change
the IV infusion to a maintenance dose of _____ and
continue transporting to the emergency department.

CASE STUDY 17

While on duty in the emergency department triage, a woman enters and asks for some antacid for her indigestion. During assessment of the patient, you find that she has had "indigestion" in the mid chest area for 2 hours. She also complains of a toothache. She is pale and slightly clammy, with a BP of 248/112, HR 70, and RR 22.

17-A. You and a nurse take the patient to the examination room and put her on the bed. Following the department's pre-printed physician orders, you initiate the following:

a. _____

b. _____

c. _____

d. _____

17-B. You identify the rhythm on the monitor as _____;
see Fig. 11-37.

FIG. 11-37

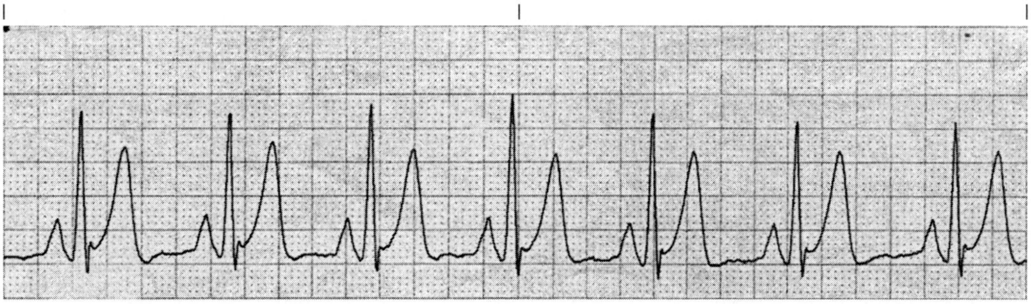

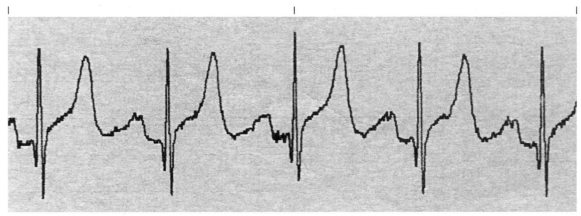

17-C. The physician agrees with your interpretation and orders a chest x-ray, laboratory blood tests, and tells you to continue the MONA protocol, which stands for (a) _____, (b) _____, (c) _____ and (d) _____.

17-D. Reassessing the patient, you see the monitor shows _____;
see Fig. 11-38. The patient's vital signs are BP 280/156, HR 50, and RR 18. The patient tells you that her "toothache" is gone but the pain in her chest has improved only slightly.

FIG. 11-38

17-E. The doctor orders an infusion of _____ to control the hypertension and pain, while waiting for laboratory confirmation of his diagnosis of an acute MI.

17-F. The laboratory results help to confirm an acute MI. The doctor orders heparin and _____ according to the institution's policies.

The patient is transferred to the care of a cardiologist and admitted to the cardiac care unit.

CASE STUDY 18

A patient is admitted to your unit with a diagnosis of intermittent dizziness.

18-A. During the initial assessment, you find a BP 110/70, HR 50, and RR 16. You identify the rhythm on the monitor as _____ as seen in Fig. 11-39.

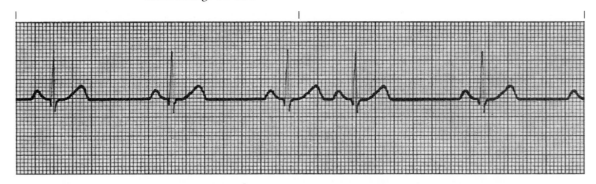

FIG. 11-39   You start oxygen at a flow rate of 2 L/min by nasal cannula and an IV of normal saline according to your department's policies.

18-B. The patient complains of sudden dizziness and shortness of breath. The monitor now shows _____ as seen in Fig. 11-40.

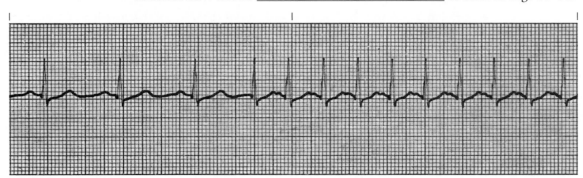

FIG. 11-40   **18-C.** The doctor enters and attempts to perform (a) _____ and orders a (b) _____.

18-D. The monitor shows no change and the patient's symptoms remain the same. The doctor now orders _____.

18-E. You administer the medication _____, followed by a 20-ml flush with normal saline solution and then elevate the arm.

18-F. Two minutes later, there has been no change in the patient's condition. The doctor orders an additional dose of the adenosine. The dose is

_____.

18-G. The monitor shows _____; see Fig. 11-41. The patient's vital signs are BP 108/64, HR 110, and RR 26.

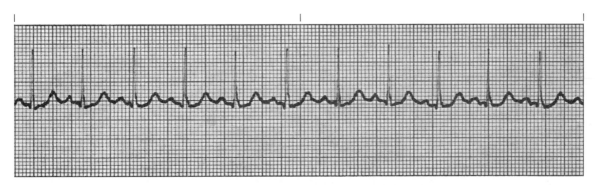

FIG. 11-41   **18-H.** The patient is flushed and has some difficulty breathing. You reassure the patient by explaining that these symptoms are normal _____ and will disappear in a few minutes.

18-I. After a few minutes, the monitor now shows _____; see Fig. 11-42.

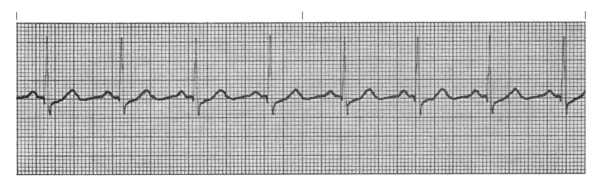

FIG. 11-42   The patient is stable with no symptoms of poor cardiac output; vital signs are: BP 110/66, HR 80, and RR 22.

CASE STUDY 19

While monitoring a patient with a recent MI, you notice the QT intervals are becoming prolonged on the monitor.

19-A. Suddenly, the rhythm changes and is now _____ ; see Fig. 11-43.

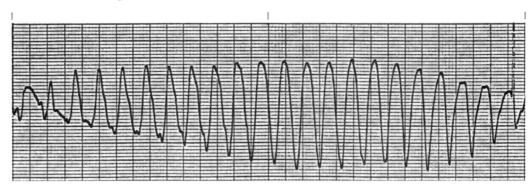

FIG. 11-43

19-B. You have pre-printed physician orders. Your first action is to

_____ .

The patient is awake, complaining of some shortness of breath and dizziness, and has pale, cool, and clammy skin. Vital signs are: BP 104/48, HR 210 to 220, and RR 26. He has oxygen at a rate of 2 L/min by nasal cannula and an IV of normal saline solution.

19-C. You increase _____ .

19-D. You administer an infusion of _____ . The rhythm changes.

19-E. You identify the dysrhythmia as _____ ; see Fig. 11-44. The patient's symptoms of poor cardiac output have improved slightly, and vital signs are BP 110/52, HR 40, and RR 22.

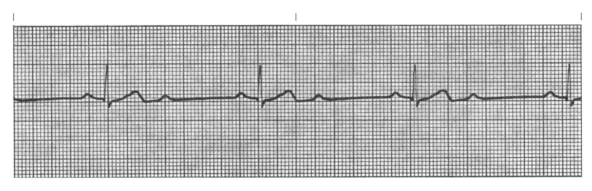

FIG. 11-44   **19-F.** You change the IV to a maintenance dose of _____ .

19-G. The doctor arrives and decides to put in a pacemaker. Until the surgery, you attach a _____ . The patient's cardiac output improves and he is now stable with vital signs of BP 112/64, HR 72, and RR 22.

CASE STUDY 20

20-A. You are monitoring a patient in your unit and notice the monitor shows
_____ as seen in Fig. 11-45.

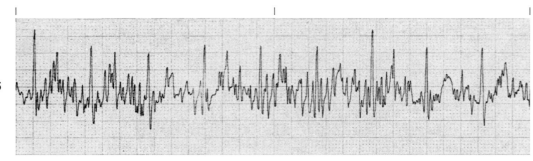

FIG. 11-45

20-B. You immediately _____, then adjust the leads.

20-C. The monitor now shows a new rhythm, _____,
as seen in Fig. 11-46.

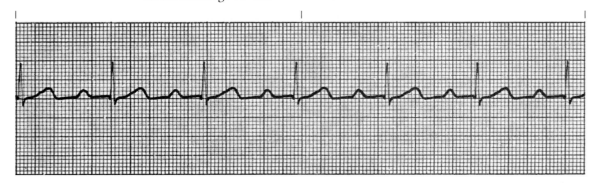

FIG. 11-46   The patient is alert and oriented with no signs of poor cardiac output. Vital
signs are BP 118/63, HR 70, and RR 16.

20-D. You _____ and continue to monitor the patient.

CASE STUDY 21

You are treating a 75-kg patient in the emergency department for a superficial head laceration. During your assessment of the patient, he states that he "blacked out" and hit his head. His vital signs are BP 110/70, HR 70, and RR 16. He has no signs of poor cardiac output.

21-A. You connect the patient to a heart monitor. The rhythm is
_____; see Fig. 11-47.

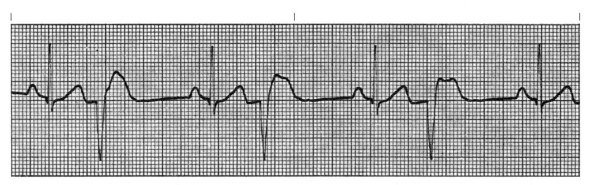

FIG. 11-47   **21-B.** You notify the doctor. Following the department's pre-printed physician orders, you start (a) _____ and (b)_____.
The doctor orders a 12-Lead ECG, blood tests, and the following medication: (c) _____.

The PVCs slow to 1 to 2 per minute. You reassess the patient and find him clammy and pale. His vital signs are BP 88/42, HR 70, and RR 22.

21-C. You stop the procainamide because of the patient's _____.

Continuing to assess the patient, you find that his color is better, his skin is dry, and vital signs are BP 94/60, HR 70, and RR 18.

21-D. The monitor now shows _____; see Fig. 11-48.

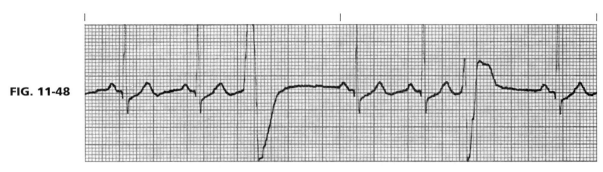

FIG. 11-48

21-E. The doctor orders lidocaine at the following dose: _____.

21-F. After the lidocaine, the monitor shows _____, as seen in Fig. 11-49.

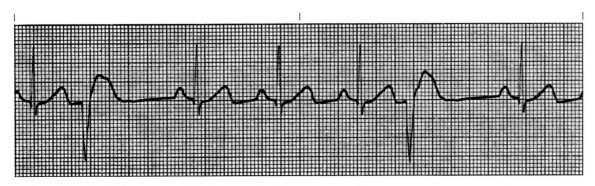

FIG. 11-49   **21-G.** Suddenly the monitor shows a new rhythm, seen in Fig. 11-50, which you identify as _____.

FIG. 11-50

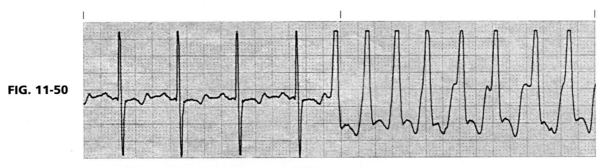

21-H. The doctor orders amiodarone at a dose of (a) _____ repeated in 2 to 3 minutes at a dose of (b)_____.

21-I. You reassess the patient, finding vital signs BP 88/60, HR 40, and RR 14. The dysrhythmia has converted to _____, as seen in Fig. 11-51.

FIG. 11-51

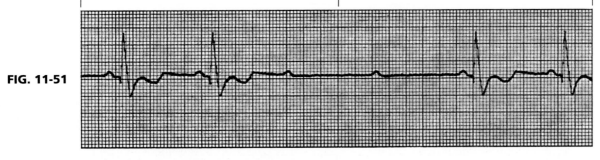

21-J. The doctor initiates a _____.

21-K. You slow the amiodarone infusion to _____.

The patient's cardiac output is improved, BP 108/50, HR 70, and RR 16. He is admitted.

CASE STUDY 22

Your ambulance responds to a call of "man down" in a shopping mall. On the scene, a store manager comes up to you and tells you she has attended CPR and special training classes.

22-A. After seeing the man collapse, she assessed the victim and then applied the _____ when she found he had no pulse.

22-B. After the machine had defibrillated three times, the manager followed the AED's directions and began _____. After several minutes of CPR, the man began to breath on his own and had a pulse.

Your partner has assessed the patient and attached him to a portable cardiac monitor. Vital signs are BP 60/30, HR 30, and RR 10. The patient is unresponsive and pale.

22-C. The dysrhythmia on the monitor is _____; see Fig. 11-52.

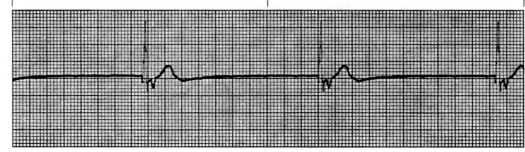

FIG. 11-52

22-D. Using your pre-printed physician orders, you immediately begin the following treatments:
  a. _____
  b. _____
  c. _____

22-E. The patient now has vital signs of BP 100/52, HR 50, and RR 14, and the monitor now shows the new rhythm seen in Fig. 11-53 _____.

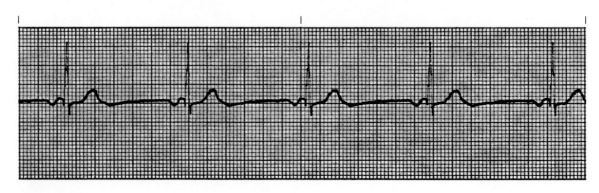

FIG. 11-53

22-F. You apply a (a) _____ pacemaker. This changes
the dysrhythmia to a (b) _____; see Fig. 11-54.

FIG. 11-54

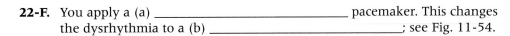
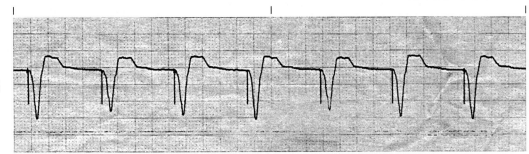

22-G. It is important with this rhythm that even if it is not 100%
(a) _____ the rhythm must have 100%
(b) _____.

The patient's cardiac output improves with BP 108/62, HR 70, and RR 16. You
transport him to the hospital for further treatment.

ANSWER SECTION

CHAPTER 1

Review Question Answers

1. False
2. True
3. False
4. False
5. Atria; ventricles
6. (in any order)
   a. Endocardium
   b. Myocardium
   c. Epicardium
7. (in any order)
   a. Tricuspid valve
   b. Pulmonic valve
   c. Mitral valve
   d. Aortic valve
8. a. Arteries
   b. Veins
   c. Capillaries
9. b
10. b
11. Alveoli
12. d
13. d

14. d
15. b
16. a. Depolarization occurs as the electrical impulse travels through the cardiac cells, causing potassium to leave the cell and sodium to enter the cell, which causes the cell to become positively charged. This is the phase of contraction.
    b. Repolarization is the recovery stage. The potassium is reentering the cells and the sodium is leaving the inside of the cell. The cells are returning to the ready or negatively charged state.
17. Vena cava → right atrium → tricuspid valve → right ventricle →pulmonic valve → pulmonary arteries →lungs →pulmonary veins → left atrium → mitral valve→ left ventricle → aortic valve → aorta → rest of body, including the heart.
18. Sinoatrial (SA) node →Internodal and intraatrial → Atrioventricular (AV) node → Bundle of His → Bundle branches (BB) → Purkinje's fibers →Ventricular muscle

Crossword Puzzle Answers

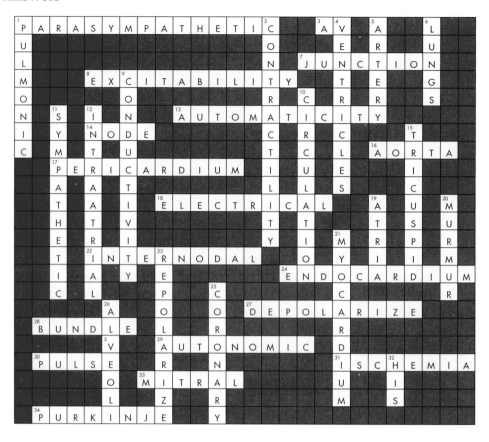

CHAPTER 2

Review Question Answers

1. True
2. False
3. True
4. True
5. d
6. c
7. d
8. (in any order)
   a. P wave
   b. PR interval
   c. QRS
   d. ST segment
   e. T wave
   f. QT interval
   g. Baseline to the beginning of the next P wave (the resting stage of the heart where no electrical activity is occurring)
9. d.
10. Less than one half the R to R interval of that complex to the R wave of the following complex

11. Count the number of R waves in 6 seconds using the indicator lines on the rhythm strip. Multiply the number of R waves by 10 to get the heart rate per minute. **OR**
Measure 6 inches of strip (1 inch equals 1 second); count the number of R waves on the 6-inch strip; multiply the number of R waves by 10 to get the heart rate. **OR**
Count the number of R waves in 30 large squares (equals 6 seconds); multiply the number of R waves by 10 to get the heart rate.

12. a. 300 divided by 3 equals 100; 100 is the heart rate; or 3 large squares equals 15 small squares; 1500 divided by 15 equals heart rate of 100
    b. 300 divided by 4.4 equals 68.18; heart rate approximately 68; or 4 large squares and 2 small squares equals 22 small squares; 1500 divided by 22 equals 68.18 or heart rate approximately 68

13. (in any order)
    a. Are all PR intervals equal?
    b. Are all PR intervals within normal limits of 0.12 to 0.20 second?

14. (in any order)
    a. Are QRS complexes present?
    b. Do all QRS complexes look alike?
    c. Is there a QRS after each P wave?
    d. Are the R to R intervals equal?
    e. Are all QRS complexes within normal limits of 0.04 to 0.12 second?

15. d

16. Absolute refractory period occurs when the cardiac cells have depolarized and can not transmit any electrical stimulus. Relative refractory period occurs when some of the cardiac cells have repolarized to the point where they can be depolarized again, if the electrical stimulus is strong enough.

Rhythm Strip Review Answers

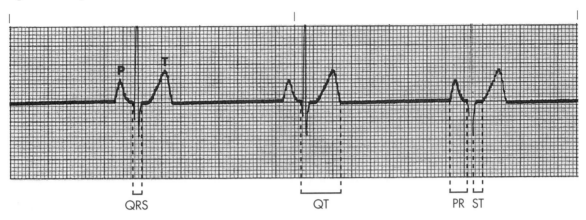

1. Identify P wave, PR interval, QRS complex, ST segment, T wave, and QT interval
   MEASURE PR interval: 0.20
   QRS: 0.08–0.10
   QT interval: Normal
   Rhythm: Regular
   Heart rate: 30

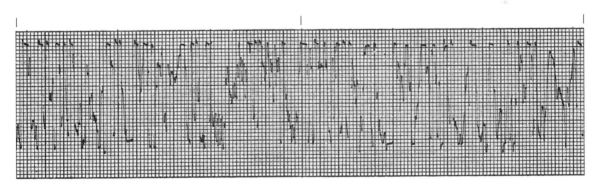

2. Identify P wave, PR interval, QRS complex, ST segment, T wave, and QT interval
   MEASURE PR interval: Not measurable
   QRS: Not measurable
   QT interval: Not measurable
   Rhythm: Not measurable
   Heart rate: Not measurable

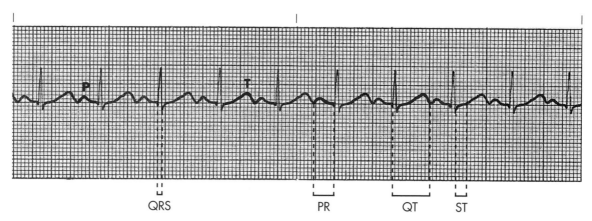

3. Identify P wave, PR interval, QRS complex, ST segment, T wave, and QT interval
   MEASURE PR interval: 0.20–0.24   Rhythm: Regular
   QRS: 0.04–0.06   Heart rate: 100
   QT interval: Prolonged

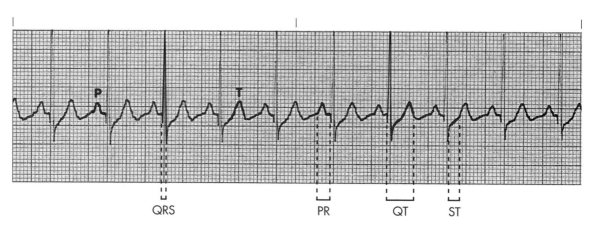

4. Identify P wave, PR interval, QRS complex, ST segment, T wave, and QT interval
   MEASURE PR interval: 0.12–0.14   Rhythm: Regular
   QRS: 0.06   Heart rate: 100
   QT interval: Normal

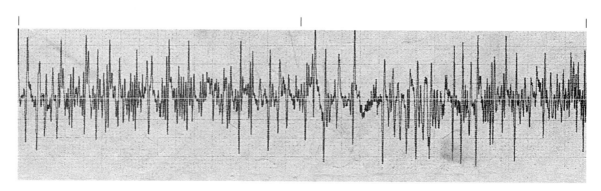

5. Identify P wave, PR interval, QRS complex, ST segment, T wave, and QT interval
   MEASURE PR interval: Not measurable   Rhythm: Not measurable
   QRS: Not measurable   Heart rate: Not measurable
   QT interval: Not measurable

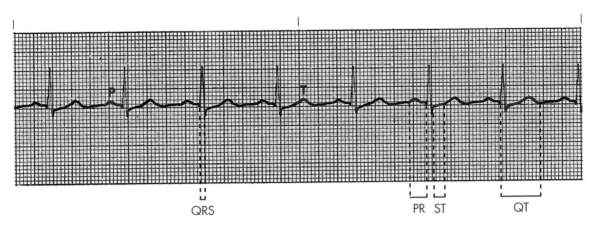

QRS   PR ST   QT

6. Identify P wave, PR interval, QRS complex, ST segment, T wave, and QT interval

    MEASURE PR interval: 0.20   Rhythm: Regular
           QRS: 0.06   Heart rate: 80
           QT interval: Normal

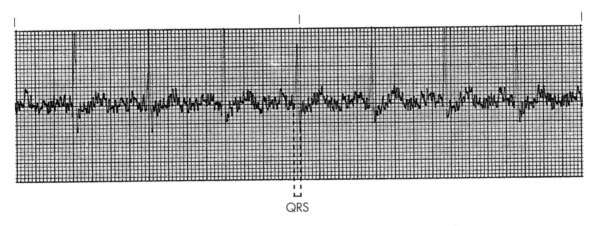

QRS

7. Identify P wave, PR interval, QRS complex, ST segment, T wave, and QT interval

    MEASURE PR interval: Not measurable   Rhythm: Regular
           QRS: 0.04–0.08   Heart rate: 70
           QT interval: Not measurable

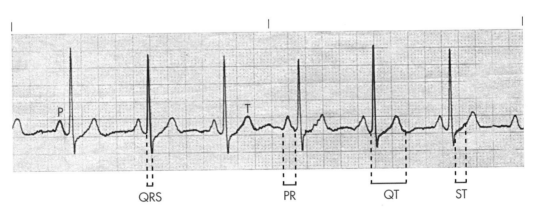

QRS   PR   QT   ST

8. Identify P wave, PR interval, QRS complex, ST segment, T wave, and QT interval

    MEASURE PR interval: 0.16   Rhythm: Regular
           QRS: 0.06–0.08   Heart rate: 60–70
            QT interval: Normal

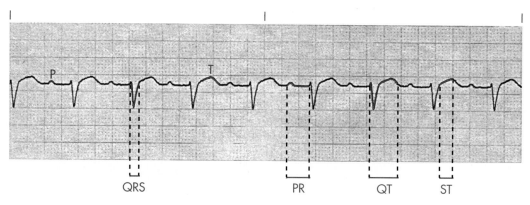

9. Identify P wave, PR interval, QRS complex, ST segment, T wave, and QT interval

MEASURE PR interval: 0.28
QRS: 0.08–0.10
QT interval: Normal

Rhythm: Regular
Heart rate: 90

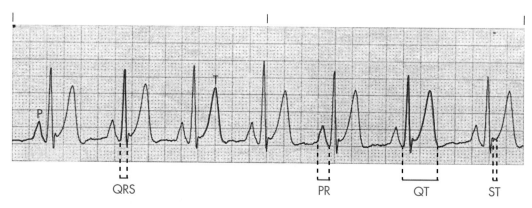

10. Identify P wave, PR interval, QRS complex, ST segment, T wave, and QT interval

MEASURE PR interval: 0.16
QRS: 0.08
QT interval: Normal

Rhythm: Regular
Heart rate: 70

CHAPTER 3

Review Question Answers

1. True
2. True
3. False
4. False
5. True
6. 101 to 150
7. 0.12
8. Two or more
9. b
10. a
11. c
12. c
13. c
14. Variable ventricular response occurs when the impulse that depolarized the ventricle is conducted from the atria at irregular intervals. This results in changing ratios, such as 3:1, 4:1, 2:1, etc.

15. SA node to atria (by the intraatrial pathways) and to the AV node (by the internodal pathways), to the bundle of His and bundle branches, to the Purkinje's fibers, to the ventricular muscle cells

16. Upright P wave before each QRS; all P waves look alike; PR interval measuring 0.12 to 0.20 second; QRS measuring 0.04 to 0.12 second, follows each P wave; all QRS complexes look alike; upright T wave; QT interval less than half the R to R interval; all P to P intervals and R to R intervals are equal; and the heart rate is between 60 to 100 per minute.

17. a. less than 60 impulses per minute
b. greater than 150 impulses per minute
c. varies; usually 60 to 100 impulses per minute

18. a. 250 to 350 per minute
b. 350 to 500 or more per minute

19. The pause of a sinus exit block is exactly two or
    more cardiac cycles of the underlying rhythm.
    The pause would fit into exactly two, three, four,
    or more cardiac cycles of the underlying rhythm.
    The pause of a sinus arrest is more than two or
    more cardiac cycles. It will not fit exactly into
    two, three, or four cardiac cycles of the
    underlying rhythm.

Rhythm Strip Review Answers

1. PRI: 0.16
   QRS: 0.06–0.08
   Interpretation: Normal Sinus Rhythm
   Rhythm: Regular
   Heart rate: 80

2. PRI: Not measurable
   QRS: 0.04–0.08
   Interpretation: Atrial flutter with a 3:1 Block
   Rhythm: Regular
   Heart rate: 90
   (atrial flutter rate: 270–280; 3 × 90 = 270)

3. PRI: 0.16–0.20
   QRS: 0.04–0.06
   Interpretation: Sinus tachycardia with prolonged QT intervals
   Rhythm: Regular
   Heart rate: 110

4. PRI: 0.20
   QRS: 0.06–0.08
   Interpretation: Sinus bradycardia with one PAC (4th complex)
   Rhythm: Irregular
   Heart rate: 50

5. PRI: 0.10–0.16
   QRS: 0.06–0.08
   Rhythm: Irregular
   Heart rate (calculated by 3-second method):
       first 3 seconds: 100 (sinus rhythm)
       second 3 seconds: 160 (PAT or PSVT)
   Interpretation: Sinus rhythm to PAT or PSVT (5th complex is a PAC)

6. PRI: 0.20
   QRS: 0.06–0.08
   Interpretation: Sinus bradycardia with peaked P waves
   Rhythm: Regular
   Heart rate: 40

7. PRI: 0.10–0.12
   QRS: 0.12–0.14
   Interpretation: Sinus bradycardia with Wolff-Parkinson-White syndrome
   Rhythm: Regular
   Heart rate: 50

8. PRI: 0.14–0.16
   QRS: 0.08
   Interpretation: Sinus tachycardia with prolonged QT intervals
   Rhythm: Regular
   Heart rate: 110

9. PRI: Not measurable
   QRS: 0.06-0.08
   Interpretation: Controlled atrial fibrillation
   Rhythm: Irregular
   Heart rate: 70 (atrial fibrillation rate: 350–500)

10. PRI: Not measurable
    QRS: 0.06–0.08
    Interpretation: Atrial flutter with varying block
    Rhythm: Irregular
    Heart rate: 70 (atrial flutter rate: 250–350)

11. PRI: Not measurable
    QRS: 0.04–0.06
    Interpretation: Supraventricular tachycardia with depressed ST segments
    Rhythm: Regular
    Heart rate: 190

12. PRI: 0.16–0.18
    QRS: 0.04–0.06
    Interpretation: Sinus arrhythmia
    Rhythm: Irregular
    Heart rate: 70

13. PRI: 0.16
    QRS: 0.06
    Interpretation: Sinus bradycardia
    Rhythm: Regular
    Heart rate: 40

14. PRI: Not measurable
    QRS: 0.06–0.08
    Interpretation: Controlled atrial fibrillation
    Rhythm: Irregular
    Heart rate: 90 (atrial fibrillation rate: 350–500)

15. PRI: 0.20
    QRS: 0.04–0.06
    Interpretation: Sinus arrest
    Rhythm: Irregular
    Heart rate: 70

Crossword Puzzle Answers

```
          F                   U
          I         3   4     P A U S E
          R   B     H   N     R       V
        P A R R H Y T H M I A   T
      P A C     I     T   E   G   F
      A   E     L     H   R   H   L
      T   M     L     M   E   T   U
          A     A         N       T
    S     K     T     P A T I E N T
    I     E X I T     R           E
    N S   R     O     R     P O O R
    U           N     E
    S                 S
                      A T R I A L
```

Word Puzzle Answers

```
D A F H A L B P A U S E K N Q D M H U
Y C D E T A L H H S W O W S K O G B I
S C R A R I O N F P T P C H E L U A U
R E L R I D C F W A V E A E M A X Z J
H S E T A R K I P C L L D W Y S B Q Z
Y S T G L A W B V X T P Q J D T A E V
T O A M W C S R Q R H W Z I S Q E Z O
H R S E D Y R I T O B A B P X A E U Y
M Y I D D E L T A H V A F P A U J U
I U N O N A T L P I C E Q A H O M I G
A M U N S R T A L H X H L R R R L Z G
M H S A L B U T E I H E Y I C L E C U
X Y N S U K L I Z K P N F C S D N N I
H G T X R B F O W D C K P X A R F R J
E G F S R I G N O W O A I Q L R Y Z I
S G D T I Q D N L K G E G M V A D G O
Y J V K N G I V P I H I G A O X G I V
I V X R G Z E X D L M L X U R O G U A
J O Y C Y K M O M M J Z O J J Y Z U J
```

CHAPTER 4

Review Question Answers

1. False
2. True
3. False
4. False
5. 40 to 60
6. d
7. 101 to 150
8. (in any order)
   a. appearing behind (retrograde P wave)
   b. in a reverse or backwards movement (electrical impulse travels in a retrograde manner from the AV junction throughout the atria)
9. d
10. (in any order)
    a. inverted
    b. buried or hidden
    c. retrograde
11. (in any order)
    a. inverted P wave originates high in the AV junctional area
    b. buried P wave originates in the mid AV junctional area
    c. retrograde P wave originates low in the AV junctional area
12. a
13. P waves vary in size and shape, may originate anywhere in the atria, above the bundle of His; may include junctional complexes. PR intervals vary but are usually less than 0.20 second if present. QRS complexes usually measure less than 0.12 second. P to P intervals and R to R intervals vary so the rhythm is irregular.
14. Junctional tachycardia has a rate of 101 to 150 electrical impulses per minute. The rate of an accelerated junctional dysrhythmia is 61 to 100 electrical impulses per minute.

Rhythm Strip Review Answers

1. PRI: 0.16
   QRS: 0.06–0.08
   Rhythm: Irregular
   Heart rate: 70
   Interpretation: Sinus rhythm with one PJC (7th complex)
2. PRI: Not measurable
   QRS: 0.04–0.06
   Rhythm: Regular
   Heart rate: 30
   Interpretation: Junctional bradycardia (with retrograde P waves)
3. PRI: 0.16–0.18
   QRS: 0.04–0.06
   Rhythm: Regular
   Heart rate: 50
   Interpretation: Junctional dysrhythmia (with inverted P waves)
4. PRI: Not measurable
   QRS: 0.04–0.06
   Rhythm: Regular
   Heart rate: 70
   Interpretation: Accelerated junctional dysrhythmia (with hidden P waves)
5. PRI: Not measurable
   QRS: 0.08
   Rhythm: Regular
   Heart rate: 110
   Interpretation: Junctional tachycardia (with retrograde P waves)
6. PRI: 0.14—not measurable
   QRS: 0.04–0.06
   Rhythm: Irregular
   Heart rate: 40
   Interpretation: Wandering junctional pacemaker
7. PRI: 0.08—not measurable
   QRS: 0.06–0.08
   Rhythm: Irregular
   Heart rate: 80–90
   Interpretation: Wandering atrial pacemaker with depressed ST segments

CHAPTER 5

Review Question Answers

1. True
2. False
3. False
4. True
5. c
6. b
7. c
8. 0.20
9. Third-degree heart block
10. Longer, QRS complex
11. It has no pattern and may lead to third-degree heart block, or if the block is severe enough, the rate may be too bradycardic to maintain life.
12. (in any order)
    a. Underlying rhythm
    b. Ratio of P waves to each QRS complex
    c. Frequency, or how often the dysrhythmia occurs

Rhythm Strip Review Answers

1. PRI: 0.20–0.32   Rhythm: Irregular
   QRS: 0.04–0.08   Heart rate: 50 (atrial rate: 80)
   Interpretation: Second-degree heart block, type I, with bradycardic rate

2. PRI: 0.32–0.36   Rhythm: Regular
   QRS: 0.04–0.06   Heart rate: 60
   Interpretation: Sinus rhythm with first-degree heart block

3. PRI: 0.22–0.24   Rhythm: Regular
   QRS: 0.06   Heart rate: 40 (atrial rate: 70)
   Interpretation: Second-degree heart block, type II (2:1 block), with bradycardic rate

4. PRI: 0.16   Rhythm: Irregular
   QRS: 0.16–0.20   Heart rate: 40 (atrial rate: 60)
   Interpretation: Second-degree heart block, type II (3:1 block), with bradycardic rate, BBB, and inverted T waves

5. PRI: 0.20–0.32   Rhythm: Irregular
   QRS: 0.06–0.08   Heart rate: 50 (atrial rate: 80)
   Interpretation: Second-degree heart block, type I, with bradycardic rate

6. PRI: 0.24   Rhythm: Regular
   QRS: 0.06   Heart rate: 20 (atrial rate: 50)
   Interpretation: Second-degree heart block, type II (2:1 block), with bradycardic rate

7. PRI: 0.18   Rhythm: Irregular
   QRS: 0.20   Heart rate: 30 (atrial rate: 60)
   Interpretation: Second-degree heart block, type II (varying block), with bradycardic rate, BBB, and depressed (inverted) T waves

8. PRI: 0.16–0.20   Rhythm: Regular
   QRS: 0.16–0.20   Heart rate: 60
   Interpretation: Sinus rhythm with BBB and elevated ST segments

9. PRI: Not measurable (No true PRI)   Rhythm: Regular
   QRS: 0.14   Heart rate: 30 (atrial rate: 70; P wave hidden in first T wave)
   Interpretation: Third-degree heart block

10. PRI: 0.24–0.28   Rhythm: Regular
    QRS: 0.04   Heart rate: 70
    Interpretation: Sinus rhythm with first-degree heart block

11. PRI: 0.22–0.24   Rhythm: Regular
    QRS: 0.08   Heart rate: 20 (atrial rate: 60)
    Interpretation: Second-degree heart block, type II (2:1 block), with bradycardic rate

12. PRI: Not measurable (No true PRI)   Rhythm: Regular
    QRS: 0.12   Heart rate: 30 (atrial rate: 50)
    Interpretation: Third-degree heart block

Crossword Puzzle Answers

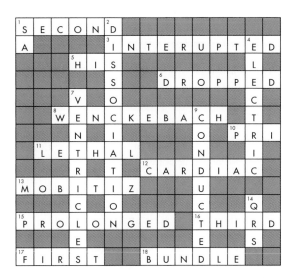

Word Puzzle Answers

R N J K U H Y T A D N N D L J Z J P K Q N
N P W C H C A B E K C N E W K Y W A I J O
F Q D T X L L T Q P P U H Z I O V T N D T
T J J N G C C Z T R S Z C W D R I H T J A
V X H I H S O F O A T P T Q Y L M W E V I
E L V R A K J G Z C R S O I E D I A R I C
N X K H S B R Y G G A B N B B B A Y U N O
T E R X F E G O P U E T B C L O P S P T S
R H M D S V C G N C H E R M O O M Q T E S
I Z D S C D E O H O H L A I F M C C I R I
C W I D N Q H D N N R X D P A W P K O M D
L V N Y D F B D J D W A Y X G J I L N I E
E C L O T Q M A H U X G C N T B B Z E T G
W V A V T A K O X C P F A S U G G E G T R
B D J D I C X E I T T U R N D X F E I E E
E R O R J R O F O I Z I D E Y A L E D N E
C U O T D M A A R O F L I O V O Z X J T G
L P N Y L Z O T N N E L A H T E L L R O Q
E A K W F U O E K U R R M A A K K J Z K Z
K B A K C T P O U F X U U X Z V J G L S R
U K J Q Y K O Q X U Z Y Y Y Q K O K Z K J

CHAPTER 6

Review Question Answers

1. False
2. True
3. True
4. False
5. False
6. 20
7. The QRS complexes of torsades de pointes begin close to the baseline, and gradually increase and decrease in amplitude, in a twisting, repeating pattern. The QRS complexes of ventricular tachycardia remain more similar in height, without the twisting and turning motion.

8. a. Different ventricular sites and different appearances
   b. Two PVCs in a row
   c. Every other complex is a PVC, with at least three episodes in a row.
9. (in any order)
   Severe heart disease, electrical shock, drug toxicity
10. b
11. d
12. d

Rhythm Strip Review Answers

1. PRI: 0.20—not measurable
   QRS: 0.06–0.16

   Rhythm: Irregular
   Heart rate: (calculated by 3-second method)
      first 3 seconds: 50 (sinus bradycardia)
      second 3 seconds: 120 (VT)

   Interpretation: Sinus bradycardia with run of ventricular tachycardia

2. PRI: Not measurable
   QRS: Not measurable
   Rhythm: Not measurable
   Heart rate: 0 (atrial rate: 0)
   Interpretation: Asystole

3. PRI: 0.16–0.20
   QRS: 0.06–0.20
   Rhythm: Irregular
   Heart rate: 80
   Interpretation: Sinus rhythm with unifocal PVCs, occurring in bigeminy (1st, 3rd, 5th, and 7th complexes)

4. PRI: 0.16
   QRS: 0.06–0.26
   Rhythm: Irregular
   Heart rate: (calculated by 3-second method)
      first 3 seconds: 60 (sinus rhythm)
      second 3 seconds: 0 (V Fib; atrial rate: 0)

   Interpretation: Sinus rhythm with multifocal PVCs (1st and 6th complexes); R on T phenomenon (6th complex), changing to ventricular fibrillation

5. PRI: 0.20
   QRS: 0.06–0.34
   Rhythm: Irregular
   Heart rate: 70
   Interpretation: Sinus rhythm with multifocal PVCs (2nd, 3rd, and 7th complexes), with one multifocal couplet (2nd and 3rd complexes)

6. PRI: Not measurable
   QRS: Greater than 0.12
   Rhythm: Regular
   Heart rate: 310 (atrial rate: 0)
   Interpretation: Torsades de pointes

7. PRI: 0.12
   QRS: 0.04–0.14
   Rhythm: Irregular
   Heart rate: 60
   Interpretation: Junctional dysrhythmia with one PVC (3rd complex)

8. PRI: Not measurable
   QRS: Not measurable
   Rhythm: Not measurable
   Heart rate: 0 (atrial rate: 0)
   Interpretation: Fine ventricular fibrillation

9. PRI: Not measurable
   QRS: 0.36–0.40
   Rhythm: Regular
   Heart rate: 30 (atrial rate: 0)
   Interpretation: Idioventricular dysrhythmia

10. PRI: Not measurable
    QRS: 0.16
    Rhythm: Regular
    Heart rate: 150 (atrial rate: 0)
    Interpretation: Ventricular tachycardia

11. PRI: Not measurable
    QRS: 0.10–0.32
    Rhythm: Irregular
    Heart rate: 100 (atrial fibrillation rate: 350–500)
    Interpretation: Controlled atrial fibrillation with one PVC (5th complex), and depressed ST segments

12. PRI: 0.20
    QRS: 0.04–0.12
    Rhythm: Irregular
    Heart rate: 70
    Interpretation: Sinus rhythm with one multifocal PVC couplet (4th and 5th complexes)

13. PRI: Not measurable
    QRS: Not measurable
    Interpretation: Coarse ventricular fibrillation

    Rhythm: Not measurable
    Heart rate: 0 (atrial rate: 0)

14. PRI: Not measurable
    QRS: Not measurable
    Interpretation: Ventricular standstill

    Rhythm: Regular
    Heart rate: 0 (atrial rate: 50)

15. PRI: Not measurable
    QRS: 0.40–0.44
    Interpretation: Agonal dysrhythmia

    Rhythm: Not measurable
    Heart rate: 10 (atrial rate: 0)

CHAPTER 7

Review Question Answers

1. False
2. True
3. False
4. False
5. False
6. (in any order)
   a. impulse generator
   b. leadwires
   c. electrodes
7. a. 75% capture indicates that one fourth or 25% of the pacer spikes on the rhythm strip are not followed by a QRS complex.
   b. 50% paced indicates that only one half or 50% of the complexes on the rhythm strip are generated by the mechanical pacemaker. The other half of the impulses are initiated by the heart.
8. 3
9. d
10. d
11. 3
12. An aberrantly conducted complex is a complex that does not follow the normal pathway of the underlying rhythm and appears different than the normal complexes. It may be smaller than the normal complexes and usually appears as only a single complex.

13. (in any order)
    a. atrial pacemaker stimulates only the atria
    b. ventricular pacemaker stimulates only the ventricles
    c. sequential (dual chamber) pacemaker stimulates both the atria and ventricles in a sequential manner
14. (in any order)
    a. transcutaneous—applied by means of sticky pads, which contain electrodes, to the chest and back of the patient.
    b. transvenous—insert through a large vein by means of a large needle directly into the right atria.
15. (in any order)
    a. fixed-rate set to generate an electrical impulses at regular intervals, usually between 70 and 80 impulses per minute.
    b. demand-set to generate electrical impulses only when the patient's heart rate falls below a certain point, usually 60 beats per minute.

Rhythm Strip Review Answers

1. PRI: Not measured
   QRS: 0.06–0.08
   Rhythm: Regular
   Heart rate: 70
   Interpretation: Atrial pacemaker with 100% pacing and 100% capture
2. PRI: 0.20
   QRS: 0.06–0.08
   Rhythm: Regular
   Heart rate: 90
   Interpretation: Sinus rhythm with an aberrant beat (5th complex), and prolonged QT intervals
3. PRI: Not measured
   QRS: 0.10
   Rhythm: Regular
   Heart rate: 80
   Interpretation: Sequential pacemaker with 100% pacing and 100% capture
4. PRI: Not measured
   QRS: 0.10-0.12
   Rhythm: Regular
   Heart rate: 70
   Interpretation: Ventricular pacemaker with 100% pacing and 100% capture
5. PRI: 0.16-0.18
   QRS: 0.04-0.10
   Rhythm: Irregular
   Heart rate: 120
   Interpretation: Sinus tachycardia with one aberrant beat (10th complex), and prolonged QT intervals

6. PRI: Not measured
   QRS: 0.12
   Rhythm: Regular
   Heart rate: 70
   Interpretation: Sequential pacemaker with 100% pacing and 100% capture
7. PRI: Not measured
   QRS: 0.12–0.14
   Rhythm: Regular
   Heart rate: 70
   Interpretation: Ventricular pacemaker with 100% pacing and 100% capture
8. PRI: 0.20
   QRS: 0.04–0.08
   Rhythm: Regular
   Heart rate: 90
   Interpretation: Sinus rhythm with three aberrant beats (1st, 6th, and 7th complexes), and prolonged QT intervals
9. PRI: Not measured
   QRS: Not measurable
   Rhythm: Regular
   Heart rate: 0; Pacemaker rate: 70
   Interpretation: Pacemaker with 100% pacing and 0% capture
10. PRI: Not measured
    QRS: 0.04–0.06
    Rhythm: Regular
    Heart rate: 70
    Interpretation: Atrial pacemaker; 100% pacing, 100% capture
11. PRI: 0.20—not measured
    QRS: 0.06–0.22
    Rhythm: Irregular
    Heart rate: 60
    Interpretation: Ventricular pacemaker with 50% pacing and 66% capture
12. PRI: Not measured
    QRS: 0.08–0.16
    Rhythm: Irregular
    Heart rate: 50
    Interpretation: Ventricular pacemaker with 60% pacing and 100% capture

Crossword Puzzle Answers

¹S			²P	U	L	³S	E	L	E	S	S	
⁴P	E	⁵A				E						
I		I				Q						
K		⁶C	O	N	D	U	C	T	E	D		
E		D				E						
	⁷T		⁸G	E	N	E	R	A	T	O	R	¹⁰E
¹¹B	E	A	T			Y		⁹B				S
	M		¹²A	I			E		¹³A		C
¹⁴P	A	C	E	M	A	K	E	R		T		A
	O		D		L			R		T		P
	R			¹⁵Q		¹⁶L	E	A	D	W	I	R	E
¹⁷C	A	P	T	U	R	E			N		A	
	R			S		¹⁸L	E	T	H	A	L	
	Y											

Word Puzzle Answers

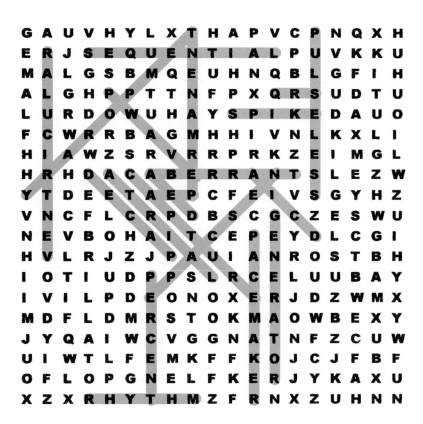

CHAPTER 10

Rhythm Strip Review Answers

1. PRI: 0.20–0.22   Rhythm: Regular
QRS: 0.06   Heart rate: 70
Interpretation: Sinus rhythm with first-degree heart block

2. PRI: 0.16   Rhythm: Irregular
QRS: 0.06–0.20   Heart rate: 80
Interpretation: Sinus rhythm with one PVC (5th complex)

3. PRI: Not measurable   Rhythm: Not measurable
QRS: Not measurable   Heart rate: 0 (atrial rate: 0)
Interpretation: Fine ventricular fibrillation

4. PRI: 0.16   Rhythm: Irregular
QRS: 0.04   Heart rate: (calculated by 3-second method)
                                 first 3 seconds: 40 (sinus bradycardia)
                                 second 3 seconds: 140 (sinus tachycardia)
Interpretation: Sinus bradycardia changing to sinus tachycardia

5. PRI: 0.20–0.58   Rhythm: Irregular
QRS: 0.06–0.08   Heart rate: 50 (atrial rate: 70)
Interpretation: Second-degree heart block, type I, with bradycardic rate and depressed ST segments

6. PRI: 0.08   Rhythm: Regular
QRS: 0.04–0.06   Heart rate: 220
Interpretation: Supraventricular tachycardia

7. PRI: 0.16–0.20   Rhythm: Irregular
   QRS: 0.06–0.16   Heart rate: 70
   Interpretation: Sinus rhythm with two unifocal PVCs (1st and 4th complexes)

8. PRI: Not measurable   Rhythm: Regular
   QRS: 0.06   Heart rate: 30
   Interpretation: Junctional bradycardia (with retrograde P waves)

9. PRI: Not measurable   Rhythm: Regular
   QRS: 0.12   Heart rate: 70 (atrial flutter rate: 260–280;
                                               $4 \times 70 = 280$)

   Interpretation: Atrial flutter with 4:1 block

10. PRI: Not measurable   Rhythm: Regular
    QRS: 0.12–0.14   Heart rate: 20 (atrial rate: 70; one P wave hidden in
                                               1st QRS complex)

    Interpretation: Third-degree heart block

11. PRI: Not measurable   Rhythm: Regular
    QRS: 0.36–0.40   Heart rate: 30 (atrial rate: 0)
    Interpretation: Idioventricular dysrhythmia

12. PRI: 0.14   Rhythm: Regular
    QRS: 0.04–0.06   Heart rate: 140
    Interpretation: Sinus tachycardia with depressed ST segments and prolonged QT intervals

13. PRI: 0.16—not measurable   Rhythm: Irregular
    QRS: 0.06–0.20   Heart rate: 50
    Interpretation: Junctional dysrhythmia (with inverted P waves) and two unifocal PVCs
       (1st and 3rd complexes)

14. PRI: Not measurable   Rhythm: Regular
    QRS: 0.16–0.20   Heart rate: 150 (atrial rate: 0)
    Interpretation: Ventricular tachycardia

15. PRI: 0.22–0.24   Rhythm: Regular
    QRS: 0.06   Heart rate: 40 (atrial rate: 70)
    Interpretation: Second-degree heart block, type II (2:1 block), with bradycardic rate

16. PRI: 0.20   Rhythm: Irregular
    QRS: 0.06   Heart rate: 60
    Interpretation: Sinus rhythm with one PAC (2nd complex)

17. PRI: 0.16–not measurable   Rhythm: R to R regular; P to P irregular
    QRS: 0.08–0.10 to not measurable   Heart rate: (calculated by 3-second method)
                                                 first 3 seconds: 60 (sinus bradycardia; atrial rate: 80)
                                                 second 3 seconds: 0 (ventricular standstill;
                                                 atrial rate: 40)
    Interpretation: Sinus rhythm changing to ventricular standstill

18. PRI: 0.16–not measurable   Rhythm: Irregular
    QRS: 0.04–0.06   Heart rate: 60
    Interpretation: Wandering junctional pacemaker

19. PRI: 0.20   Rhythm: Irregular
    QRS: 0.06–0.40   Heart rate: 80
    Interpretation: Sinus rhythm with multifocal PVCs in bigeminy (2nd, 4th, 6th, and 8th complexes)

20. PRI: Not measurable   Rhythm: Regular
    QRS: 0.06-0.10   Heart rate: 70 (atrial flutter rate: 280; $4 \times 70 = 280$)
    Interpretation: Atrial flutter with 4:1 block

21. PRI: Not measured   Rhythm: Regular
    QRS: 0.16   Heart rate: 70
    Interpretation: Ventricular pacemaker with 100% pacing and 100% capture

22. PRI: Not measurable   Rhythm: Regular
    QRS: 0.06–0.08   Heart rate: 80
    Interpretation: Artifact (60 cycle interference)

23. PRI: 0.08–not measurable   Rhythm: Irregular
    QRS: 0.06–0.08   Heart rate: 90
    Interpretation: Wandering atrial pacemaker with depressed ST segments

24. PRI: 0.20   Rhythm: Irregular
      QRS: 0.06–0.08   Heart rate: 80
      Interpretation: Sinus arrest with prolonged QT intervals

25. PRI: 0.16—not measurable   Rhythm: Irregular
      QRS: 0.06, not measurable   Heart rate: (calculated by 3-second method)
                                               first 3 seconds: 100 (sinus rhythm; atrial rate: 80)
                                               second 3 seconds: 0 (V Fib; atrial rate: 0)
      Interpretation: Sinus rhythm with a PVC (5th complex), R on T phenomenon (5th complex), changing
         to ventricular fibrillation

26. PRI: 0.16–0.48   Rhythm: Irregular
      QRS: 0.04–08   Heart rate: 50 (atrial rate: 70)
      Interpretation: Second-degree heart block, type I with bradycardic rate

27. PRI: Not measured   Rhythm: Regular
      QRS: 0.04–0.06   Heart rate: 70
      Interpretation: Atrial pacemaker with 100% pacing and 100% capture

28. PRI: 0.20   Rhythm: Irregular
      QRS: 0.06–0.24   Heart rate: 80
      Interpretation: Sinus rhythm with unifocal PVCs (5th and 8th complexes)

29. PRI: Not measurable   Rhythm: Irregular
      QRS: 0.06–0.24   Heart rate: 90 (atrial fibrillation rate: 350–500)
      Interpretation: Atrial fibrillation (with depressed ST segments), with R on T phenomenon
         (4th complex) and run of ventricular tachycardia (4th, 5th, and 6th complexes)

30. PRI: Not measurable   Rhythm: Not measurable
      QRS: 0.40   Heart rate: 10 (atrial rate: 0)
      Interpretation: Agonal rhythm

31. PRI: 0.16–0.20   Rhythm: Irregular
      QRS: 0.04–0.14   Heart rate: 110–120
      Interpretation: Sinus tachycardia (with prolonged QT intervals), with an aberrantly conducted beat
         (11th complex)

32. PRI: 0.16–0.18   Rhythm: Regular
      QRS: 0.18–0.20   Heart rate: 60
      Interpretation: Sinus rhythm with BBB, elevated ST segments, and prolonged QT intervals

33. PRI: Not measured   Rhythm: Regular
      QRS: 0.16   Heart rate: 80
      Interpretation: Sequential pacemaker with 100% pacing and 100% capture

34. PRI: 0.32   Rhythm: Regular
      QRS: 0.08   Heart rate: 80
      Interpretation: Sinus rhythm with first-degree heart block

35. PRI: 0.16–0.18   Rhythm: Irregular
      QRS: 0.06–0.40   Heart rate: 70
      Interpretation: Sinus rhythm with multifocal PVCs (3rd and 6th complexes)

36. PRI: Not measurable   Rhythm: Irregular
      QRS: 0.04   Heart rate: 60 (atrial fibrillation rate: 350–500)
      Interpretation: Controlled atrial fibrillation

37. PRI: 0.08–0.10   Rhythm: Regular
      QRS: 0.06–0.08   Heart rate: 170
      Interpretation: Supraventricular tachycardia with depressed ST segments, and prolonged QT intervals

38. PRI: 0.16–0.20   Rhythm: Irregular
      QRS: 0.06–0.08   Heart rate: 70
      Interpretation: Sinus rhythm with one PJC (6th complex)

39. PRI: 0.16   Rhythm: Irregular
      QRS: 0.16–0.20   Heart rate: 40 (atrial rate: 60)
      Interpretation: Second-degree heart block, type II (3:1 block), with inverted T waves, BBB,
         and a bradycardic rate

40. PRI: 0.16   Rhythm: Irregular
      QRS: 0.04–0.44   Heart rate: 70
      Interpretation: Sinus rhythm with unifocal PVCs (2nd and 6th complexes)

41. PRI: 0.20   Rhythm: Regular
    QRS: 0.06-0.08   Heart rate: 100
    Interpretation: Normal sinus rhythm with prolonged QT intervals
42. PRI: 0.22   Rhythm: Irregular
    QRS: 0.06–0.16   Heart rate: (calculated by 3-second method)
                                                        first 3 seconds: 80 (sinus rhythm)
                                                        second 3 seconds: 140 (VT; atrial rate: 0)
    Interpretation: Sinus rhythm with a run of ventricular tachycardia (5th, 6th, 7th, 8th, 9th, and 10th
        complexes)
43. PRI: 0.18–0.20   Rhythm: Irregular
    QRS: 0.06–0.20   Heart rate: 90
    Interpretation: Sinus rhythm with two episodes of unifocal PVC couplets (4th and 5th complexes;
        8th and 9th complexes)
44. PRI: Not measurable   Rhythm: Regular
    QRS: 0.06–0.08   Heart rate: 110
    Interpretation: Junctional tachycardia (with retrograde P waves)
45. PRI: 0.16–0.18   Rhythm: Irregular
    QRS: 0.06–0.20   Heart rate: 80
    Interpretation: Sinus rhythm with unifocal PVCs in bigeminy (1st, 3rd, 5th, and 7th complexes)
46. PRI: 0.16–0.18   Rhythm: Irregular
    QRS: 0.06   Heart rate: 50
    Interpretation: Sinus arrhythmia with bradycardic rate
47. PRI: 0.16–0.18   Rhythm: Regular
    QRS: 0.04–0.06   Heart rate: 50
    Interpretation: Junctional dysrhythmia (with inverted P waves)
48. PRI: 0.32–0.36   Rhythm: Regular
    QRS: 0.06   Heart rate 50
    Interpretation: Sinus bradycardia with first-degree heart block
49. PRI: 0.16—not measurable   Rhythm: Irregular
    QRS: 0.04–0.06   Heart rate: (by division method)
                                                        first rhythm: 80 (sinus rhythm)
                                                        second rhythm: 160 (PAT or PSVT)
    Interpretation: Sinus rhythm changing to PAT or PSVT
50. PRI: Not measurable   Rhythm: Irregular
    QRS: 0.06   Heart rate: 50
    Interpretation: Wandering junctional pacemaker
51. PRI: 0.12–0.16   Rhythm: Irregular
    QRS: 0.04–0.06   Heart rate: 50
    Interpretation: Sinus arrhythmia with bradycardic rate
52. PRI: Not measurable   Rhythm: Regular
    QRS: 0.14   Heart rate: 20 (atrial rate 70)
    Interpretation: Third-degree heart block
53. PRI: Not measurable   Rhythm: Not measurable
    QRS: Not measurable   Heart rate: 0 (atrial rate: 0)
    Interpretation: Coarse ventricular fibrillation
54. PRI: Not measurable   Rhythm: Regular
    QRS: 0.20–0.24   Heart rate: 140 (atrial rate: 0)
    Interpretation: Ventricular tachycardia
55. PRI: 0.12–not measurable   Rhythm: Irregular
    QRS: 0.06   Heart rate: 90
    Interpretation: Wandering atrial pacemaker
56. PRI: 0.20   Rhythm: Irregular
    QRS: 0.06–0.36   Heart rate: 80
    Interpretation: Sinus rhythm with multifocal PVCs (1st, 7th, and 8th complexes)
57. PRI: Not measurable   Rhythm: Not measurable
    QRS: Not measurable   Heart rate: 0 (atrial rate: 0)
    Interpretation: Asystole

58. PRI: 0.20   Rhythm: Regular
QRS: 0.06   Heart rate: 100
Interpretation: Sinus rhythm with one aberrantly conducted beat (3rd complex) and prolonged
    QT intervals

59. PRI: Not measurable   Rhythm: Irregular
QRS: 0.12–0.32   Heart rate: 100 (atrial fibrillation rate: 350–500)
Interpretation: Controlled atrial fibrillation with one PVC (4th complex)

60. PRI: Not measurable   Rhythm: Regular
QRS: 0.08   Heart rate: 60 (atrial flutter rate: 240–250;
                                      $4 \times 6 = 240$)
Interpretation: Atrial flutter (4:1 block)

61. PRI: Not measurable   Rhythm: Regular
QRS: Greater than 0.12   Heart rate: 220-250 (atrial rate: 0)
Interpretation: Torsades de pointes

62. PRI: 0.16–0.20   Rhythm: Regular
QRS: 0.08–0.10   Heart rate: 50
Interpretation: Sinus bradycardia with depressed ST segments and artifact

63. PRI: Not measurable   Rhythm: Irregular
QRS: 0.06–0.08   Heart rate: 90 (atrial fibrillation rate: 350–500)
Interpretation: Controlled atrial fibrillation with depressed ST segments

64. PRI: 0.14–0.30   Rhythm: Irregular
QRS: 0.06   Heart rate: 50 (atrial rate: 80)
Interpretation: Second-degree heart block, type I, with bradycardic rate

65. PRI: 0.16–0.20   Rhythm: Irregular
QRS: 0.06–0.08   Heart rate: 90
Interpretation: Sinus rhythm with one aberrantly conducted beat (7th complex), peaked P waves,
    and artifact

66. PRI: Not measured   Rhythm: Irregular
QRS: 0.06–0.22   Heart rate: 60
Interpretation: Ventricular pacemaker with 50% pacing and 66% capture, and artifact

67. PRI: Not measurable   Rhythm: Regular
QRS: 0.36–0.40   Heart rate: 40 (atrial rate: 0)
Interpretation: Idioventricular dysrhythmia

68. PRI: Not measurable   Rhythm: Regular
QRS: 0.08–0.10   Heart rate: 100
Interpretation: Sinus rhythm with artifact

69. PRI: Not measurable   Rhythm: Regular
QRS: 0.08   Heart rate: 100
Interpretation: Accelerated junctional dysrhythmia (with hidden P waves)

70. PRI: Not measurable   Rhythm: Not measurable
QRS: Not measurable   Heart rate: 0 (atrial rate: 0)
Interpretation: Ventricular fibrillation (fine VF → coarse VF → fine VF)

71. PRI: 0.16   Rhythm: Regular
QRS: 0.08–0.12   Heart rate: 50
Interpretation: Sinus bradycardia

72. PRI: Not measurable   Rhythm: Irregular
QRS: 0.04–0.08   Heart rate: 90 (atrial flutter rate: 250–350)
Interpretation: Atrial flutter with variable block and artifact

73. PRI: Not measured   Rhythm: Regular
QRS: 0.04–0.06   Heart rate: 70
Interpretation: Atrial pacemaker with 100% pacing and 100% capture

74. PRI: 0.14–0.20   Rhythm: Regular
QRS: 0.04–0.08   Heart rate: 90
Interpretation: Sinus rhythm with depressed ST segments

75. PRI: Not measurable   Rhythm: Regular
QRS: 0.16   Heart rate: 60
Interpretation: Junctional dysrhythmia with artifact

76. PRI: Difficult to measure
    QRS: 0.10–0.36
    Interpretation: Sinus rhythm with BBB, two multifocal PVCs (2nd and 4th complexes), and 60-cycle interference
Rhythm: Irregular
Heart rate: 80

77. PRI: Not measurable
    QRS: 0.26–0.28
    Interpretation: Ventricular tachycardia
Rhythm: Regular
Heart rate: 160 (atrial rate: 0)

78. PRI: 0.16
    QRS: 0.08
    Interpretation: Normal sinus rhythm with elevated ST segments and elevated (peaked) T waves
Rhythm: Regular
Heart rate: 70

79. PRI: 0.16–0.20
    QRS: 0.04–0.08
    Interpretation: Wandering atrial pacemaker rhythm with depressed ST segments
Rhythm: Irregular
Heart rate: 90

80. PRI: 0.28
    QRS: 0.08–0.10
    Interpretation: Sinus rhythm with first-degree heart block
Rhythm: Regular
Heart rate 90

81. PRI: 0.16
    QRS: 0.04
    Interpretation: Second-degree heart block, type II (3:1 block), with a bradycardic rate
Rhythm: Regular
Heart rate: 40 (atrial rate: 100)

82. PRI: 0.16
    QRS: 0.06–0.08
    Interpretation: Normal sinus rhythm with depressed ST segments
Rhythm: Regular
Heart rate: 60

83. PRI: 0.12–0.14
    QRS: 0.04–0.06
    Interpretation: Sinus tachycardia
Rhythm: Regular
Heart rate: 100–110

84. PRI: 0.10–0.12
    QRS: 0.06
    Interpretation: Sinus rhythm with depressed ST segments
Rhythm: Regular
Heart rate: 70

85. PRI: Not measurable
    QRS: 0.12–0.36
    Interpretation: Atrial fibrillation with controlled ventricular response, depressed ST segments, and one PVC (7th complex)
Rhythm: Irregular
Heart rate: 100 (atrial fibrillation rate: 350–500)

86. PRI: 0.20
    QRS: 0.06–0.10
    Interpretation: Sinus rhythm with depressed ST segments and one PAC (4th complex)
Rhythm: Irregular
Heart rate: 90

87. PRI: 0.16
    QRS: 0.08
    Interpretation: Sinus rhythm with peaked P waves and elevated (peaked) T waves
Rhythm: Regular
Heart rate: 60

88. PRI: Not measurable
    QRS: Greater than 0.12
    Interpretation: Torsades de pointes
Rhythm: Regular
Heart rate: 220 (atrial rate: 0)

89. PRI: Not measurable
    QRS: 0.08
    Interpretation: Atrial fibrillation with slow ventricular response
Rhythm: Irregular
Heart rate: 50 (atrial fibrillation rate: 350–500)

90. PRI: Not measurable
    QRS: 0.04–0.06
    Interpretation: Atrial flutter with varying block and wandering baseline
Rhythm: Irregular
Heart rate: 100 (atrial flutter rate: 250–350)

91. PRI: 0.12–0.14
    QRS: 0.08–0.10
    Interpretation: Normal sinus rhythm with prolonged QT intervals
Rhythm: Regular
Heart rate: 100

92. PRI: Not measurable
    QRS: Not measurable
    Interpretation: Artifact
Rhythm: Regular
Heart rate: 90 (atrial rate: not measurable)

93. PRI: 0.12–0.16
    QRS: 0.12
    Interpretation: Sinus rhythm
Rhythm: Regular
Heart rate: 80

94. PRI: 0.16   Rhythm: Irregular
    QRS: 0.06–0.16   Heart rate: 100
    Interpretation: Sinus rhythm with three aberrantly conducted PACs (1st, 6th, and 10th complexes) and depressed ST segments

95. PRI: 0.14–0.16   Rhythm: Regular
    QRS: 0.08–0.10   Heart rate: 80
    Interpretation: Normal sinus rhythm

96. PRI: 0.14   Rhythm: Regular
    QRS: 0.08   Heart rate: 50
    Interpretation: Junctional dysrhythmia (with inverted P waves), with depressed (inverted) T waves, and depressed ST segments

97. PRI: Not measurable   Rhythm: Regular
    QRS: 0.06–0.08   Heart rate: 250
    Interpretation: Supraventricular tachycardia with depressed ST segments

98. PRI: 0.20   Rhythm: Regular
    QRS: 0.12–0.14   Heart rate: 100
    Interpretation: Sinus rhythm with depressed ST segments and prolonged QT intervals

99. PRI: Not measurable   Rhythm: Regular
    QRS: 0.08   Heart rate: 70
    Interpretation: Accelerated junctional dysrhythmia (with hidden P waves), and depressed ST segments

100. PRI: Not measurable   Rhythm: Irregular
    QRS: Not measurable   Heart rate: Not measurable (atrial rate: 0)
    Interpretation: Ventricular tachycardia (possible torsades de pointes) changing to fine ventricular fibrillation

101. PRI: 0.14–0.20 when present   Rhythm: Irregular
    QRS: 0.10–0.12   Heart rate: 50
    Interpretation: Wandering atrial pacemaker rhythm with bradycardic rate

102. PRI: Not measurable   Rhythm: (Atrial: regular)
    QRS: 0.10   Heart rate: 10 (atrial rate: 40)
    Interpretation: Ventricular standstill with one escape beat

103. PRI: Not measurable   Rhythm: Irregular
    QRS: 0.14–0.16   Heart rate: 200 (atrial rate: 0)
    Interpretation: Ventricular tachycardia

104. PRI: 0.20–0.40   Rhythm: Irregular
    QRS: 0.08   Heart rate: 60 (atrial rate: 80)
    Interpretation: Second-degree heart block, type I, with elevated ST segments

105. PRI: Not measurable   Rhythm: Regular
    QRS: Not measurable   Heart rate: 0; Pacemaker rate: 70
    Interpretation: Pacemaker rhythm with 100% pacing and 0% capture

106. PRI: Not measurable   Rhythm: Not measurable
    QRS: Not measurable   Heart rate: 0 (atrial rate: 0)
    Interpretation: Coarse ventricular fibrillation

107. PRI: 0.10   Rhythm: Irregular
    QRS: 0.08–0.10   Heart rate: 70
    Interpretation: Sinus rhythm with three PACs (2nd, 4th, and 6th complexes)

108. PRI: 0.16   Rhythm: Regular
    QRS: 0.08–0.24   Heart rate: 100
    Interpretation: Sinus rhythm with unifocal PVCs in trigeminy (1st, 4th, 7th, and 10th complexes)

109. PRI: Not measurable   Rhythm: Not measurable
    QRS: Not measurable   Heart rate: Not measurable
    Interpretation: Artifact (loose leads, patient movement)

110. PRI: 0.12–0.16   Rhythm: Regular
    QRS: 0.04–0.06   Heart rate: 110
    Interpretation: Sinus tachycardia with prolonged QT intervals

111. PRI: Not measurable   Rhythm: Not measurable
    QRS: 0.26   Heart rate: 10 (atrial rate: 0)
    Interpretation: Agonal rhythm (possibly going into asystole)

112. PRI: 0.24

    QRS: 0.10

Rhythm: Regular

Heart rate: 40 (atrial rate: 70)

    Interpretation: Second-degree heart block, type II (2:1 block), with a bradycardic rate and artifact

113. PRI: 0.16

    QRS: 0.08–0.24

Rhythm: Irregular

Heart rate: (overall heart rate:140)

    Interpretation: Sinus rhythm with multifocal PVCs (2nd and 6th complexes), a run of ventricular tachycardia (8-12 complexes), and one junctional escape beat (13th complex)

114. PRI: 0.12–0.16

    QRS: 0.06–0.14

Rhythm: Irregular

Heart rate: (calculated by 3-second method)

        first 3 seconds: 120 (sinus tachycardia)

        second 3 seconds: 180 (PAT or PSVT)

    Interpretation: Sinus tachycardia with two PACs (3rd and 5th complexes), changing to PAT or PSVT, with depressed ST segments throughout

115. PRI: Not measurable

    QRS: Greater than 0.12

Rhythm: Regular

Heart rate: 220 (atrial rate: 0)

    Interpretation: Ventricular tachycardia (possible torsades de pointe)

116. PRI: 0.10—not measurable

    QRS: 0.08–0.16

Rhythm: Irregular

Heart rate: 170

    Interpretation: Supraventricular tachycardia with two escape beats (13th and 16th complexes)

117. PRI: Not measurable

    QRS: 0.06–0.08

Rhythm: Regular

Heart rate: 150

    Interpretation: Sinus tachycardia with depressed ST segments and wandering baseline

118. PRI: 0.12–0.16

    QRS: 0.04–0.06

Rhythm: Regular

Heart rate: 70

    Interpretation: Sinus rhythm with wandering baseline

119. PRI: Not measurable

    QRS: 0.06–0.08

Rhythm: Regular

Heart rate: 30

    Interpretation: Junctional bradycardia (with retrograde P waves), with depressed ST segments

120. PRI: 0.14–0.20

    QRS: 0.08–0.22

Rhythm: Irregular overall

Heart rate: (calculated by 3-second method)

        first 3 seconds: 80 (sinus rhythm)

        second 3 seconds: 160 (VT)

    Interpretation: Sinus rhythm with R on T phenomenon (5th complex), followed by ventricular tachycardia

121. PRI: 0.20

    QRS: 0.04–0.06

Rhythm: Irregular

Heart rate: 60

    Interpretation: Sinus rhythm with three PACs (2nd, 4th, and 6th complexes)

122. PRI: 0.14–0.16

    QRS: 0.04–0.06

Rhythm: Irregular

Heart rate: 60

    Interpretation: Sinus arrhythmia

123. PRI: Not measurable

    QRS: 0.08–0.18

Rhythm: Irregular

Heart rate: 90

    Interpretation: Junctional dysrhythmia with unifocal PVCs in bigeminy (2nd, 4th, 6th, and 8th complexes)

124. PRI: Not measurable

    QRS: 0.06–0.10

Rhythm: Irregular

Heart rate: 80 (atrial flutter rate: 250–350)

    Interpretation: Atrial flutter with variable block

125. PRI: Not measurable

    QRS: Not measurable

Rhythm: Irregular

Heart rate: 0 (atrial rate: 50)

    Interpretation: Ventricular standstill

126. PRI: Not measurable

    QRS: Not measurable

Rhythm: Not measurable

Heart rate: 10 (atrial rate: 0)

    Interpretation: Coarse ventricular fibrillation changing to agonal rhythm

127. PRI: 0.12–not measurable

    QRS: 0.06–0.08

Rhythm: Regular

Heart rate: 90

    Interpretation: Sinus rhythm with prolonged QT intervals and artifact (possible patient movement)

128. PRI: 0.14–0.16

    QRS: 0.06–0.16

Rhythm: Irregular

Heart rate: 50

    Interpretation: Sinus bradycardia with unifocal PVCs in bigeminy (1st, 3rd, and 5th complexes)

129. PRI: 0.16—not measurable · Rhythm: Irregular
QRS: 0.04–0.08 · Heart rate: 130 (atrial fibrillation rate: 350–500)
Interpretation: Atrial fibrillation with rapid ventricular response and depressed ST segments

130. PRI: 0.40–0.48 · Rhythm: Regular
QRS: 0.12–0.16 · Heart rate: 50
Interpretation: Sinus bradycardia with first-degree heart block, depressed ST segments and BBB

131. PRI: Not measurable · Rhythm: Regular
QRS: 0.10 · Heart rate: 40
Interpretation: Junctional dysrhythmia (with hidden P waves)

132. PRI: Difficult to measure to 0.16 · Rhythm: Regular
QRS: 0.06 · Heart rate: 90
Interpretation: Sinus rhythm with prolonged QT intervals and artifact

133. PRI: 0.16–0.18 · Rhythm: Irregular
QRS: 0.06–0.16 · Heart rate: 80
Interpretation: Sinus rhythm with depressed ST segments and one PVC (3rd complex)

134. PRI: Not measurable · Rhythm: Regular
QRS: 0.06–0.08 · Heart rate: 40
Interpretation: Junctional dysrhythmia (with hidden P waves)

135. PRI: 0.16 · Rhythm: Regular
QRS: 0.04–0.06 · Heart rate: 70
Interpretation: Normal sinus rhythm

136. PRI: Not measurable · Rhythm: Regular
QRS: 0.04–0.06 · Heart rate: 140
Interpretation: Sinus tachycardia with prolonged QT intervals

137. PRI: Not measurable · Rhythm: Irregular
QRS: 0.06–0.08 · Heart rate: 70 overall (atrial fibrillation rate: 350-500; atrial flutter rate: 250–350)
Interpretation: Controlled atrial fibrillation changing to atrial flutter with variable block

138. PRI: Not measured · Rhythm: Regular
QRS: 0.14–0.18 · Heart rate: 70
Interpretation: Ventricular pacemaker with 100% pacing and 100% capture

139. PRI: 0.18–0.20 · Rhythm: Regular
QRS: 0.10 · Heart rate: 70
Interpretation: Sinus rhythm with elevated (peaked) T waves

140. PRI: Not measurable · Rhythm: Not measurable
QRS: Not measurable · Heart rate: 0 (atrial rate: 0)
Interpretation: Fine ventricular fibrillation

141. PRI: 0.18—not measurable · Rhythm: Irregular
QRS: 0.06–0.08 · Heart rate: 100
Interpretation: Wandering atrial pacemaker

142. PRI: 0.20–0.40 · Rhythm: Irregular
QRS: 0.08 · Heart rate: 60 (atrial rate: 80)
Interpretation: Second-degree heart block, type I, with elevated ST segments

143. PRI: Not measurable · Rhythm: Not measurable
QRS: Not measurable · Heart rate: 0 (atrial rate: 0)
Interpretation: Coarse ventricular fibrillation

144. PRI: 0.16–0.18 · Rhythm: Regular
QRS: 0.06–0.08 · Heart rate: 60
Interpretation: Normal sinus rhythm with depressed ST segments

145. PRI: Not measurable · Rhythm: Regular
QRS: Not measurable · Heart rate: 0 (atrial rate: 70)
Interpretation: Ventricular standstill

146. PRI: Not measurable · Rhythm: Not measurable
QRS: 0.18–0.20 · Heart rate: 20 (atrial rate: 0)
Interpretation: Agonal rhythm with 60 cycle interference

147. PRI: 0.14–0.16 · Rhythm: Regular
QRS: 0.06 · Heart rate: 30
Interpretation: Sinus bradycardia with slightly depressed ST segments

148. PRI: Not measurable   Rhythm: Not measurable
QRS: Not measurable   Heart rate: 0 (atrial rate: 0)
Interpretation: Asystole

149. PRI: Not measured   Rhythm: Regular
QRS: 0.10   Heart rate: 70
Interpretation: Sequential pacemaker rhythm with elevated ST segments, and with 100% pacing and 100% capture

150. PRI: Not measurable   Rhythm: Regular
QRS: 0.28–0.32   Heart rate: 40 (atrial rate: 90; P wave hidden in ST segment of 1st and 4th ventricular complexes)
Interpretation: Third-degree heart block

151. PRI: 0.12   Rhythm: Regular
QRS: 0.04–0.06   Heart rate: 120 (calculated using first 3 seconds)
Interpretation: Sinus tachycardia

152. PRI: 0.16   Rhythm: Regular
QRS: 0.04–0.08   Heart rate: 90
Interpretation: Sinus rhythm with depressed ST segments

153. PRI: Not measurable   Rhythm: Not measurable
QRS: Not measurable   Heart rate: 0 (atrial rate: 0; calculated by 3-second method)
Interpretation: Coarse ventricular fibrillation

154. PRI: 0.20   Rhythm: Regular
QRS: 0.04   Heart rate: 60
Interpretation: Sinus rhythm with one PVC (4th complex)

155. PRI: 0.20–0.36   Rhythm: Irregular
QRS: 0.04–0.08   Heart rate: 70 (atrial rate: 90; P wave hidden in 1st, 3rd, and 5th T waves)
Interpretation: Second-degree heart block, type I

156. PRI: 0.12   Rhythm: Regular
QRS: 0.04–0.08   Heart rate: 180
Interpretation: Supraventricular tachycardia

157. PRI:0.20–0.24   Rhythm: Regular
QRS: 0.08–0.12   Heart rate: 90
Interpretation: Sinus rhythm with intermittent first-degree heart block and depressed ST segments, and prolonged QT intervals

158. PRI: 0.28   Rhythm: Regular
QRS: 0.08–0.12   Heart rate: 100
Interpretation: Sinus rhythm with first-degree heart block

159. PRI: Not measurable   Rhythm: Irregular
QRS: 0.04–0.08   Heart rate: 70 (atrial fibrillation rate: 350–550)
Interpretation: Controlled atrial fibrillation with depressed ST segments

160. PRI: Not measurable   Rhythm: Regular
QRS: 0.20–0.24   Heart rate: 230 (atrial rate: 0)
Interpretation: Ventricular tachycardia

161. PRI: 0.24   Rhythm: Irregular
QRS: 0.06–0.20   Heart rate: 90
Interpretation: Sinus rhythm with first-degree heart block and a run of V Tach (4th, 5th, 6th, and 7th complexes)

162. PRI: 0.32   Rhythm: Regular
QRS: 0.16–0.20   Heart rate: 60
Interpretation: Sinus rhythm with BBB, first-degree heart block, and elevated ST segments

163. PRI: 0.32   Rhythm: Regular
QRS: 0.08   Heart rate: 90
Interpretation: Sinus rhythm with first-degree heart block, and depressed ST segments

164. PRI: 0.14–0.16   Rhythm: Regular
QRS: 0.12   Heart rate: 40 (atrial rate: 80)
Interpretation: Second-degree heart block, type II (2:1 block), with a bradycardic rate

165. PRI: 0.16—not measurable
QRS: 0.12
Rhythm: Irregular
Heart rate: 90 (atrial fibrillation rate: 350–500)
Interpretation: Controlled atrial fibrillation

166. PRI: 0.20–0.28
QRS: 0.08–0.12
Rhythm: Irregular
Heart rate: 70 (atrial rate: 80)
Interpretation: Second-degree heart block, type I, with elevated ST segments and peaked P waves

167. PRI: 0.20
QRS: 0.04–0.08
Rhythm: Irregular
Heart rate: 80
Interpretation: Sinus rhythm with one PJC (5th complex), depressed ST segments, and inverted T waves

168. PRI: 0.28
QRS: 0.04–0.06
Rhythm: Regular
Heart rate: 40
Interpretation: Sinus bradycardia with first-degree heart block and elevated (peaked) T waves

169. PRI: 0.12
QRS: 0.06–0.20
Rhythm: Irregular
Heart rate: 70
Interpretation: Sinus rhythm with inverted T waves and unifocal PVCs in bigeminy (1st, 3rd, 5th, and 7th complexes)

170. PRI: Not measurable
QRS: 0.04
Rhythm: Regular
Heart rate: 90
Interpretation: Accelerated junctional dysrhythmia (with retrograde P waves)

171. PRI: Not measurable
QRS: 0.20
Rhythm: Regular
Heart rate: 100 (atrial rate: 0)
Interpretation: Accelerated idioventricular dysrhythmia (possible VT)

172. PRI: Not measurable
QRS: 0.14
Rhythm: Regular
Heart rate: 20 (atrial rate: 60–70; P wave may be hidden in 1st ventricular complex)
Interpretation: Third-degree heart block

173. PRI: 0.16–0.18
QRS: 0.04
Rhythm: Regular
Heart rate: 50
Interpretation: Junctional dysrhythmia (with inverted P waves)

174. PRI: Not measurable
QRS: 0.04–0.06
Rhythm: Regular
Heart rate: 30
Interpretation: Junctional bradycardia (with retrograde P waves)

175. PRI: 0.20
QRS: 0.06–0.08
Rhythm: Irregular
Heart rate: 70
Interpretation: Sinus arrhythmia with elevated ST segments

176. PRI: 0.20
QRS: 0.08
Rhythm: Irregular
Heart rate: 80
Interpretation: Sinus rhythm with elevated ST segments, one PAC (5th complex), and one PJC (8th complex)

177. PRI: Not measurable
QRS: 0.04–0.06
Rhythm: Irregular
Heart rate: 100 (atrial fibrillation rate: 350–500)
Interpretation: Controlled atrial fibrillation with depressed ST segments

178. PRI: Not measurable
QRS: 0.10–0.12
Rhythm: Regular
Heart rate: 40 (atrial rate: 50; P wave hidden in 1st T wave)
Interpretation: Third-degree heart block

179. PRI: Not measurable
QRS: 0.20–0.24
Rhythm: Regular
Heart rate: 170
Interpretation: Wolff-Parkinson-White syndrome (mimicking VT)

180. PRI: Not measurable
QRS: 0.16–0.20
Rhythm: Regular
Heart rate: 30 (atrial rate: 0)
Interpretation: Idioventricular dysrhythmia

181. PRI: 0.16–0.20
QRS: 0.06
Rhythm: Irregular
Heart rate: 60 (calculated by 3-second method)
Interpretation: Sinus rhythm with PJC (4th complex), and depressed ST segments

182. PRI: Not measurable
QRS: 0.04–0.06
Rhythm: Irregular
Heart rate: 170; (atrial fibrillation rate: 350–500)
Interpretation: Uncontrolled atrial fibrillation

183. PRI: 0.16–0.20   Rhythm: Regular
QRS: 0.04–0.06   Heart rate: 40
Interpretation: Sinus bradycardia with depressed ST segments

184. PRI: 0.20—not measurable   Rhythm: Irregular
QRS: 0.04–0.20   Heart rate: 80 (calculated by 3-second method)
Interpretation: Sinus rhythm with a PVC (4th complex), changing to junctional dysrhythmia

185. PRI: 0.08   Rhythm: Regular
QRS: 0.14–0.16   Heart rate: 50
Interpretation: Wolff-Parkinson-White syndrome with bradycardia and delta wave

186. PRI: 0.20–not measurable   Rhythm: Irregular
QRS: 0.12–0.20   Heart rate: 107–160; (Sinus tachycardia rate: 107 by
                                                  division method; VT rate: 160 by 3-second strip)
Interpretation: Sinus tachycardia with prolonged QT intervals, changing to ventricular tachycardia

187. PRI: Not measurable   Rhythm: Irregular
QRS: 0.04–0.20   Heart rate: 90; (atrial flutter rate: 250–350)
Interpretation: Atrial flutter (varying block), with two PVCs (4th and 7th complexes)

188. PRI: 0.18–0.20   Rhythm: Irregular
QRS: 0.06–0.20   Heart rate: 80
Interpretation: Sinus rhythm with elevated ST segments and unifocal PVCs in bigeminy (1st, 3rd, 5th,
    and 7th complexes)

189. PRI: Not measurable   Rhythm: Regular
QRS: 0.20–0.24 (measured from R wave to notch   Heart rate: 40 (atrial rate: 100; P waves hidden in
    in ST segment)   1st and 2nd QRS complexes, and in 3rd T wave)
Interpretation: Third-degree heart block with elevated ST segments and elevated (peaked) T waves

190. PRI: Not measurable   Rhythm: Irregular
QRS: 0.04–0.08   Heart rate: 100 (atrial flutter rate: 250–350)
Interpretation: Atrial flutter with varying block

191. PRI: 0.08–0.12   Rhythm: Irregular
QRS: 0.08–0.10   Heart rate: 60
Interpretation: Sinus arrhythmia

192. PRI: 0.20—not measured   Rhythm: Irregular
QRS: 0.04–0.20   Heart rate: 70
Interpretation: Sinus rhythm with biphasic T waves and one PVC (4th complex), and two pacer spikes
    (5th and 6th complexes): 33% pacing and 100% capture

193. PRI: Not measured   Rhythm: Regular
QRS: 0.20   Heart rate: 70
Interpretation: Ventricular pacemaker with 100% pacing and 100% capture

194. PRI: Not measured   Rhythm: Regular
QRS: 0.08–0.16   Heart rate: 50
Interpretation: Ventricular pacemaker with bradycardia; with 60% pacing and 100% capture

195. PRI: Not measured   Rhythm: Regular
QRS: 0.16   Heart rate: 30 to 0
Interpretation: Ventricular pacemaker with 100% pacing and 37% capture

196. PRI: Not measured   Rhythm: Regular
QRS: 0.08–0.18   Heart rate: 70
Interpretation: Ventricular pacemaker with 86% pacing and 75% capture

197. PRI: Not measured   Rhythm: Regular
QRS: 0.12–0.18   Heart rate: 60
Interpretation: Atrial pacemaker with 100% pacing and 86% capture

198. PRI: Not measured   Rhythm: Regular
QRS: 0.16   Heart rate: 70
Interpretation: Ventricular pacemaker with 100% pacing and 100% capture

199. PRI: Not measured   Rhythm: Regular
QRS: 0.16   Heart rate: 70
Interpretation: Sequential pacemaker with 100% pacing and 100% capture

200. PRI: Not measurable   Rhythm: Irregular
QRS: 0.14–0.20   Heart rate: 210 (atrial fibrillation rate: 350–500)
Interpretation: Uncontrolled atrial fibrillation and Wolff-Parkinson-White syndrome (mimicking
    ventricular tachycardia)

CHAPTER 11

Case Study 1

1-A Sinus tachycardia

1-B (in any order)
- a. Reassure the patient and listen to her fears. Inform her of the possibility that anxiety and caffeine can cause a rapid heartbeat and palpitations.
- b. Notify the physician.
- c. Continue to monitor the patient.

1-C Normal sinus rhythm

Case Study 2

2-A Sinus bradycardia

2-B
- a. Assess airway, breathing, and circulation.
- b. Provide oxygen and apply pulse oximetry.
- c. Start an IV.
- d. Notify the physician.
- e. Administer atropine 0.5 to 1 mg IV push.

2-C Atropine 0.5 to 1 mg IV push at 3 to 5 minute intervals until the maximum dose of 3 mg has been given

2-D Transcutaneous pacemaker if available; prepare for transvenous pacing

2-E Paced rhythm

2-F
- a. 100%
- b. Paced

Case Study 3

3-A Sinus rhythm with unifocal PVCs

3-B Junctional dysrhythmia with unifocal PVCs

3-C
- a. Assess airway, breathing, and circulation.
- b. Provide oxygen and apply pulse oximetry.
- c. Start an IV.

3-D Administer atropine 0.5 to 1 mg IV push.

3-E Sinus rhythm with multifocal PVCs in bigeminy

3-F
- a. Procainamide 20 to 50 mg/minute IV, or lidocaine 50 to 100 mg (1 mg/kg) IV push over 2 to 3 minutes
- b. Procainamide 1 to 4 mg/minute, or continuous infusion of lidocaine 1 to 4 mg/minute

3-G (in any order)
- a. More than 6 PVCs in one minute
- b. Multifocal PVCs
- c. Couplets
- d. R on T phenomenon
- e. Runs of ventricular tachycardia

Case Study 4

4-A Supraventricular tachycardia

4-B
- a. Valsalva maneuver (bearing down)
- b. Carotid massage

4-C
- a. Provide oxygen and apply pulse oximetry.
- b. Start an IV.
- c. Administer adenosine 6 mg IV push rapidly; flush with 20 cc of normal saline solution, followed by elevation of extremity.

4-D Repeat adenosine 12 mg IV push rapidly; flush with 20 cc of normal saline solution, followed by elevation of extremity.

4-E Verapamil 2.5 to 5 mg IV push, over 2 minutes

4-F Synchronized

4-G Normal sinus rhythm

Case Study 5

5-A Sinus tachycardia

5-B
- a. Place the patient in a position of rest.
- b. Provide oxygen and apply pulse oximetry.
- c. Offer cool fluids to drink, or start an IV.
- d. Continue monitoring the patient.

5-C Sinus rhythm with prolonged QT interval

Case Study 6

6-A Second-degree heart block, type II; 3:1 block

6-B
- a. Assess airway, breathing, and circulation.
- b. Provide oxygen and apply pulse oximetry.
- c. Start an IV.

6-C Third-degree heart block

6-D Transcutaneous pacemaker

Case Study 7

7-A Ventricular fibrillation

7-B Assess the patient

7-C
- a. Check the telemetry leads and electrodes, change any electrode that is dry, and reconnect any leads that are loose.
- b. Inform the physician about the R on T phenomenon.
- c. Continue observing the patient.

Case Study 8

8-A Normal sinus rhythm

8-B Pulseless electrical activity (PEA)

8-C
- a. Begin CPR.
- b. Provide 100% oxygen by bag-valve mask device and intubate as soon as possible.
- c. Start an IV.
- d. Consider common causes of PEA.
- e. Administer epinephrine 1 mg IV push; repeat according to protocol.
- f. Reassess the patient.
- g. Give atropine 1 mg IV push if dysrhythmia is bradycardic; repeat according to protocol until the maximum dose has been given.

8-D Cardiac tamponade

8-E Any three of the following:
  a. Hypovolemia; give fluids
  b. Hypoxia; increase ventilations and oxygen
  c. Tension pneumothorax; perform needle decompressions
  d. Acidosis; give sodium bicarbonate according to ABGs
  e. Hypokalemia or hyperkalemia; treat according to laboratory results
  f. Drug overdose; treat according to protocol
  g. Cardiac tamponade; pericardiocentesis
  h. Hypothermia; treat according to protocol
  i. Coronary or pulmonary thrombosis; treatment based on patient's condition

8-F Second-degree heart block, type I (Wenckebach)

8-G Observe the patient for any change in the dysrhythmia or in cardiac output.

Case Study 9

9-A Torsades de pointes

9-B Any five of the following:
Pale, cool, clammy skin; nausea and vomiting; dizziness, weakness, faintness; SOB; sudden change in blood pressure; dyspnea; severe chest pain; cyanosis; confusion or disorientation; decreased urinary output; unresponsiveness

9-C a. Provide oxygen and apply pulse oximetry.
  b. Start an IV.
  c. Administer magnesium sulfate 1 to 2 g IV in 50 to 100 cc D_5W solution over 5 to 60 minutes according to protocol.
  d. Reassess the patient.
  e. Consider overdrive pacing.
  f. If patient becomes pulseless, initiate V Fib algorithm.

9-D Sinus rhythm with first-degree heart block

Case Study 10

10-A Second-degree heart block, type I (Wenckebach)

10-B a. Notify the physician.
  b. Continue to monitor the patient.

10-C Second-degree heart block, type II; 2:1 block

10-D a. Increase oxygen and apply pulse oximetry.
  b. Administer atropine 0.5 to 1 mg IV push; repeat every 3 to 5 minutes until maximum dosage is given.
  c. Continue to observe and assess the patient while you prepare a transcutaneous pacemaker for use, if available.
  d. Administer dopamine 10 to 20 μg/kg/minute by continuous IV infusion.
  e. Epinephrine 1 mg IV push

10-E Sinus rhythm

Case Study 11

11-A Cardiac output

11-B Sinus rhythm with a PVC

11-C a. Provide oxygen and apply pulse oximetry.
  b. Start an IV.
  c. Begin "MONA" protocol.

11-D Ventricular fibrillation

11-E a. Begin CPR; continue CPR except during defibrillation.
  b. Administer 100% oxygen by bag-valve mask device and intubate as soon as possible.
  c. Start an IV if not already established.
  d. Defibrillate. Multiple defibrillation attempts may be necessary throughout treatment. Initially, three consecutive shocks at 200, 200 to 300, and 360 joules should be used. Then defibrillate at 360 joules during the remaining treatment.
  e. Reassess the patient before and after each defibrillation or medication.
  f. Administer epinephrine 1 mg IV push, or vasopressin 40 units IV push, one time only; repeat epinephrine according to protocol. Defibrillate at 360 joules within 30 to 60 seconds of giving epinephrine or vasopressin.
  g. Administer amiodarone 300 mg IV push; repeat according to protocol until the maximum dose has been given; if lidocaine is used instead, follow the lidocaine protocol.
  h. Continue defibrillation between drugs.
  i. Give magnesium sulfate 1 to 2 g in 10 cc D_5W solution IV push for severe ventricular fibrillation unresponsive to defibrillation and epinephrine or vasopressin.
  j. Give procainamide 20 to 50 mg/minute IV or lidocaine 50 to 100 mg (1 mg/kg) IV push over 2 to 3 minutes.
  k. When the patient has a pulse, start an infusion drip of the medication that was successful in ending the V Fib.

11-F Sinus rhythm with bundle branch block

Case Study 12

12-A Sinus bradycardia

12-B a. Do nothing. It is normal for young adults to have a bradycardic rate during sleep.
  b. Continue to observe the patient and monitor for any changes.

Case Study 13

13-A Sinus rhythm with PVC

13-B Paroxysmal atrial tachycardia or paroxysmal supraventricular tachycardia

13-C a. Provide oxygen and apply pulse oximetry.
  b. Start an IV.
  c. Perform vagal maneuvers.
  d. Administer adenosine 6 mg IV push rapidly, flush with 20 cc of normal saline solution, followed by elevation of extremity.
  e. Reassess the patient and repeat adenosine 12 mg IV push rapidly, if necessary and according to protocol; flush with 20 cc of normal saline solution, followed by elevation of extremity.
  f. Administer amiodarone 300 mg IV push.
  g. Give calcium channel blocker IV, according to protocol.
  h. Give beta blocker IV, according to protocol.
13-D Junctional tachycardia

Case Study 14
14-A Poor cardiac output
14-B Atrial fibrillation with slow ventricular response
14-C a. Provide oxygen and apply pulse oximetry, if available.
  b. Start an IV.
  c. Administer atropine 0.5 to 1 mg IV push.
  d. Continue to observe and monitor the patient.
  e. Prepare for transcutaneous pacing, if available.
14-D Sinus rhythm with R on T phenomenon and a run of ventricular tachycardia
14-E a. Procainamide 20 to 50 mg/min IV, or amiodarone 300 mg IV push; if lidocaine is used instead, follow lidocaine protocol
  b. Same drug as above

Case Study 15
15-A Sinus rhythm with elevated (peaked) T waves and elevated ST segments
15-B a. Provide oxygen and apply pulse oximetry.
  b. Start an IV.
  c. Order a 12-Lead ECG.
  d. Begin "MONA" protocol.
15-C a. Nitroglycerin
  b. Morphine sulfate
15-D Infusion pump
15-E Fibrinolytic therapy
15-F Assess and monitor

Case Study 16
16-A Sinus bradycardia
16-B a. Provide oxygen and apply pulse oximetry.
  b. Start an IV.
  c. Administer atropine 0.5-1 mg IV push.
16-C Sinus bradycardia with unifocal PVCs in bigeminy

16-D Repeat atropine 1 mg IV push
16-E Sinus rhythm with one PVC
16-F Sinus rhythm with two sets of unifocal PVC couplets
16-G Procainamide 20 to 50 mg/minute IV
16-H Normal sinus rhythm
16-I Procainamide 1 to 4 mg/minute continuous infusion

Case Study 17
17-A a. Put the patient on a cardiac monitor.
  b. Provide oxygen and apply pulse oximetry.
  c. Start an IV.
  d. Obtain a 12-Lead ECG.
17-B Sinus rhythm with elevated ST segments and elevated (peaked) T waves
17-C a. Morphine
  b. Oxygen
  c. Nitroglycerin
  d. Aspirin
17-D Sinus bradycardia with elevated ST segments and elevated (peaked) T waves
17-E Nitroglycerin 10 to 20 µg/minute, titrated to pain relief and decrease of elevated blood pressure
17-F Fibrinolytic therapy

Case Study 18
18-A Sinus bradycardia with PAC
18-B PAT or PSVT
18-C a. Vagal maneuvers or stimulation
  b. 12-Lead ECG
18-D Adenosine, 6 mg IV
18-E Rapidly
18-F 12 mg
18-G Sinus tachycardia
18-H Side effects
18-I Normal sinus rhythm

Case Study 19
19-A Torsades de pointes
19-B Assess the patient.
19-C The oxygen to 4 to 6 L/nasal cannula
19-D Magnesium sulfate 1 to 2 g in 50 to 100 cc D_5W solution IV, titrated over 5 to 60 minutes
19-E Second-degree heart block, type II; 2:1 block
19-F Magnesium sulfate 0.5 to 1 g/hour IV, titrated to control torsades de pointes
19-G Transcutaneous pacemaker

Case Study 20
20-A Artifact
20-B Assess the patient.
20-C Sinus rhythm with first-degree block
20-D Notify the physician.

Case Study 21

21-A Sinus rhythm with unifocal PVCs in bigeminy

21-B a. Provide oxygen and apply pulse oximetry.
      b. Start an IV.
      c. Administer procainamide 20 to 50 mg/minute IV

21-C Hypotension

21-D Sinus rhythm with multifocal PVCs

21-E Lidocaine 50 to 100 mg (1 mg/kg) IV push over 2 to 3 minutes

21-F Sinus rhythm with unifocal PVCs

21-G Sinus rhythm with R on T phenomenon progressing to ventricular tachycardia

21-H a. Amiodarone 300 mg IV push
      b. Amiodarone 150 mg IV push

21-I Second-degree heart block, type II, with one episode of a 3:1 block

21-J Transcutaneous pacemaker

21-K 0.5 mg/minute for 18 hours or maximum dose of 2.2 grams

Case Study 22

22-A Automated External Defibrillator (AED)

22-B CPR

22-C Junctional bradycardia

22-D a. Provide oxygen and apply pulse oximetry.
      b. Start an IV.
      c. Administer atropine 0.5 to 1 mg IV push.

22-E Junctional dysrhythmia

22-F a. Transcutaneous
      b. Paced rhythm

22-G a. Paced
      b. Capture

GLOSSARY

Aberrant Different than normal; may refer to individual complexes or entire rhythm

Aberrantly Conducted Complexes Single complexes that appear different than the underlying rhythm because they do not follow the same conduction pathway

ABGs (Arterial Blood Gases) A blood test used to assess a patient's respiratory function

Absolute Bradycardia Cardiac rhythm with a rate less than 60 electrical beats per minute

Absolute Refractory Period Time in the cardiac cycle when the myocardial cells have not completed repolarization and cannot conduct an electrical impulse; from Q wave to the first half of the T wave

Accelerated Idioventricular Dysrhythmia A lethal dysrhythmia that occurs when the electrical impulses originate from a single site in the ventricles at a rate between 41–100 impulses per minute

Accelerated Junctional Dysrhythmia Dysrhythmia that occurs when all the electrical impulses originate from a single site within the atrioventricular junctional area at a rate between 61 and 100 impulses per minute

Accessory Pathway An additional or abnormal electrical conduction pathway; also called the Bundle of Kent or Kent Bundle; found in WPW syndrome

Acidosis The presence of too much hydrogen in the body, usually caused by an increase in the amount of acid; may result from respiratory problems, kidney failure or diabetes

Acute Sudden, recent onset of signs and symptoms

Acute Coronary Syndrome (ACS) A term used to include angina, MI, silent ischemia, and sudden death

Agonal Rhythm Dying heart; ventricular rate less than 20; see *idioventricular rhythm*

Amplitude Height of a wave or complex measured in millivolts (mV)

Anaphylaxis A severe allergic response to a substance, such as drugs or an insect bite; may be fatal; symptoms may include dyspnea, swollen/obstructed airway, shock, hives, or rash

Antegrade Movement in a forward motion; frequently used with the forward (downward) movement of an electrical current from the atria to the ventricle

Angina Chest pain caused by lack of oxygen to the heart muscle; the pain may also be felt in the left arm, jaw and shoulder; is usually relieved by rest or medication such as nitroglycerin

Anticoagulant Drug that prevents or delays the formation of clots

Antipyretic Medication used to reduce fever

Aorta Largest artery in the body

Aortic Valve Located between the left ventricle and the aorta

Arrhythmia Absence of cardiac rhythm; also frequently used to mean dysrhythmia

Artifact Abnormality in an EKG tracing that does not originate in the heart, such as static electricity, patient movement, or loose leads

Asystole Absence of electrical activity in the cardiac muscle; also called cardiac standstill

Atria Upper chambers of the heart

Atrial Fibrillation (A Fib) Dysrhythmia that originates from many atrial sites; the atria are making ineffective quivering movements, not actual contractions; only the ventricles are contracting

Atrial Flutter Dysrhythmia in which flutter (F) waves are formed instead of P waves

Atrial Rhythm Any rhythm that originates from a pacemaker cell within the atria other than the SA node

Atrioventricular Node (AV Node) Acts as a backup pacemaker of the heart

Atrium One of the two upper chambers of the heart

Automated External Defibrillator (AED) Portable device that identifies lethal dysrhythmias and provides defibrillation when necessary

Automatic Implantable Cardioverter Defibrillator (AICD) Surgically implanted overdrive pacer/defibrillator that can identify and treat some rapid lethal dysrhythmias, such as ventricular tachycardia

Automaticity Ability of cardiac pacemaker cells to generate or initiate an electrical impulse

Autonomic Nervous System Nerves that maintain the heart and blood vessels in a normal state; divided into the sympathetic and parasympathetic systems

Atrioventricular Dissociation (AV Dissociation) Occurs when the atria and ventricles function independently, as in third-degree block

Bag-valve Mask Device that is used to assist with artificial ventilation, and in the delivery of 100% oxygen to patients

Baseline Imaginary line on the rhythm strip from which all waves and deflections are measured; also known as isoelectric line

Beta Blockers (β-Blockers) Drugs used to treat hypertension, atrial, and ventricular dysrhythmias

Bigeminy Every other QRS complex is abnormal (usually premature); a minimum of three occurrences is needed to identify a dysrhythmia with bigeminy

Biphasic Any S-shaped wave that lies both above and below the baseline of the rhythm strip

Blood Pressure Measurement of pressure within the blood vessels; measured in millimeters of mercury (mm Hg)

Bolus Rapid infusion of IV fluids or medications; also called IV push

Bradyasystole A pulseless dysrhythmia that appears on the monitor as a bradycardia

Bradycardia Cardiac dysrhythmia that has a slower than normal heart rate; usually less than 60 impulses per minute

Bronchi Large airway tubes that branch off the trachea and enter the lungs; part of the respiratory system

Bronchioles Small airway tubes that extend from the bronchi into the lobes of the lungs

Bronchus One large airway tube that branches off the trachea and enters one lung

Bundle Branches (BB) Part of the conduction system of the heart; located below the bundle of His, leading to the Purkinje's fibers; divided into left and right bundle branches

Bundle Branch Block (BBB) Dysrhythmia in which the electrical impulse is blocked at one or both bundle branches; the QRS complex has a notched appearance and is usually greater than 0.12 second

Bundle of His Part of the conduction system of the heart; located below the AV junctional area and above the bundle branches

Bundle of Kent (Kent Bundle) An additional or abnormal electrical conduction pathway; found in WPW syndrome

cc Measure of liquids; 1000 cc = 1 liter; 1 cc = 1 ml

Calcium Channel Blockers A group of drugs used to treat heart diseases

Caliper Instrument used to measure R to R and P to P intervals on a rhythm strip

Capture Ability of cardiac muscle to respond to an electrical stimulus from a mechanical pacemaker and conduct the electrical impulse throughout the cardiac muscle

Cardiac Pertaining to the heart

Cardiac Arrest Lack of electrical and/or mechanical activity in the heart; blood is not being pumped throughout the body and the patient does not have a pulse

Cardiac Cycle Period from the beginning of one cardiac contraction to the beginning of another; usually includes a P wave, PR interval, QRS complex, T wave, and baseline

Cardiac Irritability Ability of cardiac cells to respond to an electrical impulse; used interchangeably with excitability

Cardiac Output The amount of blood pumped by the left ventricle in one minute

Cardiac Tamponade The presence of blood or excess fluid in the pericardial sac that decreases the heart's ability to contract and expand effectively

Cardiovascular Pertaining to the heart and blood vessels

Cardioversion Procedure that uses controlled electrical currents to correct tachycardic dysrhythmias such as uncontrolled atrial fibrillation, or ventricular tachycardia with a pulse; also known as synchronized cardioversion

Cardiovert Process of cardioversion

Chronic Symptoms that begin slowly and last for a long period of time

Circulatory System Body system that includes the heart, lungs, blood vessels, and blood

Compensatory Pause Pause that follows a premature beat, allowing the underlying rhythm to begin again at its normal rate; may be either complete or incomplete pause

Complex Segment of the rhythm strip that refers to a group of waves; such as the Q, R and S waves

Component Any part of a cardiac cycle seen on the monitor or rhythm strip; includes the P wave, the PR interval, the QRS complex, the ST segment, the T wave, and/or the QT interval

Conduct Transmit; send; carry an electrical impulse from cell to cell

Conduction System Series of cardiac cells that transmit an electrical impulse throughout the heart muscle in a sequential manner, from the SA node to the ventricular muscle

Conductivity Ability of cardiac cells to transmit electrical impulses

Contractility Ability of cardiac cells to shorten, causing cardiac muscle contraction

Contraction Tightening or squeezing action of a muscle; the contraction of the cardiac muscle pumps blood throughout the body

Coronary Pertaining to the heart; is also used to mean a heart attack

Coronary Arteries Arteries that supply oxygenated blood to the heart muscle

Coronary Artery Disease (CAD) Progressive blockage of one or more coronary arteries, resulting in lack of oxygen to the heart muscle

Coronary Occlusion Blockage or extreme narrowing of one or more coronary arteries

Couplet Two premature complexes occurring in a row; also known as coupling or a pair

CPK-MB Isoenzymes A blood test that assists in evaluating patients with suspected acute coronary syndrome

Cyanosis Bluish or grayish color of the skin, mucous membranes, and/or nail beds; caused by lack of oxygen in the tissue

Defibrillation (Shock) Procedure that uses electrical current to correct ventricular fibrillation or pulseless ventricular tachycardia; may also be called unsynchronized cardioversion

Deflection Movement of a wave or complex away from the baseline on a rhythm strip or monitor screen

Delta wave An extra "bump" on the slurred section of a QRS complex; results from the depolarization of the ventricles by way of an accessory pathway before the normal conduction reaches the ventricles; seen in Wolff-Parkinson-White syndrome

Depolarization Conduction of an electrical impulse through the heart muscle; normally causes a cardiac contraction

Depressed Wave Wave that is below the baseline

Dilate Enlargement or widening of a blood vessel

Dysrhythmia Abnormal cardiac rate or rhythm; frequently used interchangeably with arrhythmia

Ectopy (ectopic complex) Complex initiated from a site other than the SA node

Electrical Impulse Electrical stimulus generated by pacemaker cells in the myocardium, which causes depolarization of the myocardial cells; normally initiated by the SA node

Electrocardiogram (EKG, ECG) A graphic record of electrical impulses of the heart

Electrode Conduction pad that connects the patient to a telemetry monitor or an EKG machine; also the tip of the pacemaker leadwire

Electrophysiology Study of the ability of cells and tissue to use electrical currents

Embolism A substance such as a blood clot that moves through the circulatory system, until it becomes lodged against the wall of a smaller blood vessel

Endocardium The inner layer, or lining of the heart

Epicardium Thin, protective membrane that covers the outside of the heart

Escape Beat Complex initiated from a site other than the SA node; usually is the heart's attempt to maintain a normal rate or rhythm; is also the complex that ends the pause of a sinus exit block

Excitability Ability of cardiac cells to respond to an electrical impulse; used interchangeably with irritability

Fibrillation Uncontrolled, uncoordinated, and ineffective quivering movements of cardiac muscle

Fibrinolytic Therapy Group of drugs used to dissolve clots in the coronary arteries, which have caused ischemia and infarction; used following an acute MI

First-degree Heart Block Dysrhythmia caused by a delay in the conduction system between the atria and the bundle of His; PR intervals measure greater than 0.20 second

Flutter Wave (F Wave) Wave formed instead of a P wave during a rapid, flutter dysrhythmia

Foci Two or more pacemaker sites

Focus Single site of origin of an electrical impulse

Generate Initiate; begin an electrical impulse

Gram (g, gm) Measurement of weight used in the metric system; frequently used in drug dosages; 1 gram = 1000 milligrams

Ground Electrode Electrode used to help prevent artifact

Heart Rate (HR) The number of times the ventricles beat in one minute; pulse or heart beat

Hypersensitivity Usually used to mean an allergy to a medication

Hypertension Blood pressure measurement above normal

Hypotension Blood pressure measurement below normal

Hypovolemia Decreased amount of blood in the heart chambers and blood vessels

Hypoxia Decreased amount of oxygen in the body tissues or organs

Idioventricular Dysrhythmia Dysrhythmia in which the atria, AV junction, bundle of His, and bundle branches are no longer functioning; only the ventricular muscle is attempting to function

Incompatible One substance that cannot be mixed with another; for example, Nipride is incompatible with saline solution

Infarction Death of tissue; as in myocardial infarction

Infiltration Occurs when an IV catheter slips out of a vein, and solution infuses into the tissue

Infusion Pump Device that regulates the rate of administration and dosage of IV medications or fluids

Inherent Normal, natural, or inborn; for example, the inherent heart rate of the atria is 60-100 beats per minute

Initiate Generate or start an electrical impulse

Internodal Pathways Multiple electrical conduction pathways between the SA node and the AV node

Interval Period of time used to measure the distance between waves or complexes on the rhythm strip, such as PR interval or P to P interval

Intraatrial Pathways Multiple electrical conduction pathways between the right and left atrium

Intravenous Administration of medication or fluids into a vein

Irritability Ability of cardiac cells to respond to an electrical impulse; used interchangeably with excitability

Ischemia Lack of oxygen in tissue cells due to decreased blood supply

Isoelectric Line Imaginary line on the rhythm strip from which all waves and deflections are measured; also known as the baseline

Joules Measurement of electrical current used in either cardiac defibrillation (unsynchronized cardioversion) or synchronized cardioversion

Junctional Bradycardia Junctional dysrhythmia in which the heart rate is less than 40 impulses per minute

Junctional Rhythm Dysrhythmia occurring when the electrical impulses are generated by a site in the AV junctional area; inherent heart rate is 40–60 impulses per minute

Junctional Tachycardia Junctional dysrhythmia with a heart rate between 101 and 150 impulses per minute

Kilogram (kg) Measurement of weight used in the metric system; 1 kg = 2.2 pounds

Lead Identifies different types of electrode placement, such as Lead I or Lead II

Leadwire Wire that connects the electrode to a monitor or telemetry unit; also wire leading from a pacemaker generator to the myocardium

Lethal Death producing

Loss of Capture QRS complex does not follow a pacemaker spike; myocardium does not respond to the electrical stimulus from the pacemaker, and does not depolarize (contract)

Medically Unstable Patient's condition in which any combination of the following signs and symptoms of poor cardiac output occurs: pale, cool, clammy skin; N/V; SOB; sudden change in blood pressure; chest pain, or change in level of consciousness

Microgram (μg, mcg) Measurement of weight used in the metric system; used in drug dosages; 1 μg = 0.001 milligrams; 1000 μg = 1 milligram

Milligram (mg) Measurement of weight used in the metric system; frequently used in drug dosages; 1 mg = 0.001 gram; 1000 mg = 1 gram

Milliliter (ml) Measurement of liquid volume used in the metric system; 1 ml = 1 cc; 1 ml = 0.001 liter; 1 liter = 1000 ml or 1000 cc (approximately 1 quart)

Millimeter (mm) Measurement of distance used in the metric system; 1 mm is equal to one small horizontal square on rhythm strip graph paper; as a measurement of time, 1 mm = 0.04 second

Millivolt (mV) Measurement of amplitude; 0.1 mV equals one small vertical square on the rhythm strip graph paper

Mitral Valve Heart valve located between the left atrium and the left ventricle

Mobitz I Progressive heart block that occurs when the atrial impulse is interrupted at the AV junction; also called second-degree heart block, type I or Wenckebach

Mobitz II Intermittent interruption in the electrical conduction system at or below the AV junction; occurs suddenly and without warning; also called second-degree heart block, type II or classical

MONA Morphine, Oxygen, Nitroglycerin, Aspirin; treatment protocol for acute coronary syndrome

Multifocal (polymorphic, multiform) Complexes that originate from different pacemaker sites and look different from each other; usually refers to ventricular complexes

Murmur Abnormal sound made by blood flowing through a valve that is not functioning correctly

Myocardial Infarction (MI) Death of part of the cardiac muscle caused by a blockage in one or more of the cardiac arteries; also called heart attack, coronary, or acute coronary syndrome (ACS)

Myocardium Middle layer of cardiac muscle

Needle Decompression The removal of extra fluid or blood from between the heart and the pericardial sac, using a needle and syringe; also known as pericardiocentesis

Nodal Term that has been used to mean AV junctional area

Normal Sinus Rhythm (NSR) Normal conduction rhythm; electrical impulses are generated by the SA node at an inherent heart rate of 60 to 100 impulses per minute

Overdrive Pacing Use of a mechanical pacemaker to take over the pacing of the cardiac cells, altering the heart rate to produce a more normal or stable rhythm

Oxygen (O₂) Gas necessary for cell life; drug used to increase oxygen available to tissue cells; decreases shortness of breath and pain caused by ischemia

P to P Interval Measurement of time from one P wave to the following P wave

P wave Small wave seen before the QRS; it represents the depolarization of both the right and left atria

Pacemaker Cardiac cells that initiate an electrical impulse, causing cardiac depolarization (contraction); the SA node is the normal pacemaker of the heart; also refers to an artificial or mechanical pacemaker

Pacemaker Cells Any cardiac cell that is capable of initiating an electrical impulse

Pacer Abbreviated term for an artificial pacemaker

Pacer Spike A vertical line seen on the rhythm strip that represents the electrical impulse from a mechanical pacemaker

Pacing Use of mechanically generated electrical impulses that follow the electrical conduction system of the heart, and usually stimulate the cardiac muscle to contract; also refers to the percent of complexes initiated by a mechanical pacemaker

Palpitations Sensation of being able to feel own heart beating or "skipping beats"; frequently associated with rapid heart rates ("racing heart")or premature complexes

Parasympathetic Nervous System Nerves that decrease the rate of cardiac contractions, usually after stress or emergencies, allowing the body to restore energy

Paroxysmal Sudden onset of a rapid cardiac dysrhythmia

Paroxysmal Atrial Tachycardia (PAT) Dysrhythmia with a sudden onset; the electrical impulses are generated at a rate greater than 150 impulses per minute; the current term for this dysrhythmia is paroxysmal supraventricular tachycardia (PSVT)

Paroxysmal Supraventricular Tachycardia (PSVT) Dysrhythmia with a rate between 151 to 250 impulses per minute; originates suddenly from the atria or AV junctional area; also known as PAT

Pericardial Sac Tough, loose-fitting, fibrous sac that contains the heart

Pericardiocentesis Removal of extra fluid or blood from pericardial sac by a physician, using needle decompression

Peripheral Pertaining to the arms and legs

Permanent Pacemaker Mechanical pacemaker that is surgically implanted under the patient's skin

Platelets blood cells that aid in the clotting of blood

Pleural Sac A protective sac that surrounds each lung

Polarization Cardiac ready state; the cells are ready to receive an electrical impulse

Poor Cardiac Output Patient condition in which the heart is not pumping out enough blood for the body to function properly; any combination of the following symptoms may be seen: pale, cool, and clammy skin; difficulty breathing; sudden change in blood pressure; chest pain, or change in level of consciousness

Potassium (K) Chemical found in the body that aids in the conduction of electricity through the cells

PR Interval (PRI) Time required for an electrical impulse to travel through the atria and AV junction; measured from the beginning of the P wave to the beginning of the QRS complex

Premature Atrial Contraction (PAC) Atrial complex that occurs earlier than the next expected complex of the underlying rhythm

Premature Junctional Contraction (PJC) Complex initiated from the junctional area that occurs earlier than the next expected complex of the underlying rhythm

Premature Ventricular Contraction (PVC) Complex initiated from an area below the AV junction that occurs earlier than the next expected complex of the underlying rhythm

Pre-printed Physician's Orders A new term for physician standing orders

Pulmonary Pertaining to the lungs

Pulmonic Valve Valve between the right ventricle and the pulmonary artery

Pulse Wave of pressure caused by the pumping action of the left ventricle that can be counted; usually defined as heart beats per minute; heart rate (HR)

Pulseless Electrical Activity (PEA) Dysrhythmia that occurs when there is electrical activity in the heart, but the cardiac muscle does not contract in response to the electrical stimulus; the patient does not have a pulse

Pulse Oximetry Device used to measure the percentage of oxygen saturation in the blood

Purkinje's Fibers Muscular fibers found in the ventricles; part of the electrical conduction system of the heart

QRS Complex Group of one Q, R, and S wave that represents the depolarization of both the right and left ventricles

QT Interval Time required for the depolarization and repolarization of ventricular muscle cells; measured from the beginning of the Q wave to the end of the T wave

Quadrigeminy Every fourth QRS complex is abnormal (usually premature); should have a minimum of three occurrences to be identified

R on T Phenomenon Occurs when the R wave of a premature ventricular contraction falls on the T wave of the preceding complex; can lead to a lethal dysrhythmia

R to R Interval Measurement of time from one R wave to the next R wave

Radiofrequency Catheter Ablation Procedure used in WPW to destroy the abnormal pathway in the electrical conduction system

Refractory Period Time between the end of a contraction and the return of the cardiac cells to the ready state; divided into absolute and relative refractory periods

Relative Refractory Period Time during the cardiac cycle when cardiac cells have repolarized to the point that some cells can be stimulated to contract again, if the stimulation is strong enough; from the last half of the T wave to the end of the T wave

Repolarization Cardiac recovery phase; the cells are returning to the ready state

Responsiveness Term used in assessment of patient condition, such as responsive to painful stimulation or lack of responsiveness; used interchangeably with consciousness

Retrograde Occurs after or behind; traveling in a reverse or backward direction

Run of Ventricular Tachycardia (Run of VT) Group of three or more premature ventricular contractions in a row; usually has duration of less than 30 seconds

Salvo A run of ventricular tachycardia; may also be called a burst of PVCs

Second-degree Heart Block, Type I Progressive heart block that occurs when the atrial impulse is interrupted at the AV junction; also called Wenckebach or Mobitz I

Second-degree Heart Block, Type II Intermittent interruption in the electrical conduction system at or below the AV junction; occurs suddenly and without warning; also called Mobitz II or classical

Septum Thick, muscular wall that separates the right and left chambers of the heart

Shock Physical condition caused by poor cardiac output; also used as an informal term for cardiac defibrillation

Sick Sinus Syndrome (SSS) A term that has been used in the past to describe a sinus rhythm with a pause; is currently used for any dysrhythmia caused by a disruption in the atrial electrical conduction pathway

Sinoatrial Node (SA Node) Located in the upper right atrium; normal pacemaker of the heart

Sinus Arrest Dysrhythmia that occurs when the SA node fails to initiate an electrical impulse; therefore the atrium does not depolarize, causing a pause in the cardiac rhythm

Sinus Arrhythmia Dysrhythmia that occurs when the heart rate changes with respirations; meets all criteria of normal sinus rhythm except it is NOT regular

Sinus Bradycardia Dysrhythmia that occurs when all electrical impulses originate from the SA node, but at a rate slower than 60 impulses per minute

Sinus Exit Block Dysrhythmia that occurs when the SA node initiates an electrical impulse that is blocked and not conducted to the atria, creating a pause in the cardiac rhythm; the pause is ended by an escape beat

Sinus Rhythm Any cardiac rhythm that originates from the SA node; heart rate is usually between 60–100 impulses per minute

Sinus Tachycardia Dysrhythmia that occurs when all electrical impulses originate from the SA node, but at a rate of 101-150 impulses per minute

Sodium (NA) Chemical found in the body that aids in the conduction of electricity through the cells

Spike A vertical line seen on the rhythm strip that represents the electrical impulse from a mechanical pacemaker; also known as pacer spike

Stable No serious signs or symptoms of poor cardiac output

Stroke Volume The amount of blood pumped by the left ventricle with each contraction or beat; usually about 70 cc

ST Segment A wave component that starts at the end of the S wave and stops at the beginning of the T wave

Supraventricular Tachycardia (SVT) Dysrhythmia that has all the characteristics of paroxysmal atrial tachycardia, but the onset is not seen; general term describing any rapid dysrhythmia (heart rate greater than 150) originating from above the bundle of His

Sympathetic Nervous System Nerves that prepare the body to react in times of stress or emergencies by increasing the heart rate and force of cardiac contractions

Symptomatic Showing signs of poor cardiac output; see *medically unstable*

Synchronized Cardioversion Procedure used to correct unstable rapid dysrhythmias using electrical current timed to discharge or "fire" only on the R wave, avoiding the relative refractory period

Systolic Blood Pressure Pressure measured during ventricular contractions

T wave Complex component that represents repolarization of the ventricles

Tachycardia Dysrhythmia in which the heart rate is faster than normal; usually greater than 100 beats per minute

Telemetry System of electrodes, leads, monitors, and graph paper that receives and displays cardiac electrical impulses

Tension Pneumothorax The presence of air in the pleural space around a lung; usually caused by an injury to the chest wall; may cause respiratory arrest if not treated

Third-degree Heart Block Dysrhythmia in which both the atria and the ventricles are beating independently; functioning as two separate hearts; also known as complete heart block or complete AV dissociation

Thrombolytic Therapy Drugs used to dissolve clots in coronary arteries; may reduce the number of deaths from MI; currently used term is fibrinolytic therapy

Thrombosis The development of a blood clot within a blood vessel

Titrate Small adjustment of IV fluids or medications to improve vital signs, treat dysrhythmias, or relieve pain

Torsades De Pointes Dysrhythmia that resembles VT; has increasing and decreasing amplitude along the baseline; usually occurs in rhythms with a prolonged QT interval

Toxicity Condition of harmful physical changes, resulting from amounts of a substance that would usually not cause problems

Trachea A round airway tube, which is about 4½ inches long, extending from the larynx (voice box) to the bronchi; part of the respiratory system

Transmit Conduct or carry electrical impulses through the cardiac muscle; usually using normal conduction pathways

Tricuspid valve Valve located between the right atria and right ventricle

Trigeminy Every third QRS complex is abnormal (usually premature); should have a minimum of three occurrences to be identified as trigeminy

Troponins A blood test that assists in evaluating patients with suspected acute coronary syndrome

Underlying Rhythm Basic cardiac rhythm in which dysrhythmias or abnormal complexes can be identified

Unifocal (Monomorphic, Uniform) Complexes that originate from a single pacemaker site and look alike; usually refers to ventricular complexes

Unstable See *medically unstable* or *poor cardiac output*

Unsynchronized Cardioversion A term meaning defibrillation

Vagal Stimulation Stimulation of the vagus nerve in order to decrease heart rate by using physical maneuvers, such as Valsalva maneuver or carotid massage

Valsalva Maneuver Forceful bearing down, as if trying to have a bowel movement; sometimes used to treat PAT/PSVT

Valves Flap-like structures in the heart that are composed of endocardial tissue; they open and close in response to the pumping action of the myocardium, preventing the backflow of blood

Vasodilation Increased size in the diameter of a blood vessel

Vena Cava Superior and inferior; largest veins in the body

Venous Pertaining to the veins

Ventilations Use of a bag-valve-mask to assist in the patient's breathing

Ventricles Lower right and left chambers of the heart

Ventricular Fibrillation (V Fib) Dysrhythmia that originates from many ventricular sites; the ventricles make ineffective, quivering movements, not actual contractions; the patient does not have a pulse

Ventricular Muscle Layer of specialized tissue containing pacemaker cells; the muscle of the left ventricle is thicker since it pumps blood throughout the entire body

Ventricular Rate Number of times the left ventricle contracts in one minute; inherent rate is 20-40; should equal the pulse rate

Ventricular Standstill Dysrhythmia that occurs when no ventricular activity exists, only atrial complexes; the patient does not have a pulse

Ventricular Tachycardia (VT) Dysrhythmia that contains more than three premature ventricular contractions in a row; duration of more than 30 seconds; also called sustained ventricular tachycardia

Venturi Mask A mask that mixes pure oxygen with room air to provide a flow of oxygen at specific concentrations

Voltage Measurement of electrical force

Vulnerable Period The cardiac cells have repolarized to the point that some cells can again be stimulated to depolarize again, if the stimulus is strong enough; also known as the relative refractory period

Wandering Atrial Pacemaker Dysrhythmia originating from at least three different sites above the bundle of His

Wandering Junctional Pacemaker Dysrhythmia that originates from at least three different sites within the AV junctional area

Wenckebach Progressive heart block that occurs when the atrial impulse is interrupted at the AV junction; also called second-degree heart block, type I or Mobitz I

Wolff-Parkinson-White Syndrome (WPW) Dysrhythmia involving additional or accessory pathways in the electrical conduction system; an upright P wave, shortened PR interval, and delta waves are seen

ABGs	Arterial blood gases	**min**	Minute
ACS	Acute coronary syndrome	**ml**	Milliliter
AED	Automated external defibrillator	**ml/min**	Milliliters per minute
A Fib	Atrial fibrillation	**mm**	Millimeter
AICD	Automatic implantable cardioverter defibrillator	**mm Hg**	Millimeters of mercury
		MONA	Morphine, oxygen, nitroglycerin, aspirin
AV	Atrioventricular	**mV**	Millivolt
BB	Bundle branch	**Na**	Sodium
BBB	Bundle branch block	**NS**	Normal saline
BP	Blood pressure	**NSR**	Normal sinus rhythm
Brady	Bradycardia	**N/V**	Nausea and vomiting
CAD	Coronary artery disease	**O₂**	Oxygen
cc	Cubic centimeter	**PAC**	Premature atrial contraction
CHF	Congestive heart failure	**PAT**	Paroxysmal atrial tachycardia
CO	Cardiac output	**PEA**	Pulseless electrical activity
CPR	Cardiopulmonary resuscitation	**PJC**	Premature junctional contraction
CVA	Cerebral vascular accident	**PO**	Per os (by mouth)
EKG, ECG	Electrocardiogram	**PRI**	PR interval
D₅W	Dextrose 5% in water	**PSVT**	Paroxysmal supraventricular tachycardia
F Wave	Flutter wave		
FLBs	Funny looking beats	**PVC**	Premature ventricular contraction
g, gm	Gram	**QT**	Interval between beginning of Q wave and end of T wave
HR	Heart rate		
hr	Hour		
IV	Intravenous	**RR**	Respiratory rate
K	Potassium	**SA**	Sinoatrial
kg	Kilogram	**SOB**	Shortness of breath
L	Liter	**SSS**	Sick sinus syndrome
L/min	Liters per minute	**SV**	Stroke volume
μg (mcg)	Microgram	**SVT**	Supraventricular tachycardia
mEq	Milliequivalent	**Tach**	Tachycardia
mg	Milligram	**VF, V Fib**	Ventricular fibrillation
mg/kg	Milligram per kilogram of body weight	**VR**	Ventricular rate
		VT, V Tach	Ventricular tachycardia
MI	Myocardial infarction	**WPW**	Wolff-Parkinson-White syndrome

REFERENCES

These books and materials were used as background and reference information sources.

GENERAL REFERENCES

1. American Heart Association: *2000 Handbook of emergency cardiovascular care for health-care providers,* St. Louis, 2000, Mosby.
2. American Heart Association: Guidelines 2000 for cardiopulmonary resuscitation and emergency cardiovascular care, *Circulation* 102 (8): 2000.
3. American Heart Association: *ACLS for healthcare providers,* Dallas, 2001, American Heart Association
4. American Heart Association: *ACLS for instructors,* Dallas, 2001, American Heart Association
5. Berne RM, Levy M: *Cardiovascular physiology,* ed 8, St. Louis, 2001, Mosby.
6. Conover MB: *Understanding electrocardiograph,* ed 7, St. Louis, 1996, Mosby.
7. Dubin D: *Rapid interpretation of EKGs: a programmed course,* ed 5, Tampa, Fla, 1998, Cover Publishing.
8. Huszar RJ: *Basic dysrhythmias: interpretation and management,* ed 3, St. Louis, 2002, Mosby.
9. Lewis KM: *Sensible ECG analysis,* New York, 2000, Delmar Publishers.
10. *Mosby's medical, nursing, and allied health dictionary,* ed 6, St. Louis, 2002, Mosby.
11. Sifton DW, editor: *Physician's desk reference,* ed 55: Montvale NJ, 2001, Medical Economics Production Company.
12. Skidmore-Roth L: *Mosby's nursing drug reference,* St. Louis, 2002, Mosby.
13. Smith LF, Fish FH: *Pure practice for ECGs workbook,* St. Louis, 1995, Mosby.
14. Thibodeau GA, Patton KT: *Anatomy and physiology,* ed 4, St. Louis, 1999, Mosby.
15. Thibodeau GA, Patton KT: *Structure and function of the body,* ed 11, St. Louis, 2000, Mosby.
16. Walraven G: *Basic arrhythmias,* ed 5, Upper Saddle River, NJ, 1999, Brady/Prentice Hall.

ONLINE REFERENCES

1. http://www.arrhythmia.org/general/whatis/wpw.html: Wolff-Parkinson-White (WPW) syndrome.
2. http://www.mayo.edu/cv/wwwpg cv/ep lab/treatment-of-supraventricular-ta.htm: Treatment of supraventricular tachycardias, 1999, Mayo Foundation for Medical Education and Research.
3. http://www.txai.org/spec.html: Supraventricular tachycardias.
4. http://www.americanheart.org/Heart and Stroke A A Guide/wolff.html: Wolff-Parkinson-White syndrome.
5. http://www.emedicine.com/emerg/topic644.htm: Herbert M and Tully G: Wolff-Parkinson-White syndrome from emergency medicine/cardiovascular, 2001, Boston Medical Publishing.
6. http://www.advocatehealth.com/healthinfo/articles/heartcare/common/wpwsynd.html: Wolff-Parkinson-White syndrome, Oak Brook, Ill, 2001, Advocate Healthcare.
7. http://www.mayohealth.org/mayo/askphys/qa990426.htm: Ask The Mayo Physician—WPW syndrome.
8. http://www.nlm.nih.gov/medlineplus/ency/article/000161.htm: Sick sinus syndrome.